Opioids in Anesthesia II

Opioids in Anesthesia II

Edited by
Fawzy G. Estafanous, M.D.

Chairman, Division of Anesthesiology
The Cleveland Clinic Foundation
Cleveland, Ohio

With 50 Contributing Authors

Butterworth–Heinemann
Boston   London   Singapore   Sydney   Toronto   Wellington

Recognizing the importance of preserving what has been written,
it is the policy of Butterworth–Heinemann to have the books it
publishes printed on acid-free paper, and we exert our best efforts
to that end.

Library of Congress Cataloging-in-Publication Data

Opioids in anesthesia II / edited by Fawzy G. Estafanous ; with
   51 contributing authors.
     p.   cm.
     Includes bibliographical references.
     ISBN 0-409-90230-6
     1. Opioids—Physiological effect. 2. Narcotics—
Physiological effect. 3. Anesthesia. I. Estafanous, F. G.
(Fawzy G.) II. Title: Opioids in anesthesia 2.
    [DNLM: 1. Anesthesia. 2. Narcotics. QV 89 06182]
RD86.0640652 1990
617.9′62—dc20
DNLM/DLC
for Library of Congress   90-1342

British Library Cataloguing in Publication Data
Opioids in anesthesia.
  2
  1.Anesthetics
  I. Estafanous, Fawzy
  615.781

  ISBN 0-409-90230-6

Butterworth–Heinemann
80 Montvale Avenue
Stoneham, MA 02180

10 9 8 7 6 5 4 3 2 1

Printed in the United States of America

To my family and my friends, who have been so supportive of me

CONTENTS

CONTRIBUTING AUTHORS

Robert J. Adams, Ph.D.
Assistant Professor of Anesthesiology,
Medical College of Georgia, Augusta,
Georgia

Paul G. Barash, M.D.
Professor and Chairman, Department of
Anesthesiology, Yale University School of
Medicine, Yale–New Haven Hospital, New
Haven, Connecticut

David J. Benefiel, M.D.
Assistant Clinical Professor of Anesthesia,
University of California, San Francisco;
Director of Cardiovascular Anesthesia,
Department of Anesthesiology, Pacific
Presbyterian Medical Center, San Francisco,
California

John R. Blair, M.D.
Assistant Professor of Anesthesiology,
Medical College of Georgia, Augusta,
Georgia

Byron C. Bloor, Ph.D.
Associate Professor of Anesthesiology,
University of California, Los Angeles,
School of Medicine, Los Angeles, California

F. P. Boersma, M.D.
Anesthesiologist, Department of
Anesthesiology and Pain Clinic, Refaja
Hospital, Stadskanaal, The Netherlands

Robert A. Caplan, M.D.
Clinical Associate Professor of
Anesthesiology, University of Washington;
Attending Anesthesiologist, Virginia Mason
Medical Center, Seattle, Washington

Daniel B. Carr, M.D.
Associate Professor of Anesthesiology and
Medicine (Endocrinology), Harvard Medical
School; Co-Director, Anesthesia Pain Unit;
Director, Analgesic Peptide Research
Unit; Departments of Anesthesia and
Endocrinology, Massachusetts General
Hospital and Shriners Burns Institute,
Boston, Massachusetts

Harvey L. Edmonds, Jr., Ph.D.
Professor and Director of Research,
Department of Anesthesiology, University of
Louisville School of Medicine, Louisville,
Kentucky

Burton S. Epstein, M.D.
Seymour Alpert Professor and Chairman,
Department of Anesthesiology, George
Washington University Medical Center,
Washington, D.C.

William J. Farley, M.D.
Medical Director, Perspectives Professional
Health Program, Hampton, Virginia

Marc A. Feldman, M.D.
Assistant Professor of Anesthesiology and
Critical Care Medicine, Johns Hopkins
School of Medicine, Baltimore, Maryland

Peter S. A. Glass, M.B., Ch.B.
Assistant Professor of Anesthesiology, Duke
University Medical Center, Durham, North
Carolina

George Gore, J.D.
Partner, Arter & Hadden, Cleveland, Ohio

Paul R. Hickey, M.D.
Associate Professor of Anesthesia, Harvard Medical School; Senior Associate in Anesthesia, The Children's Hospital, Boston, Massachusetts

Thomas Higgins, M.D.
Director, Cardiothoracic Intensive Care Unit, Department of Cardiothoracic Anesthesia, The Cleveland Clinic Foundation, Cleveland, Ohio

John W. Holaday, Ph.D.
Adjunct Professor of Pharmacology and Psychiatry, Uniformed Services University of the Health Sciences, Bethesda, Maryland; Scientific Director, Medicis Corporation, Washington, D.C.

James R. Jacobs, Ph.D.
Assistant Professor of Anesthesiology and Biomedical Engineering, Duke University Medical Center, Durham, North Carolina

Gareth W. Jones, B.Sc., M.B.B.S., M.R.C.P., F.F.A.R.C.S.
Instructor of Anesthesiology, Medical College of Virginia, Virginia Commonwealth University, Richmond, Virginia

Surinder K. Kallar, M.D.
Professor of Anesthesiology; Director of Ambulatory Anesthesia, Medical College of Virginia, Virginia Commonwealth University, Richmond, Virginia

Byung Y. Kim, M.D.
Assistant Clinical Professor of Anesthesiology, Yale University School of Medicine; Director, Section of Neuroanesthesia, Yale–New Haven Hospital, New Haven, Connecticut

Luke M. Kitahata, M.D., Ph.D.
Professor of Anesthesiology, Yale University School of Medicine, Yale–New Haven Hospital, New Haven, Connecticut

Andrzej W. Lipkowski, Ph.D., D.Sc.
Assistant Professor of Chemistry, University of Warsaw, Warsaw, Poland; Research Associate, Analgesic Peptide Research Unit, Departments of Anesthesia and Endocrinology, Massachusetts General Hospital and Shriners Burns Institute, Boston, Massachusetts

Edward Lowenstein, M.D.
Anesthetist-in-Chief, Department of Anesthesia and Critical Care, Beth Israel Hospital; Professor of Anesthesia, Harvard Medical School, Boston, Massachusetts

Dennis T. Mangano, Ph.D., M.D.
Professor and Vice Chairman, Department of Anesthesia, University of California, San Francisco, California

Mervyn Maze, M.B., Ch.B.
Associate Professor of Anesthesia, Stanford University, Stanford, California; Staff Anesthesiologist, Anesthesiology Service, Palo Alto Veterans Administration Medical Center, Palo Alto, California

Robert W. McPherson, M.D.
Associate Professor of Anesthesiology and Critical Care Medicine; Director, Division of Neuro-anesthesia, Johns Hopkins School of Medicine, Baltimore, Maryland

Kathleen Moran, R.N.
Department of Neurology, University of Cincinnati Medical Center, Cincinnati, Ohio

H. Noorduin, M.Sc.
Assistant Director, Department of Clinical Research and Development, Janssen Research Foundation, Beerse, Belgium

Richard Payne, M.D.
Associate Professor of Neurology, University of Cincinnati Medical Center, Cincinnati, Ohio

Frank Porreca, Ph.D.
Associate Professor of Pharmacology, University of Arizona College of Medicine, Tucson, Arizona

Jack K. Pruett, Ph.D.
Professor of Anesthesiology, Pharmacology, and Toxicology, Medical College of Georgia, Augusta, Georgia

J. G. Reves, M.D.
Professor of Anesthesiology; Director, Heart

Center at Duke Hospital, Duke University Medical Center, Durham, North Carolina

Michael F. Roizen, M.D.
Chairman, Department of Anesthesia and Critical Care, and Professor of Medicine, University of Chicago, Chicago, Illinois

Richard B. Rothman, M.D., Ph.D.
Chief, Unit of Receptor Studies, Laboratory of Clinical Science, National Institutes of Health, Bethesda, Maryland

Ira Segal, M.D.
Assistant Professor of Anesthesia, University of Minnesota; Staff Anesthesiologist, Hennepin County Medical Center, Minneapolis, Minnesota

Brendan S. Silbert, M.B., B.S.
Anaesthetist, St. Vincent's Hospital, Melbourne, Australia; Research Associate, Analgesic Peptide Research Unit, Departments of Anesthesia and Endocrinology, Massachusetts General Hospital and Shriners Burns Institute, Boston, Massachusetts

Deanna Siliciano, M.D.
Research Fellow, Department of Anesthesia, University of California, San Francisco, California

Eric J. Simon, Ph.D.
Professor of Psychiatry and Pharmacology, New York University Medical Center, New York, New York

N. Ty Smith, M.D.
Professor of Anesthesiology, University of California, San Diego, School of Medicine, Veterans Administration Medical Center, San Diego, California

Maurice Sosnowski, M.D.
Assistant Professor of Anesthesiology, Institut J. Bordet, Université Libre de Bruxelles, Brussels, Belgium

Mary Southam, Ph.D.
Product Registration Manager, ALZA Corporation, Palo Alto, California

Theodore H. Stanley, M.D.
Professor of Anesthesiology, University of Utah School of Medicine, Salt Lake City, Utah

James B. Streisand, M.D.
Assistant Professor of Anesthesiology, University of Utah School of Medicine, Salt Lake City, Utah

Clyde A. Swift, M.D.
Assistant Clinical Professor of Anesthesiology; Codirector, One-Day Surgery, Yale University School of Medicine, Yale–New Haven Hospital, New Haven, Connecticut

A. Van Steenberge, M.D.
Anesthesiology, 11 Vliertjeslaan, 1900 Overyse, Belgium

G. Vanden Bussche, M.D.
Vice-Chairman, Department of Clinical Research and Development, Janssen Research Foundation, Beerse, Belgium

Paul F. White, Ph.D., M.D.
Professor of Anesthesiology; Director of Clinical Research, Washington University School of Medicine, St. Louis, Missouri

Scott B. Wurm, M.D.
Assistant Professor of Anesthesiology, George Washington University Medical Center, Washington, D.C.

Tony L. Yaksh, Ph.D.
Professor and Vice Chairman for Research, Department of Anesthesiology, University of California, San Diego

DISCUSSANTS

Ezzat Amin, M.D.
Chairman, Department of Anesthesia, Cairo
University, Cairo, Egypt

Helmut F. Cascorbi, M.D., Ph.D.
Department of Anesthesiology, Case
Western Reserve University School of
Medicine, University Hospitals, Cleveland,
Ohio

Werner E. Flacke, M.D.
Department of Anesthesia, UCLA Center
for Health Sciences, Los Angeles, California

Carl C. Hug, Jr., M.D., Ph.D.
Professor of Anesthesiology and
Pharmacology, Emory University School
of Medicine; Director, Cardiothoracic
Anesthesia, The Emory Clinic, Atlanta,
Georgia

Jean M. Millar, M.D.
Consultant in Charge, Day Surgery Unit,
Churchill Hospital, Headington, Oxford,
England

Gerard W. Ostheimer, M.D.
Vice Chairman of Anesthesia, Associate
Professor of Anesthesia, Harvard Medical
School, Boston, Massachusetts

John H. Petre, Ph.D.
Director of Clinical Engineering, Division of
Anesthesiology, Cleveland Clinic, Cleveland,
Ohio

Beverly K. Philip, M.D.
Director, Day Surgery Unit, Brigham and
Women's Hospital; Assistant Professor of
Anesthesia, Harvard Medical School,
Boston, Massachusetts

Steven Shafer, M.D.
Attending in Cardiovascular Anesthesia,
Texas Heart Institute, Houston, Texas

ADDITIONAL PARTICIPANTS

K.J.S. Anand

David Bevan

Simon de Lange

Joan W. Flacke

Kathy Foley

Katherine Gill

James Hart

Michael B. Howie

Ira Isaacson

Horace Loh

Nagy Mekhail

Robert Merin

Robert Miller

Brace Natcher

Michael Nugent

Allen Ream

Carl E. Rosow

Amira Safwat

Steve Slogoff

Michael Stanton-Hicks

Norman Starr

J.F. Viljoen

H. Ronald Vinik

1978,[4] who evaluated it as a monoanesthetic in cardiac surgery. It became clear from their work and that of many other investigators that the fentanyl-oxygen technique had clear advantages over the use of anesthetic doses of morphine. Major benefits are better cardiovascular stability, no histamine-related reactions, and shorter postoperative respiratory depression. Owing to these characteristics, fentanyl has become the drug of choice for perioperative analgesia.

However, because of the changes in contemporary anesthetic practice, new opioids were developed that are even more specific and better adapted to the latest applications. Modern analgesics offer a more rapid onset of action, a potency and duration of action more adapted to the clinical situation, an enhanced specificity, and a higher safety ratio.

SUFENTANIL

Sufentanil, synthesized in 1974, is a thienyl derivative of fentanyl and is characterized by a high selectivity and an affinity for μ opiate receptors approximately ten times that of fentanyl. Sufentanil is also a very potent analgesic. In animals its LED_{50} is 0.67 μg/kg, which makes it 9,000 times as potent as pethidine and 16 times as potent as fentanyl. Its safety margin, expressed as the ratio of the LD_{50} to the LED_{50}, is much higher than that of any other opioid. The safety margins obtained in animals of the most commonly used narcotic agents are 4.8 for meperidine, 70 for morphine, 277 for fentanyl, and 26,700 for sufentanil. These enormous differences obtained in rats do have their impact in the daily practice of the anesthesiologist. This was nicely illustrated in 1979 by de Castro and coworkers,[5] who showed that differences in safety margins result in differences in incidence and nature of side effects. At increasing doses of potent analgesics such as fentanyl, and especially sufentanil, cardiovascular stability was maintained, with the advantage of an increased venous return and myocardial contractility, which was

not observed with the less potent compounds such as pethidine and morphine. This indicated there was indeed a positive relationship between opioid potency and therapeutic index.

The work of de Castro has been confirmed by several other human clinical studies: de Lange (1982),[6] Sanford (1985),[7] and Flacke (1985).[8] Sufentanil, in more recent studies, has been shown to have a beneficial effect on postoperative outcome. By optimally controlling the metabolic effects of the stress response, it is possible to reduce postoperative morbidity.[9,10]

ALFENTANIL

Alfentanil, synthesized in 1976, has the most rapid onset and shortest duration of action of all opioids available to date. In animal studies alfentanil has been shown to be 140 times as potent as meperidine, 72 times as potent as morphine, and 4 times less potent than fentanyl. In the tail-flick test in rats, the peak analgesic effects of alfentanil occur 1 minute after intravenous injection, compared with 4 minutes after injection for fentanyl and 30 minutes following a morphine injection.

In addition to having a rapid onset of action, alfentanil is very short-acting; its analgesic activity lasts for 11 to 36 minutes following administration of a dosage equal to 2 to 16 times the lowest ED_{50}. After administration of comparable doses of fentanyl, the analgesic activity lasts for 30 to 120 minutes, and for morphine, activity is observed for 90 to 300 minutes.

The difference between alfentanil and fentanyl in onset and duration of action has also been illustrated in humans. Scott and Stanski[11] studied the relation between plasma concentration and electroencephalographic (EEG) changes as measured by power spectral analysis of EEG tracings. They calculated that the half-life of plasma-to-brain equilibration (hysteresis) was 1.1 minutes for alfentanil and 6.4 minutes for fentanyl. As well, the return to baseline EEG occurred much more rapidly with alfentanil than with fentanyl. These properties mean not only that alfentanil will penetrate and leave the brain more rapidly than other opioids but also that there will be less tendency for it to accumulate in fat and other tissues. Accordingly, alfentanil has many applications as an analgesic in surgical procedures, with a primary role as a supplement for analgesia in patients undergoing short surgical procedures, and as a bolus followed by infusion for the maintenance of anesthesia with nitrous oxide for longer-lasting surgery.

What about new developments? The concept of selective spinal analgesia represents a recent important advantage in the management of moderate and severe pain.

EPIDURAL SUFENTANIL

Sufentanil's high lipid solubility allows a rapid uptake of the drug into the spinal cord and a limited but also rapid vascular uptake, providing a fast onset of action. The amount of drug that is not bound to the spinal opioid receptor and that can migrate rostrally within the cerebrospinal fluid is minimal, thereby reducing the potential risk of delayed respiratory depression.

The main clinical application of sufentanil is with postoperative patients. Dose-finding studies, in which doses between 15 and 75 μg were evaluated, showed that 30 to 50 μg of sufentanil is the optimal dose. It provides excellent postoperative analgesia within minutes, which lasts for about six hours with moderate sedation. Double-blind studies comparing sufentanil with epidural morphine established that pain relief was fastest in onset and most complete during the first hours after epidural sufentanil, whereas total duration of analgesia was longest following morphine. Side effects were least frequently observed in the sufentanil patients.

In obstetrics, local anesthetics are most often used to provide pain-free delivery. The addition of a small dose of sufentanil (10 μg) to the local anesthetic significantly reduces the latency and increases the duration of analgesia. Because of this longer duration of action, the total dose of bupivacaine required can be decreased, resulting in less motor blockade at birth. Moreover, the quality of analgesia improves. The condition of the infant at birth is not influenced by the addition of these low dosages of sufentanil. The only side effect related to sufentanil is transient and mild pruritus.

The usefulness of epidural sufentanil administered by continuous infusion has also been demonstrated for the relief of cancer pain in outpatients; terminal cancer pain, in particular, is one of the thornier problems in pain management. Very often, such pain fails to respond to oral or systemic narcotics, or serious side effects require a reduction of medication, resulting in a resurgence of pain. Boersma and coworkers[12] carried out an investigation on patients who were in the terminal phase of their disease and in whom conventional oral therapy was no longer effective or was associated with serious side effects. It was shown that satisfactory analgesia can be maintained over a long treatment period; in this case, the mean infusion was three months. No complications occurred in the home situation. Moreover—and this is the main advantage of the technique—epidural sufentanil administered in this way enabled the patients to spend their last days in the familiar surroundings of their own homes.

INTRANASAL SUFENTANIL

Another possible extension of the use of sufentanil is intranasal administration. Anesthesiologists are often reluctant to give young patients preoperative medication, as the commonly used regimens either produce discomfort because of the intramuscular injection or are too long-acting and delay awakening. There is therefore a growing interest in shorter-acting compounds such as sufentanil as well as in alternative routes of administration. Intranasal drug delivery offers some important advantages, since the blood supply of the nasal cavity bypasses the liver and enters the systemic circulation directly.

TRANSDERMAL FENTANYL

In recent years, anesthesiologists have been provided with new selective narcotic analgesics as well as new devices and techniques for administering them. One of these is the transdermal controlled-release delivery system. This system was developed to overcome problems associated with the conventional method of treating postoperative or cancer pain with intermittent intramuscular opioids. The conventional regimen is uncomfortable and often fails to achieve satisfactory analgesia because of infrequent administration of the drug and variability of drug absorption. The aim of transdermal drug delivery systems is to overcome these problems by providing a simple, noninvasive parenteral drug administration through intact skin, which makes it possible to maintain narcotic concentrations in serum within the therapeutic window and thus optimize pain management by continuous analgesia. Furthermore, these systems ensure the prolonged availability of a short-acting drug after one administration and allow rapid termination of treatment, if this is required, by removal of the device from the skin surface. The chronic pain associated with various terminal malignant conditions urgently requires optimal and sustained analgesic management if a satisfactory quality of life is to be maintained.

TTS fentanyl patches are currently being evaluated with reference to the relief of postoperative and cancer pain. TTS fentanyl is a transdermal system, which has already been shown to provide a continuous controlled systemic delivery of fentanyl for up to 72 hours. Such prolonged availability of a steady-state concentration of fentanyl implies infrequent dosing, which is convenient and time-saving for health care personnel. In addition, it minimizes disturbances to the patient, the risk of overdosing, and the likelihood of medication errors or delays.

REFERENCES

1. Heiff W, Mayer EC, de la Luz Perales M. Nitrous oxide and oxygen anesthesia with curare relaxation. Califf Med 1947;66:67–69.
2. Laborit H, Hagnenard P. Practique de l'Hibernotherapie en Chirurgie et en Medicine. Paris: Masson & Cie, 1954.
3. De Castro J, Mundeleer P. La neuroleptanalgésic, nouvelle technique d'anésthésie IV non barbiturique. Anesth Analg (Paris) 1959; 16(5):1022.
4. Stanley T, Webster LR. Anesthetic requirements and cardiovascular effects of fentanyl-oxygen and fentanyl-diazepam-oxygen anesthesia in man. Anesth Analg 1978;57:411–416.
5. de Castro J, Van de Water A, Wouters L, et al. Comparative study of cardiovascular, neurological and metabolic side effects of eight narcotics in dogs. Acta Anaesthesiol Belg 1979;30:5–99.
6. de Lange S, Boscoe MJ, Stanley TH, et al. Comparison of sufentanil-O_2 and fentanyl-O_2 for coronary artery surgery. Anesthesiology 1982;56:112–118.
7. Santosa TJ, Smith NT, Del-Silver H, et al. A comparison of morphine, fentanyl and sufentanil anesthesia for cardiac surgery. Anesth Analg 1986;65:259–267.
8. Flacke JW, Bloor BC, Kripke BJ, et al. Comparison of morphine, meperidine, fentanyl and sufentanil in balanced anesthesia. Anesth Analg 1985;64:897–910.
9. Benefier DJ, Roizen MF, Lampe GH, et al. Morbidity after aortic surgery with sufentanil vs isoflurane anesthesia. Anesthesiology 1986; 65(3A):A516.
10. Anand KJS, Phil D, Hickey PR. Randomized trial of high-dose sufentanil anaesthesia in neonates undergoing cardiac surgery: effects on the metabolic stress response. Anesthesiology 1987;67(3A):A502.
11. Scott JC, Ponganis KV, Stanski DR. EEG quantitation of narcotic effect. The comparative pharmacodynamics of fentanyl and alfentanil. Anesthesiology 1985;62:234–241.
12. Boersma FP, Noorduin H, Van den Bussche G. Epidural sufentanil for cancer pain control in outpatients. Reg Anesth 1989;14:293–297.

PREFACE

Opioids in Anesthesia II presents the results of the most recent research and clinical experience with opioids in anesthesia and pain management. Since the publication of the previous volume in 1984, newly developed opioids have been used extensively in clinical practice, and we have become more knowledgeable about optimum applications. New routes and methods of administration have been researched extensively and the research has expanded to include the effects of opioids at the cellular level. As a result of new findings, opioids can now be used for prolonged cardiac surgery, in-and-out surgeries, and chronic pain management.

This book was prepared by the most informed researchers and clinicians. It includes the comments and remarks of the eminent physicians who participated in challenging discussions at the Cleveland Clinic. It addresses the recent issues surrounding the use of opioids in anesthesia and pain management, and provides answers to many of the questions that arise in clinical practice. It also describes the areas that need further research and investigation. Two areas of concern, chemical dependency and malpractice, are discussed candidly and professionally in a much needed forum. This book will be valuable for researchers, practitioners, and trainees.

I am privileged that Dr. Paul Janssen has provided the historical review and introduction to this book. His scientific contributions to medicine, through the development of almost all the new potent opioids and his direction of the research for their clinical use, have an important place in the history of anesthesia and pain management.

My sincere appreciation goes to all the participants in this endeavor: my secretary, Beth Grubb; Donna Jackman and Lisa Politi of the Division of Education at the Cleveland Clinic Foundation; Janssen Pharmaceutica, for their generous and unconditional support; and Butterworth Publishers, for their tremendous help.

F.G.E.

SCIENTIFIC BASIS

1 BIOCHEMISTRY OF THE OPIOID PEPTIDES

Daniel B. Carr, Andrzej W. Lipkowski, and Brendan S. Silbert

The early use of naturally occurring alkaloids as empiric treatments with little understanding of their pharmacology, and the subsequent introduction of numerous derivatives and analogues as a result of increased understanding, has many precedents. Nonetheless, the pace of progress in this field has been remarkably swift when compared, for example, to the 40-year interval between Ahlquist's identification of adrenergic receptors[1] and their study in molecular terms.[2] Further, the opioids' place in medicinal chemistry is unique, owing to their continuous widespread use from ancient times as agents of pain relief. Because other contributions in this volume discuss many physiologic and clinical implications of opioid use, our emphasis in this chapter is upon the opioids' biochemistry. In particular, since opioid structure-activity relationships have been well defined for some time and are comprehensively reviewed elsewhere,[3-6] we focus upon the processes of opioid peptide biosynthesis, metabolism, and elimination. Understanding these events is not only important for defining how opioids act in vivo[7] but is also crucial for the ongoing development of new drugs patterned after peptides themselves or inhibitors of their metabolism.

BIOSYNTHESIS OF OPIOID PROPEPTIDES

Since the discovery of the enkephalins in 1975,[8] numerous larger opioid peptides have been isolated, which have their structures based on the common N-terminal tetrapeptide fragment, Tyr-Gly-Gly-Phe- . . . . The metabolism of endogenous opioid peptides and their synthetic analogues is quite different from morphine and related (i.e., alkaloid) analgesics. Opioid and other peptides are generated from precursors, so that the concentration of a particular endogenous opioid peptide reflects two opposite processes, formation and metabolic degradation (Figure 1.1). Both these functionally opposite enzymatic processes represent important regulatory steps in opioid peptide action, since there are distinct mechanisms whereby the inactive form is converted to the physiologically active peptide and then further metabolized to inactive fragments and amino acids.

Neuropeptides are as a rule initially synthesized as large inactive protein precursors, which undergo proteolytic processing to yield biologically active peptides. All precursors possess a signal peptide, which is required for vectorial

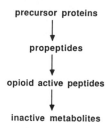

precursor proteins

↓

propeptides

↓

opioid active peptides

↓

inactive metabolites

FIGURE 1.1 Enzymatic processing liberates propeptides from larger precursor proteins. Further processing then yields opioid active peptides, which in turn are modified or degraded to yield "inactive" metabolites. Note that the absence of biological activity in one respect (e.g., analgesia) may not preclude significant effects upon other functions (e.g., immunity).

transport across the membranes of endoplasmic reticulum. The eukaryotic endoplasmic reticulum protease that cleaves the signal peptide is an integral membrane protein[9] with strong sequence homology to the signal protease isolated from bacteria.[10] The signal peptide consists predominantly of hydrophobic amino acids, but no specific sequence of amino acids is necessary for recognition by the signal protease. On the other hand, the secondary structure of the signal peptide (probably a β-turn) is important for determining the exact site of cleavage.[11] The resulting propeptides can further be proteolytically processed to smaller, biologically active fragments.

Three different precursor proteins[12] give rise to endogenous opioid peptides (Figure 1.2): prepro-opiomelanocortin (pre-POMC),[13] preproenkephalin,[14] and preprodynorphin (preproenkephalin B).[15] The expression of each precursor is controlled separately, as is the expression of a single precursor in different regions. The POMC precursor and its processing was defined by recombinant DNA methods.[16] It is the common precursor of β-endorphin and adrenocorticotropic hormone (ACTH), melanocyte stimulating hormones (MSH), and related compounds. The different distribution of met-enkephalin, as well as an absence of leu-enkephalin in the sequence of

POMC, motivated a successful search for other propeptide systems. A second precursor to be characterized was proenkephalin A, containing six copies of met-enkephalin and one copy of leu-enkephalin.[17] Recognition in hypothalamic extracts of still other distinct peptides, α-neo-endorphin[18] and dynorphin,[19] initiated a search for a third precursor. This search ended[20] in 1982 with the elucidation of the cDNA sequence encoding the third precursor, named preprodynorphin (preproenkephalin B), which contains three copies of leu-enkephalin and also gives rise to dynorphin, α-neo-endorphin, and rimorphin (dynorphin B).

Prior to their cleavage to generate opioid peptides, propeptides are modified by glycosylation, amidation, or acetylation and thereby differentiated for further metabolism. Within propeptides, the opioid sequences are flanked by pairs of basic amino acids (Lys-Lys, Lys-Arg, or Arg-Arg) or single basic amino acids followed by proline. Cleavage of propeptides at such basic sites by one or more trypsin-like endopeptidases,[21] termed prohormone-converting enzyme(s), initiates the generation of opioid peptides. Despite their functional similarities, these enzymes are distinct from either trypsin or cathepsin B.[22] An interesting feature of these enzymatic activities is that they do not cleave small synthetic substrates,[23] suggesting strong conformational dependence of these reactions. This steric dependency may underlie the relative resistance to cleavage of some basic pairs in the resultant peptides (e.g., dynorphins).

Basic residues at the amino-terminus of the resultant tryptic products are postulated to be removed by an aminopeptidase.[24] Basic residues at their carboxy-termini have been shown to be removed by carboxypeptidases, of which the best characterized is carboxypeptidase H (CPH)[25] (designated EC 3.4.17.10 and also referred to as carboxypeptidase-B-like enzyme[26] or enkephalin convertase[27]). Evidence that CPH functions in the processing of opioid peptides came from studies examining the enzymatic activity of secretory granule components. In bovine adrenal chromaffin granules, both enkephalin and C-terminally extended enke-

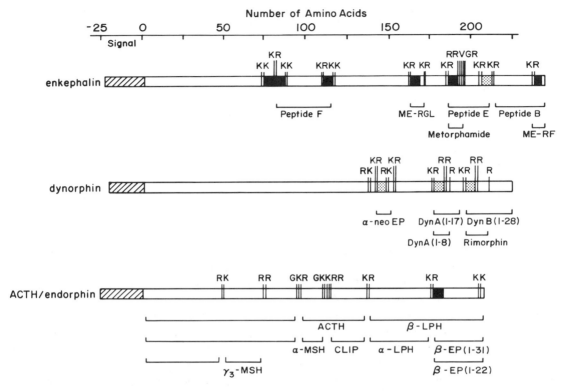

FIGURE 1.2 The three precursors for opioid peptides. Names of principal products shown on the left; other identified fragments are discussed in text. F, phenylalanine; G, glycine; K, lysine; L, leucine; R, arginine; V, valine.

phalin precursors (met-enkephalin-Arg or met-enkephalin-Lys, among others) have been detected,[28] suggesting that the enzyme activity that removes the C-terminal basic amino acids is present within these granules. CPH activity may be down-regulated by cleavage products (e.g., enkephalins) and also up-regulated (e.g., by reserpine).[25] The enzyme is stimulated by cobalt chloride and inhibited by chelating agents with a maximal activity in a pH range of 5 to 6.[29] As is true for other enzymes generating active peptides from their precursors, CPH is not selective.[30] It processes not only opioid peptides but also other neuropeptides with which opioids may interact, as well as their physiologic antagonists, tachykinins.[31]

When CPH action exposes a glycine residue at the carboxy-terminus, the transformation of the peptide into an amide may occur (Figure 1.3). Considering that amidated peptides are relatively resistant to carboxypeptidases, it is not surprising that about half of the bioactive hormones and neurohormones possess carboxy-terminus amide groups. In every tissue studied, α-amidation is catalyzed by peptidyl-glycine α-amidating mono-oxygenase (PAM). This reaction is stimulated by the presence of a reduced cofactor, ascorbic acid.[32] As for other ascorbate-stimulated enzymes, other reductants may also stimulate the reaction, notably catecholamines.[33] The optimal pH range is from 5.5 to 8.5 and depends on the amino acid at the penultimate position; a cupric ion is necessary for the enzymatic activity.[32,33] Treatment of rats with the relatively selective copper chelator N,N-diethyldithiocarbamate or its disulfide dimer, disulfiram (Antabuse), results in a dose- and time-dependent decrease in the ability of the anterior and intermediate pituitary to produce α-amidated peptides.[34] Doses of

```
            210                                          220
...-Lys-Arg-Tyr-Gly-Gly-Phe-Met-Arg-Arg-Val-Gly-Arg-Pro-Glu-...
              *                                          *
             PCA                                        PCA


          Tyr-Gly-Gly-Phe-Met-Arg-Arg-Val-Gly
                                            *
                                           PAM


          Tyr-Gly-Gly-Phe-Met-Arg-Arg-Val-NH
```
$_2$

FIGURE 1.3 Processing of adrenorphin from proenkephalin A. PCA, prohormone-converting enzyme; PAM, peptidyl-glycine α-amidating mono-oxygenase.

disulfiram equivalent to those used in humans to treat alcohol abuse brought about an accumulation of glycine-extended peptides in the pituitary.[34] In tissues producing pro-ACTH-endorphin-related peptides, levels of PAM activity and production of pro-ACTH-endorphin change in parallel,[35] whereas levels of other secretory granule-associated enzymes were unaltered. Treatment of cultured adrenal medullary cells with reserpine led to increased generation of all low-molecular-weight opioid peptides and, in particular, to a substantial increase in levels of amidorphin[36] (also termed metorphamide[37]), an α-amidated peptide produced from proenkephalin.[38,39] Enhancement of proenkephalin synthesis by exposure to high K$^+$ resulted in parallel increases in enkephalin and metorphamide.[38]

TRANSFORMATION OF PRECURSORS TO ACTIVE OPIOID PEPTIDES

Opioid propeptides contain several fragments that, after enzymatic liberation, may interact with opioid receptor families. All these peptides contain the common tetrapeptide message Tyr-Gly-Gly-Phe- . . . extended with methionine or leucine. Carboxy-terminus extension of this message by distinct peptide addresses modulates the receptor selectivity of the resultant peptides[40] and so gives rise to distinct profiles of physiologic actions. In ad-

dition, the peptides have different sensitivities to enzymatic degradation. The constellation of enzymes acting to metabolize opioid peptides at a particular tissue site is very sensitive to local biochemical changes. As a consequence, the half-life of a single peptide in differing tissues and the direction of its metabolism are very variable. Broadly speaking, the metabolism of opioid peptides may (1) yield new peptides with opioid activity; (2) generate biologically active peptides that lack opioid activity;[41] or (3) deactivate them to inactive fragments or amino acids (whose activity, strictly speaking, is best termed unknown).

In the latter regard, attention is frequently focused only on the role of one major peptide, and the physiologic role of related peptides has not always been intensively studied. However, peptides generated during metabolic processes may have important though indirect physiologic roles, e.g., to antagonize the biological response to,[42] or to act as a feedback control for, enzymatic processing of the parent molecule. They may also participate in physiologic processes not examined in our assay system.[43,44] For example, peptide α-amidation catalyzed by peptidyl-glycine α-amidating mono-oxygenase produces enzyme-resistant compounds with prolonged opioid activity.[45] Further, opioid peptide fragments may have significant actions on the immune system dissociated from their analgesic activity.[46]

Other common peptide transformations include N-terminal acetylation and O-tyrosine sulfation. The anterior pituitary generates only free N-terminal β-endorphin, but the intermediate lobe generates a combination of acetylated and nonacetylated forms.[47] The acetylation reaction seems to be a post-translational modification that occurs before or during peptide packaging in secretory granules.[48] N-acetylation produces aminopeptidase-resistant analogues, but all identified N-acetylated opioid peptides are devoid of antinociceptive activity (Table 1.1). Interestingly, all N-acetylated compounds of endorphins display nonopioid behavioral effects, suggesting separate mechanisms of behavior and antinociception of opioids. In rat pituitary, the ratio of acetylated to nonacetylated endorphin concentrations exhibits a diurnal rhythm.[41] Emotional stress selectively activates the intermediate lobe and, as a consequence, shifts the relative plasma concentrations of different forms of β-endorphin.[48] The sulfation of the tyrosine residue is catalyzed by tyrosylprotein sulfotransferase, which is widely distributed in membrane fractions of all tissues examined.[49] The sulfation of some neuropeptides strongly activates them (e.g., cholecystokinin family). However, sulfation abolishes the analgesic activity of leu-enkephalin.[50] At present, a surprisingly small amount of data is available on this process in relation to other opioid peptides.

Opioid peptides are under the continuous influence of proteolytic enzymes, the distribution and activity of which vary according to region, global exposure to stress, and biochemical conditions such as ionic milieu, pH, and temperature. The enzymes may attack an amino-terminus opioid pharmacophore portion, or carboxy-terminus fragments. Differing carboxy-terminus fragments, each capable of a distinct interaction with proteolytic systems, may be generated depending upon both the precursor molecule and the specific site at which the precursor is processed. POMC contains only one copy of β-endorphin, the carboxy-terminus cleavage products, which include β-endorphin (1-27), a potent inhibitor of parent peptide analgesia, β-endorphin (1-26), a peptide devoid of both agonist and antagonist activity, and the shorter opioids α-endorphin, γ-

endorphin, and met-enkephalin, each of which expresses a different spectrum of nonopioid effects (Table 1.1). Nonopioid peptides arising from the carboxy-terminus may express their own biological effects. β-endorphin (30-31) fragment (Gly-Gln) was shown to influence the firing of neurones[45] and immune function.[54] Des-enkephalin-γ-endorphin is the smallest fragment of β-endorphin having a neuroleptic action resulting from specific binding to nonopioid sites in the brain.[55]

The proenkephalin and prodynorphin proteins contain more than one copy of opioid pharmacophore fragments, and each of these is surrounded by different amino acid residues. Therefore, the opioid peptide mosaics that may be generated are more complicated: those expressed from proenkephalin are presented in Table 1.2. The affinities of these opioid peptides for different opioid receptor types may vary dramatically. For example, metorphamide has relative affinities to μ, κ, and δ receptors of 0.66, 0.31, and 0.03, respectively.[62] Met-enkephalin, which may be generated from metorphamide by endo-oligopeptidase A,[63] is highly selective for δ receptors: its affinities for μ, κ, and δ receptors are 0.09, 0.0, and 0.91, respectively.[62] Nevertheless, the same enzyme may also liberate met-enkephalin from dynorphin A (1-8),[63] which binds preferentially to κ receptors (affinities to μ, κ, and δ receptors are 0.22, 0.62, and 0.16, respectively).[62] Neurons termed enkephalinergic appear to store, and release upon depolarization, four different opioid peptides: met-enkephalin, leu-enkephalin, met-enkephalyl-Arg-Phe, and met-enkephalyl-Arg-Gly-Leu. These peptides are rapidly degraded by a complex of peptidases: endopeptidase 24.11, aminopeptidase, and angiotensin-converting enzyme.[64] Variation in the activity of any of these three enzymes may change the ratio of released peptides, e.g., angiotensin-converting enzyme may form met-enkephalin from heptapeptide.[65] Prodynorphin is a precursor for highly κ-selective dynorphins, but it may also serve as a source of δ-selective leu-enkephalin.[66] Consequently, detailed profiles of opioid peptide release in vivo are difficult to predict.[66]

TABLE 1.1 β-endorphin and related peptides derived in vivo from prepro-opiomelanocortin (pre-POMC)

Fragment	Amino Acid Sequence	Selected Biological Activities	Reference Number
β-endorphin (1-31) (β-EP) = POMC (235-265)	Tyr-Gly-Gly-Phe-Met-Thr-Ser-Glu-Lys-Ser-Gln-Thr-Pro-Leu-Val-Thr-Leu-Phe-Lys-Asn-Ala-Ile-Ile-Lys-Asn-Ala-His-Lys-Lys-Gly-Gln	Analgesia Behavioral effects Immunomodulator	43 46
Ac-β-EP	Ac-Tyr-Gly-Gly-Phe-Met-Thr-Ser-Glu-Lys-Ser-Gln-Thr-Pro-Leu-Val-Thr-Leu-Phe-Lys-Asn-Ala-Ile-Ile-Lys-Asn-Ala-His-Lys-Lys-Gly-Gln	No analgesic activity Behavioral effects as β-EP	48
β-EP (2-9)	Gly-Gly-Phe-Met-Thr-Ser-Glu-Lys	Antagonist of γ-EP Behavioral effects	52
α-EP = β-EP (1-16)	Tyr-Gly-Gly-Phe-Met-Thr-Ser-Glu-Lys-Ser-Gln-Thr-Pro-Leu-Val-Thr	Antagonist of γ-EP Behavioral effects Immunomodulation	51 46
β-EP (2-16)	Gly-Gly-Phe-Met-Thr-Ser-Glu-Lys-Ser-Gln-Thr-Pro-Leu-Val-Thr	Antagonist of γ-EP Behavioral effects	52
γ-EP = β-EP (1-17)	Tyr-Gly-Gly-Phe-Met-Thr-Ser-Glu-Lys-Ser-Gln-Thr-Pro-Leu-Val-Thr-Leu	Opiate activity Behavioral effects Immunomodulation	44 46 55
Acetyl-γ-EP	Ac-Tyr-Gly-Gly-Phe-Met-Thr-Ser-Glu-Lys-Ser-Gln-Thr-Pro-Leu-Val-Thr-Leu	No opiate affinity Behavioral effects as γ-EP	48 55
β-EP (2-17)	Gly-Gly-Phe-Met-Thr-Ser-Glu-Lys-Ser-Gln-Thr-Pro-Leu-Val-Thr-Leu	No opiate activity Behavioral effects as γ-EP	44 55
β-EP (6-17)	Thr-Ser-Glu-Lys-Ser-Gln-Thr-Pro-Leu-Val-Thr-Leu	No opiate activity Behavioral effects as γ-EP	44 55
β-EP (1-26)	Tyr-Gly-Gly-Phe-Met-Thr-Ser-Glu-Lys-Ser-Gln-Thr-Pro-Leu-Val-Thr-Leu-Phe-Lys-Asn-Ala-Ile-Ile-Lys-Asn-Ala	No opioid agonist or antagonist action	42
β-EP (1-27)	Tyr-Gly-Gly-Phe-Met-Thr-Ser-Glu-Lys-Ser-Gln-Thr-Pro-Leu-Val-Thr-Leu-Phe-Lys-Asn-Ala-Ile-Ile-Lys-Asn-Ala-His	Antagonist to β-EP analgesia	42
Acetyl-β-EP- (1-26) or (1-27)	Ac-Tyr-Gly-Gly-Phe-Met-Thr-Ser-Glu-Lys-Ser-Gln-Thr-Pro-Leu-Val-Thr-Leu-Phe-Lys-Asn-Ala-Ile-Ile-Lys-Asn-Ala-(His)	No analgesia Behavioral effects as β-EP	48
β-EP (30-31)	Gly-Gln	Inhibit neuron firing Immunomodulation	45 54
Met-enkephalin	Tyr-Gly-Gly-Phe-Met	Opioid activity Immunomodulation	46 53

TABLE 1.2 Opioid peptides derived from proenkephalin

Common Name	Amino Acid Sequence	Reference Number
Met-enkephalin	Tyr-Gly-Gly-Phe-Met	57
Met-enkephalyl-Lys	Tyr-Gly-Gly-Phe-Met-Lys	57
Met-enkephalyl-Arg	Tyr-Gly-Gly-Phe-Met-Arg	58
Met-enkephalyl-Arg-Phe	Tyr-Gly-Gly-Phe-Met-Arg-Phe	58
Met-enkephalyl-Arg-Gly-Leu	Tyr-Gly-Gly-Phe-Met-Arg-Gly-Leu	58
Leu-enkephalin	Tyr-Gly-Gly-Phe-Leu	57
BAM-12P	Tyr-Gly-Gly-Phe-Met-Arg-Arg-Val-Gly-Arg-Pro-Glu	59
Metorphamide/adrenorphin	Tyr-Gly-Gly-Phe-Met-Arg-Arg-Val-NH_2	37, 60
BAM-20P	Tyr-Gly-Gly-Phe-Met-Arg-Arg-Val-Gly-Arg-Pro-Glu-Trp-Trp-Met-Asp-Tyr-Gln-Lys-Arg	61
BAM-22P	Tyr-Gly-Gly-Phe-Met-Arg-Arg-Val-Gly-Arg-Pro-Glu-Trp-Trp-Met-Asp-Tyr-Gln-Lys-Arg-Tyr-Gly	61
Peptide E (BAM-25P)	Tyr-Gly-Gly-Phe-Met-Arg-Arg-Val-Gly-Arg-Pro-Glu-Trp-Trp-Met-Asp-Tyr-Gln-Lys-Arg-Tyr-Gly-Gly-Phe-Leu	57
Peptide F	Tyr-Gly-Gly-Phe-Met-Lys-Lys-Met-Asp-Glu-Leu-Tyr-Pro-Leu-Glu-Val-Glu-Glu-Glu-Leu-Ala-Asn-Gly-Gly-Glu-Val-Leu-Gly-Lys-Arg-Tyr-Gly-Gly-Phe-Met	62

ENZYMATIC DEGRADATION OF ACTIVE OPIOID PEPTIDES

The amino-terminus tetrapeptide fragment of opioid peptides is necessary for their affinity to the opioid receptor. Therefore any proteolytic process at this portion of the peptide abolishes its nociceptive effects. This process may occur by two principal mechanisms. First is the cleavage of N-terminal tyrosine by aminopeptidases. Mammalian tissues contain a wide spectrum of cytosolic and membrane-bound aminopeptidases,[67] but most of them are not regarded as the ectoenzymes that inactivate peptides in the extracellular space. Of these ectoenzymes, the best characterized is aminopeptidase N (EC 3.4.11.2, formerly designated aminopeptidase M).[68] It is sensitive to the enzymatic inhibitor bestatin but not to puromycin, another type of inhibitor. On the basis of bestatin's analgesic effect when injected into mice, it has been suggested that aminopeptidase N plays a physiologically significant role in the metabolism of endogenous opioids.[69] Puromycin, however, can produce a dose-related, naloxone-sensitive analgesia in mice,[70] suggesting that (puromycin-sensitive) aminopeptidase MII probably plays a major role in tyrosine cleavage from opioid peptides in the brain,[71] whereas aminopeptidase N plays a major role in the blood.[72,73] The membrane aminopeptidases show a broad substrate specificity and degrade a variety of polypeptides, such as angiotensins, melanostatin, and all opioid peptides. Nevertheless their potency in cleaving tyrosine from the amino-terminus of opioid peptides is strongly influenced by the size, chemical character, or conformation of carboxy-terminus extensions (Table 1.3).[74] Further, because aminopeptidases act upon a number of different peptides, these peptides in turn may modify aminopeptidase activity on the target opioid peptide: β-endorphin,[75] ACTH, somatostatin, and substance P,[76] for

TABLE 1.3 Efficacy of tyrosine cleavage from a series of dynorphin-related peptide substrates by a purified aminopeptidase

Amino Acid Sequence	Relative Activity
Tyr-Gly	1.0
Tyr-Gly-Gly	0.8
Tyr-Gly-Gly-Phe	8.6
Tyr-Gly-Gly-Phe-Leu	14.3
Tyr-Gly-Gly-Phe-Leu-NH$_2$	15.2
Tyr-Gly-Gly-Phe-Leu-Arg	6.1
Tyr-Gly-Gly-Phe-Leu-Arg-Arg-Ile	4.4
Tyr-Gly-Gly-Phe-Leu-Arg-Arg-Ile-Arg-Pro-Lys-Leu-Lys	0.3
Tyr-Gly-Gly-Phe-Leu-Arg-Arg-Ile-Arg-Pro-Lys-Leu-Lys-Trp-Asp-Asn-Gln	0.14

Source: From Udenfriend S, Kilpatrick D. Biochemistry of enkephalins and enkephalin-containing peptides. Arch Biochem Biophys 1983;221:309–323.

example, all inhibit enkephalin breakdown. Lastly, although cleavage of the amino-terminus tyrosine from opioid peptides abolishes their morphinomimetic nociceptive effects, for other nonopioid effects the presence of N-terminal tyrosine is not necessary. In consequence, aminopeptidase actions generate nonopioid peptides with a wide spectrum of non-nociceptive activity, also displayed by opioids (Table 1.1).

A second means of degradation of opioid peptides is by the membrane endopeptidase 24.11 (EC 3.4.24.11) at the Gly^3-Phe^4 peptide bond. Early studies indicated a high selectivity of this enzyme towards enkephalin, with a distribution in brain parallel to the opiate receptor, leading to its being termed enkephalinase in keeping with its presumed specificity for enkephalinergic neurons.[77] Later, it was found to be widely distributed in mammalian tissues, many of which lack enkephalin.[78] In fact, this endopeptidase acts widely to hydrolyze Gly^3-Phe^4 peptide bonds not only on enkephalin pentapeptides with free carboxyl groups but also those bearing carboxy-terminus extensions (e.g., met-enkephalin-Arg-Phe[78] or dynorphins[79]). Furthermore, substance P, which possesses a C-terminal amide group, is quite susceptible to hydrolysis by this enzyme.[80] Cholecystokinin (CCK), neurotensin, bradykinin, insulin, and other peptides are similarly susceptible.[78] The hydrolysis of enkephalin, substance P, and CCK by synaptic membranes is potently inhibited by specific inhibitors of this enzyme, suggesting that it may play a significant role in termination of these peptides in biological systems.[78] Cross-influence of different neuropeptide substrates on the activity of this endopeptidase has also been reported.[81]

It is likely that a combination of both enzyme systems, aminopeptidases and endopeptidase 24.11, is involved in the inactivation of opioid peptides. Since the ratio of activity of aminopeptidases to endopeptidases varies greatly between tissues and even within tissues, the relative importance of these two inactivation mechanisms shows marked regional differences. Other enzyme systems, too, such as angiotensin converting enzyme (EC 3.4.15.1)[64] or acetylcholinesterase,[82] may participate in this metabolic inactivation.

OPIOID PEPTIDES AND PAIN

Isolation of the endogenous opioid peptides and recognition of their rapid metabolism have spurred two broad approaches to the development of new analgesics. The first approach is to devise compounds that inhibit such degradation. Alternatively, one may prepare new opioid peptide analogues resistant to enzyme action.

The discovery of inhibitors of enzymes that metabolize opioid peptides in vivo has given rise to the attractive concept of potentiating the endogenous opioid system. Most attention has been focused in this regard on endopeptidase EC 3.4.24.11. Indeed, even a simple inhibitor of endopeptidase such as D-phenylalanine has been found to potentiate cardiac actions of met-enkephalin.[83] Based on the possibility that such compounds may not produce tolerance or dependence,[84] potent and selective inhibitors of this enzyme (e.g., thiorphan[84] or its prodrug acetorphan[85]) have been screened and found to yield analgesia in vivo. Acetorphan was the first reported endopeptidase EC 3.4.24.11 inhibitor tested in humans, relieving postmyelography headache but not experimental pain.[86] Recently an orally active inhibitor of this endopeptidase has been found to be analgesic.[87] Since endopeptidase EC 3.4.24.11 is only one among numerous enzymes participating in the metabolism of opioid peptides, several groups have proposed using nonselective inhibitors to block a number of such enzymes. This approach has given rise to kelatorphan,[88] its retro-inverso analogue,[89] and phelorphan,[90] which block not only endopeptidase but also aminopeptidase and dipeptidylaminopeptidase. Although the concept of using inhibitors of endogenous opioid peptide metabolism is attractive, none of the enzymes involved is entirely selective. Thus, even relatively specific enzyme inhibitors may affect the balance of a wide spectrum of peptide hormones and neurotransmitters, and their clinical potential should be carefully evaluated.

The development of newer, more stable analogues of natural opioid peptides with higher enzymatic stability has continued almost from the day of their discovery. The first such compound was a met-enkephalin analogue with D-alanine in position 2 and an amide on the carboxy-terminus.[91] This analogue displayed resistance to aminopeptidases as well as carboxypeptidases, and in consequence had a prolonged period of action. At this time, hundreds of analogues of all endogenous opioid peptides have been synthesized, and on this basis comprehensive structure-activity relationships have been defined.[4-6] Nevertheless, only a few authentic sequences or analogues possess biological profiles promising enough to warrant in vivo study. β-endorphin does not penetrate the blood-brain barrier but was studied early because it is more resistant to metabolic degradation than the smaller enkephalins. β-endorphin produces potent, long-lasting clinical analgesia when injected intraspinally[92] and has had some promising effects in various mental disorders.[93,94] The potential clinical utility of β-endorphin, however, seems limited because of the cost of its synthesis and confounding effects of metabolites. Enkephalin

analogues seem more promising. Most of them have limited access to the central nervous system, but modern techniques of intraspinal application help minimize this problem. A further advantage of opioid peptide analogues is their possible receptor selectivity, implying a potential targeting of analgesic actions and minimization of side effects.[95] Moreover, the degradation of peptide analogues to inactive amino acids in combination with their limited systemic access after intraspinal application may reduce potential systemic side effects. Unfortunately, certain amino acid sequences, such as those related to dynorphin A, appear to liberate excitotoxins or otherwise (e.g., by reducing spinal cord blood flow) produce sensorimotor deficits.[96-99] Frequently irreversible, such adverse effects do not appear to be a function of the opioid pharmacophore but rather to reflect sequence-specific, nonopioid mechanisms that are still undergoing clarification.

DADL, a δ-selective enkephalin analogue, has been used clinically in cases of tolerance to morphine analgesia,[100-102] apparently without adverse side effects, although it did not prevent the μ opioid withdrawal syndrome.[102] FK 33-824 (Tyr-D-Ala-Gly-(N-Me)Phe-(S=O) Met-ol) has preferential binding to μ opioid receptors and is active after intraventricular or systemic administration.[103] Both FK 33-824 and another analogue, BW 433C (Tyr-D-Arg-Gly-(4-NO$_2$)Phe-Pro-NH$_2$),[104] display non-naloxone-reversible side effects after systemic administration. Systemically administered metkephamid (Tyr-D-Ala-Gly-Phe-(N-Me)Met-NH$_2$)[105] has affinity for μ and δ opioid receptors[106] yet produced hypotension during testing in a proportion of obstetric patients, and so clinical trials have been halted.[107]

CONCLUSION

On a day-to-day basis, in part because of the complexities described earlier, opioid peptides have made few inroads into clinical practice. The application of compounds with increased receptor selectivity, for example, has been frustrating clinically.[4] This is perhaps because well-meaning efforts to match activation of opioid receptor subtypes with specific pain modalities run counter to genetic differences in opioid receptor distributions and in situ crosstalk between multiple opioid receptors and ligands within pain pathways.[108-111] Indeed, in light of apparently synergistic interactions between distinct opioid receptor types,[112,113] the design of new opioid compounds with wide receptor selectivity may be attractive. The administration of enzyme inhibitors, for the reasons reviewed, may similarly broadly enhance opioid activity within numerous receptor pathways.

This update has surveyed rapid advances in knowledge concerning the generation, processing, and metabolism of endogenous opioids, and has touched upon initial efforts to apply this knowledge clinically. Many laboratories, spanning disciplines ranging from electrophysiology to receptor genetics to enzymology, have added to this knowledge base. Physiologists and clinical pharmacologists have extended such knowledge to the in vivo setting. Anesthesiologists, accustomed to titrating opioids on a moment-to-moment basis, are uniquely privileged to witness the autonomic,[7] circulatory,[114] and analgesic results of doing so along a continuum of patient consciousness from tense awareness to deep narcotization.[115]

REFERENCES

1. Ahlquist RP. A study of the adrenotropic receptors. Am J Physiol 1948;153:586–600.
2. Kobilka BK, Kobilka TS, Daniel K, et al. Chimeric α_2-, β_2-adrenergic receptors: delineation of domains involved in effector coupling and ligand binding specificity. Science 1988;240:1310–1316.
3. Janssen PAJ. Stereochemical anatomy of morphinomimetics. In: Loh HH, Ross DH, eds. Neurochemical mechanisms of opiates and enkephalins. Adv Biochem Psychopharmacol. New York: Raven Press, 1979;20:103–129.
4. Martin WR. Pharmacology of opioids. Pharmacol Rev 1984;35:283–323.
5. Schiller PW. Conformational analysis of enkephalin and conformation-activity relationships. In: Udenfriend S, Meienhofer J, eds. The peptides. New York: Academic Press, 1984;6:220–228.
6. Morley JS, Dutta AS. Structure-activity relationships of opioid peptides. In: Rapaka RS, Barnett G, Hawks RL, eds. Opioid peptides: medicinal chemistry. Natl Inst Drug Abuse Res Monogr Ser, no. 69. Rockville, Md.: NIDA, 1986;42–64.
7. Carr DB. Opioids. In: Firestone L, ed. Molecular basis of drug action in anesthesia. Int Anesthesiol Clin. Boston: Little, Brown, 1988;26:273–287.
8. Hughes J, Smith TW, Kosterlitz HW, et al. Identification of two related pentapeptides from the brain with potent opiate agonist activity. Nature 1975;258:577–579.
9. Wolfe PB, Wickner WT. Bacterial leader peptidase, a membrane protein without a leader peptide, uses the same export pathway as presecretory proteins. Cell 1984;36:1067–1072.
10. Rice MC, Wickner WT. Mechanisms of membrane assembly and protein secretion in *Escherichia coli*. In: Gething MJ, ed. Protein transport and secretion. New York: Cold Spring Harbor Press, 1985;44.
11. Inouye M, Inouye S, Pollitt S, et al. Structural and functional analysis of the polyprotein signal peptide of *Escherichia coli*. In: Gething MJ, ed. Protein transport and secretion. New York: Cold Spring Harbor Press, 1985;54.
12. Hollt V. Multiple endogenous opioid peptides. Trends Neurosci 1983;6:24–26.
13. Mains RE, Eipper BA. Synthesis and secretion of corticotropins, melantropins, and endorphins by rat intermediate pituitary cells. J Biol Chem 1979;254:7885–7894.
14. Lewis RV, Stern AS, Kimura S, et al. An about 50,000-dalton protein in adrenal medulla: a common precursor of [Met]- and [Leu]-enkephalin. Science 1980;208:1459–1461.
15. Fischli W, Goldstein A, Hunkapiller MW, et al. Isolation and amino acid sequence analysis of a 4,000-dalton dynorphin from porcine pituitary. Proc Natl Acad Sci USA 1982;79:5435–5437.
16. Nakanishi S, Inoue A, Kita T, et al. Nucleotide sequence of cloned cDNA for bovine corticotropin-β-lipotropin precursor. Nature 1979;278:423–427.

17. Noda M, Furutani Y, Takahashi M, et al. Cloning and sequence analysis of cDNA for bovine adrenal preproenkephalin. Nature 1982;295:202–206.

18. Kangawa K, Matsuo H. α-neo-endorphin: a "big" leu-enkephalin with potent opiate activity from porcine hypothalami. Biochem Biophys Res Commun 1979;86:153–160.

19. Goldstein A, Tachibana S, Lowry PJ, et al. Dynorphin (1-13), an extraordinarily potent opioid. Proc Natl Acad Sci USA 1979;68:6666–6670.

20. Kakidani H, Furutani Y, Takahashi H, et al. Cloning and sequence analysis of cDNA for porcine α-neo-endorphin/dynorphin precursor. Nature 1982;298:245–249.

21. Gainer H, Russell JT, Loh YP. The enzymology and intracellular organization of peptide precursor processing: the secretory vesicle hypothesis. Neuroendocrinology 1985;40:171–184.

22. Loh YP, Brownstein MJ, Gainer H. Proteolysis in neuropeptide processing and other neural functions. Annu Rev Neurosci 1984;7:189–222.

23. Chang TL, Gainer H, Russell JT, et al. Proopiocortin converting enzyme activity in bovine neurosecretory granules. Endocrinology 1982;11:1607–1614.

24. Gainer H, Russell JT, Loh YP. An aminopeptidase activity in bovine pituitary secretory vesicles that cleaves the N-terminal arginine from β-lipotropin (60-65). FEBS Lett 1984;175:135–139.

25. Hook VYH. Regulation of carboxypeptidase H by inhibitory and stimulatory mechanisms during neuropeptide precursor processing. Cell Mol Neurobiol 1988;8:49–55.

26. Hook VYH, Loh YP. Carboxypeptidase-B-like converting enzyme activity in secretory granules of rat pituitary. Proc Natl Acad Sci USA 1984;81:2776–2780.

27. Lynch DR, Strittmatter SM, Venable JC, et al. Enkephalin convertase: localization to specific neuronal pathways. J Neurosci 1986;6:1662–1676.

28. Stern AS, Lewis RV, Kimura S, et al. Opioid hexapeptides and heptapeptides in adrenal medulla and brain: possible implications on the biosynthesis of enkephalins. Arch Biochem Biophys 1980;205:606–613.

29. Fricker LD, Snyder SH. Enkephalin convertase: purification and characterization of a specific enkephalin-synthesizing carboxypeptidase localized to adrenal chromaffin granules. Proc Natl Acad Sci USA 1982;79:3886–3890.

30. Fricker LD. Carboxypeptidase E. Annu Rev Physiol 1988;50:309–321.

31. Hook VYH, Affolter, HU. Identification of zymogen and mature forms of human carboxypeptidase H. FEBS Lett 1988;238:338–342.

32. Eipper BA, Mains RE, Glembotski CC. Identification in pituitary tissue of a peptide α-amidation activity that acts on glycine-extended peptides and requires molecular oxygen, copper, and ascorbic acid. Proc Natl Acad Sci USA 1983;80:5144–5148.

33. Bradbury AF, Smyth DG. C-terminal amide formation in peptide hormones. In: Hakanson R, Thorell J, eds. Biogenetics of neurohormonal peptides. London: Academic Press, 1985;171–186.

34. Mains RE, Park LP, Eipper BA. Inhibition of peptide amidation by disulfiram and diethyldithiocarbamate. J Biol Chem 1986;261:11938–11941.

35. Mains RE, Eipper BA. Secretion and regulation of two biosynthetic enzyme activities, peptidyl-glycine α-amidating mono-oxygenase, and a carboxypeptidase by mouse pituitary corticotropic tumor cells. Endocrinology 1984;115:1683–1690.

36. Matsuo H, Miyata A, Mizuno K. Novel C-terminally amidated opioid peptide in human phaeochromocytoma tumor. Nature 1983;305:721–723.

37. Weber E, Esch FS, Bohlen P, et al. Metorphamide: isolation, structure, and biological activity of an amidated opioid octapeptide from bovine brain. Proc Natl Acad Sci USA 1983;80:7362–7366.

38. Eiden LE, Zamir N. Metorphamide levels in chromaffin cells increase after treatment with reserpine. J Neurochem 1986;46:1651–1654.

39. Lindberg I. Reserpine-induced alteration in processing of proenkephalin in cultured chromaffin cells. J Biol Chem 1986;261:16317–16322.

40. Schwyzer R. Estimated membrane structure and receptor subtype selection of an opioid alkaloid-peptide hybrid. Int J Pept Protein Res 1988;32:476–483.

41. Haynes LW. Endorphins—natural selection for nonopiate actions. Trends Pharmacol Sci 1985;6:149–150.

42. Hammonds RG, Nicolas P, Li CH. β-endor-

phin (1-27) is an antagonist of β-endorphin analgesia. Proc Natl Acad Sci USA 1984; 81:1389–1390.

43. Reid RL, Yen SSC. β-endorphin stimulates the secretion of insulin and glucagon in humans. J Clin Endocrinol Metab 1981;52:592–594.

44. van Ree JM, Caffe AR, Woltering G. Nonopiate β-endorphin fragments and dopamine. III γ-type endorphins and various neuroleptics counteract the hypoactivity elicited by injection of apomorphine into the nucleus accumbens. Neuropharmacology 1982; 21:1111–1117.

45. Parish DC, Smyth DG, Normanton JR, et al. Glycyl glutamine, an inhibitory neuropeptide derived from β-endorphin. Nature 1983;306:267–270.

46. Sibinga NES, Goldstein A. Opioid peptides and opioid receptors in cells of the immune system. Annu Rev Immunol 1988;6:219–249.

47. Smyth DG, Massey DE, Zakarian S, et al. Endorphins are stored in biologically active and inactive forms: isolation of α-N-acetyl-peptides. Nature 1979;279:252–254.

48. Smyth DG. Regulation of processing in multifunctional prohormones: a new hypothesis. Biochem Soc Trans 1985;13:38–39.

49. Akil H, Shiomi H, Mathews J. Induction of the intermediate pituitary by stress: synthesis and release of a nonopioid form of β-endorphin. Science 1985;227:424–426.

50. Huttner WB. Tyrosine sulfation and the secretory pathway. Annu Rev Physiol 1988; 50:363–367.

51. Unsworth CD, Hughes J, Morley JS. O-sulphated leu-enkephalin in brain. Nature 1982;295:519–522.

52. van Ree JM. Nonopiate β-endorphin fragments and dopamine. II β-endorphin (2-9) enhances apomorphine-induced stereotypy following subcutaneous and intrastriatal injection. Neuropharmacology 1982;21:1103–1109.

53. Koida M, Ano J, Takenaga K, et al. A novel enzyme in rat brain converting β-endorphin into methionine enkephalin: affinity-chromatography and specificity. J Neurochem 1979;33:1233–1237.

54. McCain HW, Bilotta J, Lamster IB. Endorphinergic modulation of immune function: potent action of the dipeptide glycyl-L-glutamine. Life Sci 1987;41:169–176.

55. Ronken E, Tonnaer JADM, De Boer TD, et al. Autoradiographic evidence for binding sites for des-enkephalin-γ-endorphin (ORG 5878) in rat forebrain. Eur J Pharmacol 1989;162:189–191.

56. Udenfriend S, Kilpatrick D. Biochemistry of enkephalins and enkephalin-containing peptides. Arch Biochem Biophys 1983;221:309–323.

57. Matsuo H. Isolation and identification of opioid peptides. In: Rapaka RS, Hawks RL, eds. Opioid peptides: molecular pharmacology, biosynthesis, and analysis. Natl Inst Drug Abuse Res Monogr Ser, no. 70. Rockville, Md.: NIDA, 1986;92–108.

58. Mizuno K, Minamino N, Kangawa K, et al. A new endogenous opioid peptide from bovine adrenal medulla: isolation and amino acid sequence of a dodecapeptide (BAM-12P). Biochem Biophys Res Commun 1980; 95:1482–1488.

59. Miyata A, Mizuno K, Minamino N, et al. Regional distribution of adrenorphin in rat brain: comparative study with PH-8P. Biochem Biophys Res Commun 1984;120:1030–1036.

60. Mizuno K, Minamino N, Kangawa K, et al. A new family of endogenous "big" met-enkephalin from bovine adrenal medulla: purification and structure of docosa- (BAM-22P) and eicosapeptide (BAM-20P) with very potent opiate activity. Biochem Biophys Res Commun 1980;97:1283–1290.

61. Kimura S, Lewis RV, Stern AS, et al. Probable precursors of [Leu]enkephalin and [Met]enkephalin in adrenal medulla: peptides of 3–5 kilodaltons. Proc Natl Sci USA 1980;77:1681–1685.

62. Kosterlitz HW, Corbett AD, Gillan MGC, et al. Recent developments in bioassay using selective ligands and selective in vitro preparations. In: Rapaka RS, Hawks RL, eds. Opioid peptides: molecular pharmacology, biosynthesis, and analysis. Natl Inst Drug Abuse Res Monogr Ser, no. 70. Rockville, Md.: NIDA, 1986;223–236.

63. Toffoleto O, Metters KM, Oliveira EB, et al. Enkephalin is liberated from metorphamide and dynorphin A (1-8) by endo-oligopeptidase A but not by metalloendopeptidase EC 3.4.24.15. Biochem J 1988;252:35–38.

64. Patey G, Cupo A, Mazarguil H, et al. Release of proenkephalin-derived opioid peptides from

rat striatum in vitro and their rapid degradation. Neuroscience 1985;15:1035–1044.

65. Benuck M, Berg MJ, Marks N. Met-enkephalin-Arg-Phe metabolism: conversion to met-enkephalin by brain and kidney dipeptidyl carboxypeptidases. Biochem Biophys Res Commun 1981;99:630–636.

66. Traynor JR. Prodynorphin as a source of leuenkephalin. Trends Pharmacol Sci 1987;8:47–48.

67. Hui KS, Hui MPP, Lajtha A. Major rat brain membrane-associated and cytosolic enkephalin-degrading aminopeptidases: comparison studies. J Neurosci Res 1988;20:231–240.

68. Gros C, Giros B, Schwartz JC. Identification of aminopeptidase M as an enkephalininactivating enzyme in rat cerebral membranes. Biochemistry 1985;24:2179–2185.

69. De La Baume S, Gros C, Yi CC, et al. Selective participation of both "enkephalinase" and aminopeptidase activities in the metabolism of endogenous enkephalins. Life Sci 1983;31:1753–1756.

70. Herman ZS, Stachura Z, Laskawiec G, et al. Antinociceptive effects of puromycin and bacitracin. Pol J Pharmacol Pharm 1985;37:133–140.

71. McLellan S, Dyer SH, Rodriguez G, et al. Studies on the tissue distribution of the puromycin-sensitive enkephalin-degrading aminopeptidases. J Neurochem 1988;51:1552–1559.

72. Hersh LB, Aboukhair N, Watson S. Immunohistochemical localization of aminopeptidase M in rat brain and periphery: relationship of enzyme localization and enkephalin metabolism. Peptides 1987;8:523–532.

73. Weinberger SB, Martinez JL. Characterization of hydrolysis of [Leu]enkephalin and D-Ala^2-[L-leu]enkephalin in rat plasma. J Pharmacol Exp Ther 1988;247:129–135.

74. Berg MJ, Marks N. Formation of des-Tyr-dynorphins (5-17) by a purified cytosolic aminopeptidase of rat brain. J Neurosci Res 1984;11:313–321.

75. Hui KS, Graf L, Lajtha A. β-endorphin inhibits met-enkephalin breakdown by a brain aminopeptidase: structure-activity relationships. Biochem Biophys Res Commun 1982;105:1482–1487.

76. Graf L, Hui KS, Neidle A, et al. Neuropeptides may regulate neuropeptide metabolism in the brain. Neuropeptides 1982;2:169–173.

77. Malfroy B, Swerts JP, Llorens C, et al. Regional distribution of a high-affinity enkephalin degrading peptidase (enkephalinase) and effects of lesions suggest localization in the vicinity of opiate receptors in brain. Neurosci Lett 1979;11:329–334.

78. Turner AJ, Matsas R, Kenny AJ. Are there neuropeptide-specific peptidases? Biochem Pharmacol 1985;34:1347–1356.

79. Marks N, Benuck M, Berg MJ. Enzymes in the metabolism of opioid peptides: isolation, assay, and specificity. In: Rapaka RS, Hawks RL, eds. Opioid peptides: molecular pharmacology, biosynthesis, and analysis. Natl Int Drug Abuse Res Monogr Ser, no. 70. Rockville, Md.: NIDA, 1986;66–91.

80. Matsas R, Kenny AJ, Turner AJ. The metabolism of neuropeptides: the hydrolysis of peptides, including enkephalins, tachykinins, and their analogues, by endopeptidase 24.11. Biochem J 1984;223:433–440.

81. Deschodt-Lanckman M, Strosberg AD. In vitro degradation of the C-terminal octapeptide of cholecystokinin by "enkephalinase A". FEBS Lett 1983;152:109–113.

82. Chubb IW, Ranieri E, White GH, et al. The enkephalins are amongst the peptides hydrolyzed by purified acetylcholinesterase. Neuroscience 1983;10:1369–1377.

83. Rhee HM. Prolongation of cardiovascular actions of methionine enkephalin by d-phenylalanine in intact rabbits. Ann NY Acad Sci 1988;529:314–316.

84. Roques BP, Fournie-Zaluski MC, Soroca E, et al. The enkephalinase inhibitor thiorphan shows antinociceptive activity in mice. Nature 1980;288:286–288.

85. Lecomte JM, Constetin J, Vlaiculescu A, et al. Pharmacological properties of acetorphan, a parenterally active "enkephalinase" inhibitor. J Pharmacol Exp Ther 1986;237:937–944.

86. Floras P, Bidabe AM, Caille JM, et al. Double-blind study of effects of enkephalinase inhibitor on adverse reactions to myelography. Am J Neuroradiol 1983;4:653–655.

87. Chipkin RE, Berger JG, Billard W, et al. Pharmacology of SCH-34,826, an orally active enkephalinase inhibitor analgesic. J Pharmacol Exp Ther 1988;245:829–838.

88. Fournie-Zaluski MC, Coulaud A, Bouboutou R, et al. New bidentates as full inhibitors of enkephalin-degrading enzymes: synthesis

and analgesic properties. J Med Chem 1985;28:1158–1169.

89. Hernandez JF, Soleilhac JM, Roques BP, et al. Retro-inverso concept applied to the complete inhibitors of enkephalin-degrading enzymes. J Med Chem 1988;31:1825–1831.

90. van Amsterdam JGC, van Buuren KJH, Blad MWM, et al. Synthesis of enkephalinase B inhibitors, and their activity on isolated enkephalin-degrading enzymes. Eur J Pharmacol 1987;135:411–418.

91. Pert CB, Pert A, Chang JK, et al. [D-Ala²]-met-enkephalinamide: a potent, long-lasting synthetic pentapeptide analgesic. Science 1976;194:330–332.

92. Oyama T, Jin T, Yamaya R, et al. Profound analgesic effects of β-endorphin in man. Lancet 1980;1:122–125.

93. Berger PA, Watson SJ, Akil H, et al. β-endorphin and schizophrenia. Arch Gen Psychiatry 1980;37:635–640.

94. Marx JL. Brain opiates in mental illness. Science 1981;214:1013–1015.

95. Pasternack GW. Multiple morphine and enkephalin receptors and the relief of pain. JAMA 1988;259:1362–1367.

96. Herman B, Goldstein A. Antinociception and paralysis induced by intrathecal dynorphin A. J Pharmacol Exp Ther 1985;232:27–32.

97. Stevens CW, Weinger MB, Yaksh TL. Intrathecal dynorphins suppress hindlimb electromyographic activity in rats. Eur J Pharmacol 1987;138:299–302.

98. Long JB, Petras JM, Mobley WC, et al. Neurological dysfunction after intrathecal injection of dynorphin A (1-13) in the rat. II Nonopioid mechanisms mediate loss of motor, sensory, and autonomic function. J Pharmacol Exp Ther 1988;246:1167–1173.

99. Stewart P, Isaac L. Localization of dynorphin-induced neurotoxicity in rat spinal cord. Life Sci 1989;44:1505–1514.

100. Moulin DE, May MB, Kaiko RF, et al. The analgesic efficacy of intrathecal D-Ala²-D-Leu⁵-enkephalin in cancer patients with chronic pain. Pain 1985;23:213–221.

101. Onofrio BM, Yaksh TL. Intrathecal δ receptor ligand produces analgesia in man. Lancet 1983;1:1386–1387.

102. Krames ES, Wilkie DJ, Gershow J. Intrathecal D-Ala²-D-Leu⁵-enkephalin (DADL) restores analgesia in patient analgetically tolerant to intrathecal morphine sulfate. Pain 1986;24:205–209.

103. Stacher G, Bauer P, Steinringer H, et al. Effects of the synthetic enkephalin analogue FK 33-824 on pain threshold and pain tolerance in man. Pain 1979;7:159–172.

104. Posner J, Dean K, Jeal S, et al. Tolerance and pharmacokinetics of a novel opioid peptide BW 443C in healthy volunteers. Br J Clin Pharmacol 1987;24:266p.

105. Calimlim JF, Wandell WM, Sriwatanakul K, et al. Analgesic efficacy of parenteral metkephamid acetate in treatment of postoperative pain. Lancet 1982;1:1374–1375.

106. Frederickson RCA, Smithwick EL, Shuman R, et al. Metkephamid, a systemically active analog of methionine-enkephalin with potent opioid δ receptor activity. Science 1981;211:603–604.

107. Frederickson RCA, Chipkin RE. Endogenous opioids and pain: status of human studies and new treatment concepts. Prog Brain Res 1988;77:407–417.

108. Mansour A, Khachaturian H, Lewis ME, et al. Anatomy of CNS opioid receptors. Trends Neurosci 1988;11:308–314.

109. Millan MJ. Multiple opioid systems and pain. Pain 1986;27:303–347.

110. Yaksh TL. Opioid receptor systems and the endorphins: a review of their spinal organization. J Neurosurg 1987;67:157–176.

111. Hollt V, Sanchez-Blazquez P, Garzon J. Multiple opioid ligands and receptors in the control of nociception. Philos Trans R Soc Lond [Biol] 1985;308:299–310.

112. Rothman RB, Danks JA, Jacobson AE, et al. Leucine enkephalin noncompetitively inhibits the binding of [³H]-naloxone to the opiate μ recognition site: evidence for δ-μ binding site interactions in vitro. Neuropeptides 1985;6:351–363.

113. Yamamoto T, Ohno M, Ueki S. A selective κ opioid agonist, U-50,488H, blocks the development of tolerance to morphine analgesia in rats. Eur J Pharmacol 1988;156:173.

114. Carr DB, Saini V, Verrier RL. Opioids and cardiovascular function: neuromodulation of ventricular ectopy. In: Kulbertus HE, Franck G, eds. Neurocardiology. New York: Ventura, 1988;223–245.

115. Carr DB, Murphy MT. Anesthesia, surgery, and the endorphin system. In: Napolitano L, Chernow B, eds. The stress response in anesthesia and surgery. Int Anesthesiol Clin. Boston: Little, Brown, 1988;26:199–205.

Chapter 1 Discussion

EZZAT AMIN: In this presentation, the authors have shown that the biologically active endogenous opioid peptides are generated from their respective inactive precursors by enzymatic processes. Also, the metabolism of opioid peptides is achieved by enzymatic degradation to yield inactive peptides and amino acids. Different proteolytic enzymes (peptidases) are responsible for the generation and metabolic degradation of the peptides. However, these peptidases are nonspecific.

The following implications can be derived:

1. The concentration of a particular opioid peptide reflects the balance between the two opposite enzymatic processes responsible for its generation and metabolic degradation. This represents an important regulatory mechanism of the biological action of opioid peptides.
2. There are two broad approaches to the development of new analgesics:
   a. To devise compounds that inhibit the enzymatic degradation of opioid peptides so that the body can use its own opioids as analgesics.
   b. To prepare stable analogues of the natural opioid peptides that can resist enzymatic degradation.

These approaches may usher in the era of nonaddictive analgesics.

CARL C. HUG, JR.: For many decades, the study of opioid pharmacology proceeded along two primary pathways: (1) description of their effects in whole bodies and isolated organs, and (2) synthesis of new compounds with characterization of structure-activity relationships. The latter was spurred on by the desire to find an analgesic devoid of the most dangerous side effects of morphine, ventilatory depression and addiction liability, a goal not yet realized.[1]

Given the high potency of morphine and its surrogates, the existence of specific receptors in the central nervous system was taken for granted. The receptor hypothesis was firmly established by the synthesis of even more potent compounds exhibiting stereoselectivity in their actions and by the identification of a specific morphine antagonist, nalorphine.

Anesthesiologists were prominent in these early developments. Eckenhoff et al. were first to report the use of nalorphine as an antidote for morphine poisoning.[2] Beecher and Lasagna demonstrated that nalorphine possessed analgesic properties in surgical patients despite its antagonistic abilities, which gave rise to the notion of mixed agonist-antagonist opioids.[3]

The receptor theory was furthered by the observations of Martin,[4] who hypothesized the existence of multiple types of opioid receptors. Then, in 1973, three groups of investigators independently described saturable, stereospecific opioid binding sites in mammalian nervous tissues.[5-7] Two years later, Kosterlitz, Hughes and coworkers isolated substances from the brain (enkephalins) that exhibited morphinelike actions on the guinea pig ileum (used to screen for opioid activity),[8] and other investigators reported that the pituitary gland contained substances (endorphins) with opioidlike activity.[9] In the past 14 years information about opioid peptide transmitters and receptors has exploded forth from basic research laboratories around the world.

Yet much remains to be learned by basic scientists and clinicians about the pharmacology of morphine and the other opioids. Ventilatory depression remains linked to analgesia; tolerance continues to develop to opioids without any understanding of the basic mechanisms; interactions of opioids with other types of drugs are only beginning to be explored; and addiction continues to claim many in our society, including some in the medical profession.

There is another aspect of opioid pharmacology to which I would like to draw your attention because it has the potential of offering at least partial solutions to today's problems with the clinical use of opioids as well as offering a means of linking observations in the basic science laboratory to the clinical use of opioids. I am referring to pharmacokinetics.

Traditionally, pharmacology is divided into pharmacodynamics (what the drug does to the body) and pharmacokinetics (what the body does to the drug). The latter is often thought of in terms of rather boring descriptions of drug metabolism and excretion or in terms of complicated and abstract mathematical equations describing the uptake, distribution, and elimination of drugs. Although such information is fundamental, it is the application of that information that holds promise for more efficient and safer use of the opioids in patients and for unraveling at least some of the issues related to side effects, toxicity, drug interactions, tolerance, and addiction.

2 OPIOID PEPTIDES AND THEIR RECEPTORS

Eric J. Simon

The purpose of this chapter is to provide an overview of the state of our knowledge concerning the properties and functions of endogenous opioid peptides and their receptors. Clearly, such an active field cannot be exhaustively reviewed in the space of a chapter, and I have chosen aspects that I feel will be of interest and serve as background for the general topic of "Opioids in Anesthesia" and in which I have expertise. I shall have little to say about the importance and role of the endogenous opioid system in anesthesia, since that is the central topic of this volume and many authors are far better qualified than I to deal with this topic.

DISCOVERY OF OPIATE RECEPTORS AND ENDOGENOUS OPIOID PEPTIDES

Opium is probably the oldest known medically useful material. Its psychological effects and usefulness in controlling pain and diarrhea were known to the ancient Sumerians (4000 B.C.) and Egyptians (2000 B.C.). The main active ingredient in opium, an extract derived from the poppy *Papaver somniferum,* is the alkaloid morphine, which is still the most effective and widely used medication against pain. The wide variety of pharmacologic activities of morphine have long fascinated scientists, who have desired to understand the mechanisms that underlie these activities. The most interesting actions of morphine and related drugs are those affecting the central nervous system, such as the control of pain and the phenomena of tolerance and physical and psychological dependence, which together make up the major undesirable side effect of the opiate drugs, namely, narcotic addiction.

An important insight concerning the actions of opiates came as a result of the large synthetic program mounted by pharmaceutical companies in the 1940s and 1950s in an attempt to produce the perfect nonaddictive analgesic, a dream not achieved to this day. In addition to producing some clinically useful drugs, this work led to the hypothesis that opiate drugs must bind to highly specific sites or receptors on nerve cells in order to exert most of their pharmacologic effects. This hypothesis was based on the finding that many of the pharmacologic effects of these drugs, including analgesia, are highly stereoselective, i.e., exhibited by one enantiomer (usually the levorotatory one) but not by its mirror image. In 1973 our laboratory[1] and two others[2,3] simultaneously published biochemical evidence for the existence of stereospecific binding sites for opiates. There is now considerable evidence that strongly supports the idea that these binding sites are receptors that mediate various pharmacologic effects of the opiate drugs.

This important finding led to yet another very exciting discovery. The observation that every vertebrate species examined, and even some invertebrates, have opiate receptors in their nervous systems led scientists to pose the question as to why such receptors are so widespread and why they have survived eons of evolution. This led to the postulate that they must have endogenous functions and, as a corollary, suggested the existence of endogenous opiatelike ligands. An exhaustive study of the known neurotransmitters and hormones did not reveal any that had high affinity for the newly found binding sites. In 1975, Hughes and Kosterlitz and their coworkers[4] published the identification of the first endogenous molecules with opiatelike (opioid) activity and high affinity for opiate receptors. They were the two pentapeptides Tyr-Gly-Gly-Phe-Met and Tyr-Gly-Gly-Phe-Leu, named methionine enkephalin and leucine enkephalin, respectively, by the authors. Since then, about 12 peptides with opioid activity have been found, including the endorphins[5,6] derived from the previously known pituitary hormone β-lipotropin, and dynorphin, a very basic peptide (containing many lysine and arginine residues) with leucine enkephalin at its N-terminal and no relationship to β-lipotropin.[7] Since these opioid peptides are thought to be the natural ligands of the receptors, the latter have been renamed opioid receptors, a term used throughout the rest of this chapter.

Molecular biological research has permitted the establishment of some order among the dozen or so opioid peptides known. As shown in Figure 2.1, it is now clear that all the known opioid peptides are derived from three large precursor proteins: proenkephalin, pro-opiomelanocortin, and prodynorphin, each coded by a separate gene. The structures of the genes are also known, and their similarities suggest that they were derived from a common ancestor gene by gene duplication (for more detailed discussion, see review[8]).

The name pro-opiomelanocortin merits an explanation, because implicit in the name is a very significant discovery,[9,10] namely, that several important and distinct biologically active peptides can be made via a common precursor. In this case, the molecules are the endorphins, adrenocorticotropic hormone (ACTH), and several forms of melanocyte-stimulating hormone, α-, β-, and γ-MSH. The protein is therefore a prohormone for all these peptides with widely different biological activities; hence the name.

It should be mentioned that two distin-

Precursors	Peptides	Structures
Proenkephalin	Met-enkephalin	Tyr-Gly-Gly-Phe-Met$_5$
	Leu-enkephalin	Tyr-Gly-Gly-Phe-Leu$_5$
	Heptapeptide	Tyr-Gly-Gly-Phe-Met-Arg-Phe$_7$
	Octapeptide	Tyr-Gly-Gly-Phe-Met-Arg-Gly-Leu$_8$
Pro-opio melanocortin	α-endorphin	Tyr-Gly-Gly-Phe-Met-Thr-Ser-Glu-Lys-Ser-Glu-Thr-Pro-Leu-Val-Thr$_{16}$
	γ-endorphin	Tyr- " " " " " " " " " " " " " " " -Thr-Leu$_{17}$
	β-endorphin	Tyr- " " " " " " " " " " " " " " " "
		Phe-Lys-Asn-Ala-Ile-Ile-Lys-Asn-Ala-His-Lys-Lys-Gly-Gly-Glu$_{31}$
Prodynorphin	α-neo-endorphin	Tyr-Gly-Gly-Phe-Leu-Arg-Lys-Tyr-Pro-Lys$_{10}$
	Dynorphin A (1-17)	Tyr-Gly-Gly-Phe-Leu-Arg-Arg-Ileu-Arg-Pro-Lys-Leu-Lys-Trp-Asp-Asn-Glu
	Dynorphin (1-8)	Tyr-Gly-Gly-Phe-Leu-Arg-Arg-Ileu$_8$
	Dynorphin B (Rimorphin)	Tyr-Gly-Gly-Phe-Leu-Arg-Arg-Gly-Phe-Lys-Val-Val-Thr$_{13}$

FIGURE 2.1   Opioid peptides and their precursors.

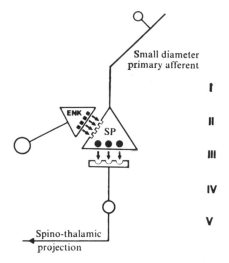

Small diameter
primary afferent

I

II

III

IV

V

ENK

SP

Spino-thalamic
projection

FIGURE 2.2 Schematic representation of a possible mechanism for opioid-induced modulation of substance P (SP) release. SP is shown localized within the terminal of a small-diameter afferent fiber, which forms an excitatory axodendritic synapse with the process of a spinal cord neuron originating in lamina IV or V and projecting rostrally. A local enkephalin-containing inhibitory interneuron (ENK), confined to laminae II and III, forms a presynaptic contact on the terminal of the primary afferent. Opioid receptor sites are located presynaptically. Roman numerals on the right refer to the laminae of Rexed. (Reprinted with permission of the authors and Macmillan Journals, Ltd, from Jessel TM, Iversen LL. Opiate analgesics inhibit substance P release from rat trigeminal nucleus. Nature 1977; 268:549–551.)

acetylcholine and dopamine, respectively. Moreover, at the postsynaptic level the activation of μ as well as δ receptors appears to inhibit dopamine-stimulated adenylate cyclase. This work also confirmed earlier studies suggesting that there may be allosteric interactions between μ and δ receptors. Thus, the inactivation of δ receptors by the irreversible blocker FIT prevented the reversal by naloxone of the μ-receptor (DAGO)-mediated inhibition of adenylate cyclase.

Electrophysiological studies (e.g., Cherubini and North[33] and Gross and Macdonald[34]) have led to the conclusion that activation of the major opioid receptors is coupled to changes in ion conductance. The μ and δ receptors seem to hyperpolarize cells by increasing potassium conductance (opening potassium channels), which in turn results in a decrease in calcium flux. Activation of the κ receptor leads directly to a reduction of calcium conductance. This effect is due to the closing of N-type of calcium channels. There is preliminary evidence that guanosine triphosphate regulatory proteins (G-proteins) may be involved in the coupling of opioid binding sites to ion channels.

On the biochemical level there is considerable evidence that μ and δ channels are linked to the enzyme adenylate cyclase in a negative fashion,[35,36] i.e., the binding of opioid ligands leads to inhibition of cyclic adenosine monophosphate synthesis. This occurs by a coupling via G-proteins. A similar second messenger pathway has recently been described for κ receptors.[37] How all this fits together and exactly how opioid binding leads to pharmacologic response still represent a "black box", the contents of which we are slowly discovering.

PHYSIOLOGIC STUDIES OF OPIOID RECEPTORS

Possible Role in Pain Modulation

The most widely studied putative role for the endogenous opioid peptides and their receptors is the modulation of pain, by analogy with the opiate alkaloids, which are excellent analgesics.

The evidence that the endogenous opioid system is important in pain modulation, while it may not constitute proof, is quite impressive. The major evidence is summarized, followed by a brief discussion of the possible role of the major types of opioid receptors.

Many of the early experiments involved attempts to show reversal of non-drug-induced analgesia by naloxone. Akil and coworkers[38] demonstrated a partial reversal by naloxone of analgesia induced by electrical brain stimulation in rats. This has also been shown in human chronic pain patients, in whom stimulation of the central gray area provides effective analgesia of relatively long duration.

Acupuncture and electroacupuncture have also been shown to be reversed by opiate antagonists,[39,40] and some fascinating experiments suggest that the opioid system may play a role in placebo analgesia, which is effective in about 30% of the population.[41]

More direct evidence for the release of opioid peptides was provided by Akil and collaborators,[42] who observed a large increase in β-endorphin release into cerebrospinal fluid in terminal cancer patients after stimulation of implanted electrodes in the central gray region of the brain.

A study by Han and coworkers[43,44] in Beijing, China, indicates that electroacupuncture in rats is a type of analgesia that involves release of opioid peptides. Using radioimmunoassays, these workers found that low-frequency electroacupuncture led to release of enkephalins into spinal perfusate, while high-frequency electroacupuncture resulted in the release of dynorphin A. These results were confirmed by experiments in which the injection of appropriate antibodies (against enkephalin or dynorphin) was shown to block electroacupuncture analgesia at the appropriate frequencies.

These experiments suggest that δ (or μ) receptors are stimulated at low frequency while κ receptors are primarily activated at high frequency. This brings us to the question of which receptors play a role in pain modulation. It was first thought that only μ receptors are involved, but this neat and simple picture was quickly dispelled. It is now generally accepted that all three major receptor types are involved in analgesia, but some evidence that they may be implicated in different kinds of pain relief is also becoming available. Thus, most reports suggest that supraspinal analgesia may be mediated via μ rather than δ or κ receptors.[45,46] This should not be taken too seriously, since

some evidence for supraspinal δ[47] and κ[48] analgesia also exists.

At the spinal level analgesia against thermal pain stimuli seems to be mediated by separate μ and δ mechanisms, while κ receptors seem to mediate analgesia preferentially active against chemically induced visceral pain.[49]

While much still needs to be learned concerning type of receptor and kind of opioid peptide involved, the evidence that the endogenous opioid system plays a role in the body's system that regulates onset, duration, and severity of pain is quite impressive.

Other Putative Functions of the Endogenous Opioid System

The endogenous opioid system has been implicated in a large number of other physiologic functions, but the evidence that it plays a primary role is not as strong as it is for pain. However, many of these functions are of considerable importance in anesthesia, and a brief discussion of some of the postulated functions is in order.

Evidence that opioid peptides may play a role in the regulation of blood pressure and other cardiovascular functions has been reported by several laboratories, most notably that of Holaday.[50] Early experiments showed that the blood pressure drop induced by several kinds of shock (blood loss, endotoxin, spinal, etc.) was reversed quite effectively by the opiate antagonist naloxone. Further investigation led to the recognition that the δ receptor seems to be the major one involved in this action of endogenous opioids. This conclusion is based on the finding that the selective δ receptor antagonist ICI 174864 was much more effective than naloxone, a μ-preferring antagonist. An interesting byproduct of this study was the finding that blocking μ receptors prevented the blocking of δ receptors and therefore the hypertensive effect. This is best explained by assuming that μ and δ sites exist in a receptor complex in which they affect each other allosterically.

It has been known for many years that morphine and related analgesics cause respiratory depression, a side effect that requires careful supervision of patients. It is therefore not surprising that similar respiratory depression is also observed for opioid peptides. This effect has not yet been intensively studied. We therefore do not know which peptides and receptor types are the major offenders.

Another effect easily predicted from our knowledge of opiate drugs is that on mood. Both euphoria and dysphoria have been observed. The type of change seems to depend both on the subject and on the environment in which the drug is administered. Such effects are observed with pharmacologic doses of opioid peptides, and a role for these peptides in the regulation of mood is postulated, but little is yet known about their involvement.

It may be useful to enumerate some of the other activities in which the endogenous opioid system is thought to be involved. A role in appetite and thirst and in sexual activity has been reported. There is a considerable literature about a role of opioid peptides in memory, which has stimulated research on the possible role of the endogenous opioid system in Alzheimer's disease. The opioids are known to modulate the secretion of a variety of hormones, ranging from prolactin to gonadotropin. There have also been studies suggesting a role in such mental diseases as schizophrenia and depression. Finally, there has been some fascinating recent evidence concerning interactions between the nervous system and the immune system. The opioid peptides may be involved in the cross-talk between these two important systems in our bodies.

This list is by no means exhaustive. It should however be emphasized that a role need not mean a primary role. The brain is so complicated that a secondary or even more remote role is difficult to rule out. However, it is safe to say that the endogenous opioid peptides and their receptors constitute a system of great importance to the function of the brain and some peripheral organs and may prove to rival in significance such classical systems as those involving neurotransmitters like acetylcholine and catecholamines.

BIOCHEMICAL CHARACTERIZATION OF THE MAJOR TYPES OF OPIOID RECEPTORS

I shall utilize the remaining pages to review some of the biochemical studies on opioid receptors, with particular emphasis on work that addresses this question: Are the major known types of opioid receptors separate molecules, or are they different (possibly interconvertible) conformations of the same molecule? This will permit me to discuss some of the more recent research from my own laboratory.

Studies on Membrane-Bound Receptors

The Kosterlitz group[15] obtained support for the existence of separate μ and δ receptors from competition binding studies in guinea pig brain homogenates. It was observed that enkephalins compete significantly better against a labeled enkephalin than against a labeled opiate alkaloid (tritiated naloxone), while the opposite was true for competition of opiates such as morphine or naloxone. When similar experiments were done to detect κ binding, this proved to be more difficult. The reasons for this early problem have been clarified. Many early studies were done in rat brain, now known to contain a very low concentration of κ sites. Moreover, the κ ligands used, ethylketocyclazocine and bremazocine, turned out to be quite nonselective, binding almost as well to μ and δ receptors as they do to κ receptors, although they act like κ agonists in vivo. The latter fact can be explained by the observation that these drugs are antagonists at the other sites. The demonstration of κ binding sites was first successful in Kosterlitz's laboratory using guinea pig brain homogenate to bind ethylketocyclazocine in the presence of saturating concentrations of selective μ and δ ligands. These results have been confirmed by competition experiments with selective κ ligands such as U-50,488H, Cambridge 20, and D-Pro[10] dynorphin (1-11) in many laboratories.

Such competition binding studies have been carried out in various brain regions of a number of species and have led, together with autoradiographic fine-mapping, to the finding that the ratio of μ:δ:κ varies widely from region to region, and for a given region from species to species. A number of regions have been found to be highly enriched in a single receptor type. Thus, the guinea pig cerebellum is highly enriched in κ receptors (80 to 90%), and rabbit cerebellum is enriched in μ receptors, as is the thalamus of several species. No region highly enriched in δ receptors is yet known. The cell culture system NG108-15, a neuroblastoma-glioma hybrid cell, is most frequently used as source of δ receptors.

Another, perhaps more convincing, approach to the differentiation of opioid receptor types is the ability to protect a given type selectively against inactivation by chemical reagents. This was first shown by Robson and Kosterlitz[51] using phenoxybenzamine and by our laboratory[52] with N-ethylmaleimide. Both reagents are irreversible inactivators of opioid receptors. The presence of μ ligands such as morphine, naloxone, or DAGO can selectively protect the μ sites, while the presence of δ or κ ligands will protect the corresponding sites. James and Goldstein[53] have further refined this approach. They utilized β-chlornaltrexamine, an opioid receptor-selective irreversible reagent to produce, by selective protection, tissues that are highly enriched in a given receptor type.

Interesting reagents that can distinguish between receptor types are ethyl alcohol and related short-chain alcohols.[54] These compounds are reversible inhibitors of opioid receptor binding and exert a much greater effect on δ sites than on μ and κ. The inhibition results from a change in the affinity constant with no effect on the number of binding sites. The decrease in affinity is the result of an increase in the dissociation rate of the ligand-receptor complex. As expected, the effect is not competitive and is probably due to a change in receptor conformation resulting from a decrease in membrane fluidity, to which the δ receptors seem to be most sensitive.

All the studies cited tend to support, but do not prove, the molecular distinctiveness of the three major opioid receptor types. To prove

whether or not receptor types are distinct molecules requires their physical separation.

Physical Separation and Purification of Opioid Binding Sites

One way to establish whether receptor types represent distinct molecular species is to separate either active binding sites or binding subunits of the receptors. This area has been reviewed quite recently;[55] therefore only papers too recent to be included in the review are cited here.

A separation of active binding sites has been achieved for κ receptors. Dr. Itzhak in our laboratory was able to separate κ sites from other opioid binding sites using sucrose density gradient centrifugation, while Chow and Zukin had success using a Sepharose column. Such a separation proved more difficult for μ and δ sites. However, a different approach, that of affinity cross-linking of labeled ligands to a membrane fraction, has been successful.

For this purpose Howard in our laboratory used radioiodinated human β-endorphin (labeled in position 27), which has high affinity for both μ and δ receptors but virtually none for κ. This ligand permitted us to examine μ and δ receptors in the same tissue. Membranes were bound with ^{125}I β-endorphin and washed thoroughly. Cross-linking was achieved using one of the commercially available (Pierce) cross-linking reagents, such as bis[2-(succinimido-oxycarbonyloxy)-ethyl]sulfone (BSCOES). This treatment resulted in the covalent linking of 40 to 50% of the ligand prebound to μ and δ receptors. The cross-linked binding sites were extracted from the membranes with SDS and separated by SDS-PAGE. Autoradiography of the gels resulted in the visualization of a number of labeled bands, the number and relative density varying from tissue to tissue. The most important result of these studies was that a band with an apparent molecular weight (Mr) of 65 kDa was present only in tissues known to contain μ receptors and its density increased with the μ:δ ratio of the tissue. A band of apparent Mr of 53 kDa correlated well with the presence and proportion of δ sites. These bands, as well as several others, were eliminated when the binding was carried out in the presence of excess unlabeled naloxone or bremazocine, indicating that they are all subunits of opioid binding sites. The identity of bands other than the 65 and 66 kDa bands is not clear.

While these results suggest that the two proteins represent separate binding subunits of μ and δ receptors, further evidence was deemed necessary. Howard obtained important evidence by performing binding prior to cross-linking in the presence of highly selective μ and δ ligands. It was found that DAGO (μ-selective) selectively suppressed the 65 kDa band at concentrations where it had little or no effect on the 53 kDa band, while DPDPE (δ-selective) preferentially suppressed the labeling of the 53 kDa band. The results strongly support the hypothesis that the 65 kDa and 53 kDa glycoprotein bands represent binding subunits of μ and δ receptors, respectively.

A similar cross-linking study has recently been performed with κ receptors in our laboratory[56] in collaboration with the laboratory of Dr. J. Cros in Toulouse. D-Pro[10] dynorphin (1-11) (DPDYN) was obtained from Dr. Gairin and radioiodinated as described by him and his collaborators. A membrane fraction from guinea pig cerebellum (85 to 90% κ) was allowed to bind the labeled DPDYN in the absence and presence of an excess of unlabeled bremazocine (nonspecific binding) as well as in the presence of μ, δ, and κ ligands. The membranes were washed and cross-linked, and the SDS extracts of the labeled membranes were submitted to SDS-PAGE followed by autoradiography. Two labeled protein bands of apparent Mr of 55 and 35 kDa were obtained. Neither band was reduced significantly when binding was performed in the presence of μ or δ ligands. However, κ ligands such as U-50,488H and DPDYN competed with ^{125}I DPDYN binding. The 55 kDa band disappeared completely, whereas the 35 kDa band was reduced in intensity but did not disappear, even at rather high concentrations of κ competitors. We conclude that the 55 kDa band is a high-affinity κ binding protein. The 35 kDa band may be a low-affinity κ site or a mixture of a κ and a nonopioid protein, the latter labeled nonspecifically.

The results so far discussed suggest that the three major types of opioid receptors are indeed separate molecular entities. We do not know whether they are separate gene products (polypeptides) or whether the differences reside in post-translational modifications, such as sugar residues or phosphorylation. This question will only be answered when the receptors have been cloned and sequenced.

Progress has been reported for the purification of all three major types of opioid receptors. The δ receptor was purified to homogeneity by Klee and coworkers from NG108-15 cells in culture in a covalently cross-linked (inactive) form. This was achieved by use of the δ-selective affinity labeling agent, ^{3}H-3-methylfentanylisothiocyanate (superFIT). A membrane fraction from NG108-15 cells was labeled with this reagent and solubilized with a detergent. Purification was achieved by chromatography on wheat germ agglutinin (WGA)-agarose, followed by chromatography on a column of immobilized antibodies to FIT (fentanylisothiocyanate). Preparative SDS-PAGE was the final purification step. A glycoprotein of Mr 58 kDa was purified 30,000-fold to a final specific activity of 21,000 pmol/mg protein of superFIT, close to the theoretical value for a single binding site per 58,000 daltons.

There has not yet been extensive purification of δ sites from central nervous system tissue, nor has an active δ binding site been purified from any source.

The first partial purification of μ receptors was reported by Bidlack and coworkers, and the first purification to homogeneity of μ binding sites was reported from our laboratory. The latter involved a two-step purification of digitonin-solubilized crude membranes from bovine striatum. The major step was ligand affinity chromatography on immobilized 6-des-oxy-naltrexylethylenediamine (NED), developed by Dr. Gioannini, which results in 3,000- to 5,000-fold purification in a single pass. This was followed by lectin affinity chromatography on immobilized WGA, earlier shown by us to retain applied opioid binding sites, which can then be eluted with N-acetylglucosamine in a yield of 40 to 50% of applied receptor. The purification is about 65,000-fold in an overall yield of 3 to 6%. SDS-PAGE of the purified μ binding site gave a single band of 65 kDa, as detected by autoradiography of a radioiodinated sample or by silver staining. Specific binding activity of the purified receptor is about 15,000 pmol/mg protein, close to the theoretical value for a protein of this size with a single binding site. It should be noted that the purified receptor binds antagonists with high affinity but agonists with very low affinity (in the micromolar range). This may be due to the absence of essential lipids or to uncoupling from G-protein. Efforts to reconstitute high-affinity agonist binding to the purified μ receptor are in progress.

Purification to homogeneity of μ receptors has since been reported by other laboratories, by Cho et al. in San Francisco and Demoliou-Mason and Barnard in England. An interesting difference between Cho's results and ours is that the μ receptor they purified requires acidic lipids for high-affinity binding, while ours does not (at least not for antagonist binding). The reason for this difference is not understood. The κ receptor has been purified fairly extensively from a nonmammalian source, the frog brain, by Simon and co-workers[57] in Hungary. Very recently a report on the purification of κ binding sites from human placenta has appeared.[58] The authors do not claim homogeneity, but specific binding activity is nearly 50% of the theoretical value. The purification procedure is remarkable inasmuch as no ligand affinity chromatography step was used. The technique consisted of covalent chromatography on an SH-containing Sepharose column followed by a WGA column. Neither column is specific for opioid receptors.

CONCLUSION

It is apparent from the foregoing discussion that we have learned a great deal about the endogenous opioid system. Its role in the regulation of pain seems to be quite firmly established. There is, however, still a considerable gap in our understanding of how this system functions. We know quite a lot about the biosynthesis and molecular genetics of the endogenous opioid peptides but very little about how they are released and how their release is controlled. The events that intervene between opioid receptor-ligand interaction and pharmacologic or physiologic response are still largely obscure. The nature and function of the receptors as well as the relationship between the various types and subtypes will only become clear when the receptors are finally cloned and fully sequenced. For reasons that are not understood the molecular biology of opioid receptors has advanced very slowly. However, it is highly probable that the amino acid sequence of one or more of these receptors will soon be available. There is considerable evidence suggesting that the opioid receptors belong to the family of G-protein-linked receptors, a family that includes the monoaminergic, muscarinic acetylcholine and substance K receptors, which have already been sequenced. All these receptors have considerable homology with the protein rhodopsin, the light receptor of the eye. They all have seven hydrophobic regions, which appear to be transmembrane segments, i.e., the receptor seems to traverse the cell membrane seven times.

It is disappointing that our knowledge in this area has not yet led to the discovery of novel, clinically useful products, but it should be remembered that the lag period between discovery and application can be quite long. Thus, the neurotransmitters acetylcholine and norepinephrine were known for many years before clinically useful treatments based on this knowledge became available. There is little doubt that this research has improved our understanding of pain and its modulation, and some potentially useful compounds are on the horizon. To cite one example, it now appears possible to use the body's own opioid peptides as analgesics by administering suitable inhibitors of enzymes that break them down. This approach and an understanding of the exact role of the different types of receptors in analgesia may well usher in the era of nonaddictive analgesics. It is hoped that these studies will also lead to improved ways to produce spinal and general anesthesia.

REFERENCES

1. Simon EJ, Hiller JM, Edelman I. Stereospecific binding of the potent narcotic analgesic ^{3}H-etorphine to rat brain homogenate. Proc Natl Acad Sci USA 1973;70:1947–1949.

2. Terenius L. Stereospecific interaction between narcotic analgesics and a synaptic plasma membrane fraction of rat cerebral cortex. Acta Pharmacol Toxicol (Copenh) 1973;32:317–320.

3. Pert CB, Snyder SH. Opiate receptors: demonstration in nervous tissue. Science 1973; 179:1011–1014.

4. Hughes J, Smith TW, Kosterlitz HW, et al. Identification of two related pentapeptides from the brain with potent opiate agonist activity. Nature 1975;258:577–579.

5. Bradbury AF, Smyth DG, Snell CR, et al. C fragment of lipotropin has a high affinity for brain opiate receptors. Nature 1976;260:793–795.

6. Cox BM, Goldstein A, Li CH. Opioid activity of a peptide, β-lipotropin (61-91) derived from β-lipotropin. Proc Natl Acad Sci USA 1976; 73:1821–1823.

7. Goldstein A, Tachibana S, Lowney LI, et al. Dynorphin (1-13), an extraordinarily potent opioid peptide. Proc Natl Acad Sci USA 1979;76:6666–6670.

8. Simon EJ, Hiller JM. Opioid peptides and opioid receptors. In: Siegel GJ, Agranoff BW, Albers RW, Molinoff PB, eds. Basic neurochemistry. 4th ed. New York: Raven Press, 1989;271–285.

9. Roberts JL, Herbert E. Characterization of a common precursor to corticotropin and β-lipotropin: cell-free synthesis of the precursor and identification of corticotropin peptides in the molecule. Proc Natl Acad Sci USA 1977; 74:4826–4830.

10. Mains RE, Eipper BA, Ling N. Common precursor to corticotropins and endorphins. Proc Natl Acad Sci USA 1977;74:3014–3018.

11. Goldstein A, Barrett RW, James IF, et al. Morphine and other opiates from beef brain and adrenal. Proc Natl Acad Sci USA 1985; 82:5203–5207.

12. Donnerer J, Oka K, Brossi A, et al. Presence and formation of codeine and morphine in the rat. Proc Natl Acad Sci USA 1986;83:4566–4567.

13. Martin WR, Eades CG, Thompson JA, et al. The effects of morphine- and nalorphine-like drugs in the nondependent and morphine-dependent chronic spinal dog. J Pharmacol Exp Ther 1976;197:517–532.

14. Gilbert PW, Martin WR. The effects of morphine- and nalorphine-like drugs in the nondependent, morphine-dependent, and cyclazocine-dependent chronic spinal dog. J Pharmacol Exp Ther 1976;198:66–82.

15. Lord JAH, Waterfield AA, Hughes J, et al. Endogenous opioid peptides: multiple agonists and receptors. Nature 1977;267:495–499.

16. Zukin RS, Zukin SR. Demonstration of ^{3}H-cyclazocine binding to multiple opiate receptor sites. Mol Pharmacol 1981;20:246–254.

17. Herkenham M. Mismatches between neurotransmitter and receptor localization in brain: observations and implications. Neuroscience 1987;23:1–38.

18. Handa BW, Lane AC, Lord JAH, et al. Analogues of β-LPH$_{61-64}$ possessing selective agonist activity at μ opiate receptors. Eur J Pharmacol 1981;70:531–540.

19. Chang K-J, Killian A, Hazum E, et al. Morphiceptin: a potent and specific agonist for morphine μ receptors. Science 1981;212:75–77.

20. Mosberg HI, Hurst R, Hruby VJ, et al. Bis-penicillamine enkephalins possess highly improved specificity toward δ opioid receptors. Proc Natl Acad Sci USA 1983;80:5871–5874.

21. Delay-Goyet P, Seguin C, Gacel G, et al. ^{3}H-D-Ser^2(O-Ter-butyl), Leu^5-enkephalyl-Thr^6 and D-Ser^2(O-Ter-butyl), Leu^5-enkephalyl-Thr^6(O-Ter-butyl): two new enkephalin analogs with both a good selectivity and a high affinity toward δ opioid binding sites. J Biol Chem 1988;263:4124–4130.

22. Von Voigtlander PF, Lahti RA, Ludens JH. U-50,488: a selective and structurally novel non-μ (κ) opioid agonist. J Pharmacol Exp Ther 1983;224:7–12.

23. Lahti RA, Mickelson MM, McCall JM, et al. [^{3}H]-U-69,593: a highly selective ligand for the opioid κ receptor. Eur J Pharmacol 1985; 109:281–284.

24. Leighton BE, Johnson MA, Meecham KG, et al. Pharmacological profile of PD 117302, a

selective κ opioid agonist. Br J Pharmacol 1987;92:915–922.

25. Goldstein A, Nestor JJ Jr, Naidu A, et al. DAKLI: a multipurpose ligand with high affinity and selectivity for dynorphin (κ opioid) binding sites. Proc Natl Acad Sci USA 1988; 85:7375–7379.

26. Gairin JE, Guarderes C, Mazarguil H, et al. D-Pro¹⁰ dynorphin (1-11) is a highly potent and selective ligand for κ opioid receptors. Eur J Pharmacol 1985;106:457–458.

27. Gulya K, Pelton JT, Hruby VJ, et al. Cyclic somatostatin octapeptide analogues with high affinity and selectivity toward μ opioid receptors. Life Sci 1986;30:2221–2229.

28. Cotton R, Giles MG, Miller L, et al. ICI 174864: a highly selective antagonist for the opioid δ receptor. Eur J Pharmacol 1984; 97:331–332.

29. Portoghese PS, Sultana M, Takemori AE. Naltrindole, a highly selective and potent non-peptide δ opioid receptor antagonist. Eur J Pharmacol 1988;146:185–186.

30. Portoghese PS, Lipowski AW, Takemori AE. Binaltorphimine and nor-binaltorphimine, potent and selective κ opioid receptor antagonists. Life Sci 1987;40:1287–1292.

31. Jessel TM, Iversen LL. Opiate analgesics inhibit substance P release from rat trigeminal nucleus. Nature 1977;268:549–551.

32. Schoffelmeer ANM, Rice KC, Jacobson AE, et al. μ, δ, and κ opioid receptor-mediated inhibition of neurotransmitter release and adenylate cyclase activity in rat brain slices: studies with fentanylisothiocyanate. Eur J Pharmacol 1988;154:169–178.

33. Cherubini E, North RA, μ and κ opioids inhibit transmitter release by different mechanisms. Proc Natl Acad Sci USA 1985;82:1860–1863.

34. Gross RA, Macdonald RL. Dynorphin A selectively reduces a large transient (N-type) calcium current of mouse dorsal root ganglion neurons in cell culture. Proc Natl Acad Sci USA 1987;84:5469–5473.

35. Collier HOJ, Roy AC. Morphinelike drugs inhibit the stimulation by E. prostaglandins of cyclic AMP formation by rat brain homogenate. Nature 1974;248:24–27.

36. Sharma SK, Nirenberg M, Klee WA. Morphine receptors as regulators of adenylate cyclase activity. Proc Natl Acad Sci USA 1975; 72:590–594.

37. Atalli B, Saya D, Vogel Z. κ opiate agonists inhibit adenylate cyclase and produce heterologous desensitization in rat spinal cord. J Neurochem 1989;52:360–369.

38. Akil H, Mayer DJ, Liebeskind JC. Antagonism of stimulation-produced analgesia by naloxone, a narcotic antagonist. Science 1976; 191:961–962.

39. Pomeranz B, Chui D. Naloxone blockade of acupuncture analgesia: endorphin implicated. Life Sci 1976;19:1757–1762.

40. Mayer DJ, Price DD, Rafii A. Antagonism of acupuncture analgesia in man by the narcotic antagonist naloxone. Brain Res 1977;121:368–372.

41. Levine JD, Gordon NC, Field HL. The mechanism of placebo analgesia. Lancet 1978;2:654–657.

42. Akil H, Richardson ED, Barchas JD, et al. Appearance of β-endorphin-like immunoreactivity in human ventricular cerebrospinal fluid upon analgesic electrical stimulation. Proc Natl Acad Sci USA 1978;75:5170–5172.

43. Han JS, Xie GX, Zhou ZF. Acupuncture mechanisms in rabbits studied with microinjection of antibodies against β-endorphin, enkephalin, and substance P. Neuropharmacology 1984;23:1–5.

44. Han J-S, Xie GX. Dynorphin: important mediator for electroacupuncture analgesia in the spinal cord of the rabbit. Pain 1984;18:367–376.

45. Chaillet P, Coulaud A, Zajac JM, et al. The μ rather than the δ subtype of opioid receptors appears to be involved in enkephalin-induced analgesia. Eur J Pharmacol 1984;101:83–90.

46. Wood PL, Rackham A, Richard J. Spinal analgesia: comparison of the μ agonist morphine and the κ agonist ethylketocyclazocine. Life Sci 1981;28:2119–2125.

47. Porreca F, Heyman JS, Mosberg HI, et al. Role of μ and δ receptors in the supraspinal and spinal analgesic effects of (D-Pen², D-Pen⁵) enkephalin in the mouse. J Pharmacol Exp Ther 1987;241:393–400.

48. Carr KD, Bonnet KA, Simon EJ. μ and κ opioid agonists elevate brain stimulation threshold for escape by inhibiting aversion. Brain Res 1982;245:389–393.

49. Yaksh TL. Multiple spinal opiate receptor systems in analgesia. In: Kruger L, Liebeskind J, eds. Advances in pain research and therapy. New York: Raven Press, 1984;6:197–215.

50. Holaday JW. Cardiovascular effects of endogenous opiate systems. Annu Rev Pharmacol Toxicol 1983;23:541–594.

51. Robson LE, Kosterlitz HW. Specific protection of the binding site of D-Ala^2-D-Leu^5-enkephalin (δ receptors) and dihydromorphine (μ receptors). Proc R Soc Lond [Biol] 1979; 205:425–432.

52. Smith JR, Simon EJ. Selective protection of stereospecific enkephalin and opiate binding against inactivation by N-ethylmaleimide: evidence for two classes of opiate receptors. Proc Natl Acad Sci USA 1980;77:281–284.

53. James IF, Goldstein A. Site directed alkylation of multiple opioid receptors. I. Binding selectivity. Mol Pharmacol 1984;25:332–342.

54. Hiller JM, Angel LM, Simon EJ. Characterization of the selective inhibition of the δ subclass of opioid sites by alcohols. Mol Pharmacol 1984;25:249–255.

55. Simon EJ, Hiller JM. Solubilization and purification of opioid binding sites. In: Pasternak GW, ed. The opiate receptors. Clifton, N.J.: Humana Press, 1988;165–194.

56. Yao Y-H, Gairin J, Meunier J-C, et al. Cross-linking of κ receptors in the guinea pig cerebellum with D-Pro^{10} dynorphin (1-11). In: Cros J et al. eds. Progress in opioid research. Oxford: Pergamon Press, 1989;21–24.

57. Simon J, Benye S, Hepp J, et al. Purification of a κ opioid receptor subtype from frog brain. Neuropeptides 1987;101:19–28.

58. Ahmed MS, Zhon D-H, Cavinato AG, et al. Opioid binding properties of the purified κ receptor from human placenta. Life Sci 1989;44:861–871.

Chapter 2 Discussion

EZZAT AMIN: The author has presented evidence suggesting that the three major types of opioid receptors (μ, δ, and κ) are distinct molecular entities. However, whether they are coded by separate genes or whether the differences between them are due to post-translational modifications during their protein synthesis is not yet known. This question will only be answered when the amino acid sequence of each receptor protein is fully established.

The author has also stated that there is considerable evidence suggesting that the opioid receptors belong to the family of G-protein-linked receptors. This family includes the visual pigment rhodopsin and monoaminergic, muscarinic acetylcholine receptors. All these receptors appear to pass through the cell membrane seven times, forming seven hydrophobic transmembrane segments. The N-terminal, with its sugar residues, lies outside the cell membrane, while the phosphorylated C-terminal extends inside the cell.

It is hoped that further research in the field of molecular biology of opioid receptors will permit the full establishment of their structure, function, and molecular genetics. Such knowledge will lead to very useful clinical applications in the fields of pain relief and anesthesia.

3 INTERACTION BETWEEN ADRENERGIC AND OPIOID PATHWAYS

Byron C. Bloor, Mervyn Maze, and Ira Segal

NORADRENERGIC PATHWAYS IN THE CENTRAL NERVOUS SYSTEM

The two major norepinephrine-containing nuclei are in the locus ceruleus and the lateral tegmental area. From these cell bodies, axonal systems arise to innervate targets throughout the neuraxis. Five major noradrenergic tracts arise from the locus ceruleus, namely, the central tegmental tract, dorsal longitudinal tract, ventral tegmental-medial forebrain tract, cerebellar tract, and a descending tract into the spinal cord.[1] The major effect of activating these efferent pathways from the locus ceruleus is to inhibit spontaneous discharge of the target cell by hyperpolarizing and thereby increasing the membrane resistance. The lateral tegmental area gives rise to less discrete pathways ascending to the forebrain and diencephalon and descending via the mesencephalon into the spinal cord. Epinephrine-containing cells are found in two groups (C1 and C2).[2] These axons ascend to the hypothalamus via the periventricular system or descend to the locus ceruleus, the intermediolateral cell columns of the spinal cord, and the periventricular regions of the fourth ventricle.

Receptor Subtypes and Synaptic Location

For the purposes of this discussion we confine our remarks to the α adrenoceptors. Initially, α adrenoceptors were classified according to their synaptic location, with α_1 being designated as postsynaptic and α_2 being designated presynaptic where it exerts an autoinhibitory effect on norepinephrine release into the synapse.[3] The α_1 and α_2 receptor classifications are based on pharmacologic characterizations, not location, as it has become evident that the majority of α_2 adrenoceptors in the central nervous system (CNS) (and on the peripheral vasculature) are postsynaptic.[4] The functional role for central α_2 adrenoceptors is not precisely known.[5]

Signal Transduction and Physiologic Responses

The α-adrenergic receptors are functionally and spatially separated from their membrane-bound effector molecule. The functional coupling between receptor and effector is provided by a guanine nucleotide binding protein (or G-protein) which is sometimes referred to as a nucleotide regulatory component (N-protein) in the older literature. In the functionally uncoupled state the G-protein is bound by guanosine diphosphate (GDP). Following agonist binding to the receptor, a conformational change facilitates the release of GDP from the α subunit of the heterotrimeric G-protein. The vacant guanine nucleotide binding site is immediately occupied by guanosine triphosphate (GTP), which is abundantly present in the cytosol, causing the dissociation of the heterotrimer into an activated α subunit and a β-γ dimer. In the GTP-bound state the α subunit is now capable of activating the effector molecule.[6]

For the α_1 receptor, the effector molecule is a phosphodiesterase called phospholipase C (PLC), which hydrolyzes a membrane phospholipid substrate, phosphatidyl inositol bisphosphate (PIP_2), into diacylglycerol (DG) and inositol triphosphate (IP_3). IP_3 triggers the release of calcium from the endoplasmic reticulum into the cytosol, where it will promote the translocation of cytosolic protein kinase C to a membrane-bound location where it is activated in concert with DG. Subsequent phosphorylation of regulatory proteins produces the α-neuronal response.

For the α_2 receptor, the effector molecule may either be adenylate cyclase or an ion channel. In the case of adenylate cyclase, stimulation of the α_2 adrenoceptor will result in the inhibition of adenylate cyclase, thereby opposing the stimulatory action of compounds such as β-adrenergic receptor agonists. The decrease in cyclic adenosine monophosphate (cAMP) and cAMP-dependent protein kinase activity will attenuate the enhanced conductance through voltage-operated calcium channels, which is activated by phosphorylation mediated by cAMP-dependent protein kinase. In addition, the activated α subunit of the G-protein may directly regulate conductance through ion channels, specifically potassium (increasing) and calcium (decreasing) con-

ductances without any intervening second messenger system.[7]

The functional consequence of α_1 stimulation in the CNS, i.e., activation of protein kinase C and a rise in the intracellular calcium transient, is not precisely known, although it is thought to be excitatory in nature and may be involved in arousal-vigilance behavioral responses. With respect to α_2 stimulation, the decrease in calcium conductance in the presynaptic neuron, whether produced directly or indirectly by changes in potassium conductance, will have the net effect of decreasing neurotransmitter release, both of the excitatory (norepinephrine, glutamine substance P, etc.) and the inhibitory (GABA) neurons. Thus, the net result may be a decrease in excitatory and nociceptive pathways or a disinhibition of inhibitory interneurons. Following activation of the somatodendritic α_2 receptors, the firing rate is decreased through an increase in potassium conductance, which may be linked to changes in the level of consciousness. In essence, the postsynaptic α_2 adrenoceptor hyperpolarizes the cell, thereby decreasing neuronal excitability.

Pharmacology of α-Adrenergic Receptor Agonists and Antagonists

The factors governing the ability of the agonist to produce a response include its selectivity, potency, and efficacy. Selectivity refers to its bindability to the two major classes of α receptor subtypes (α_1 or α_2). This is of particular importance in CNS-active α-adrenergic agonists, since diametrically opposite responses are produced by these two subtypes (i.e., excitatory via α_1 and inhibitory via α_2). Thus, it can be expected that a highly selective α_2 agonist (e.g., dexmedetomidine) will tend to produce CNS depression, while a highly selective α_1 agonist (ST-587 or cirazoline) will produce excitation. A nonselective agonist may have little or no net effect. Potency can be measured directly by the amount of an agonist (or antagonist) that results in a quantitated response.

The potency of the agonist is conferred in part by the agonist's affinity for the receptor, which can be precisely quantitated by its ability to displace a radio-labeled ligand from the binding site (i.e., the affinity constant). Efficacy relates to the capability of an agonist to transduce a maximum response. The factors governing this feature are now being unraveled given our new understanding of the components necessary for signal transduction. It is now appropriate to discuss efficacy in terms of the receptor occupancy necessary to produce a full effect, with the most efficacious compounds able to produce a full response with a minimum number of the receptors being occupied. Thus, in some manner, the efficiency by which an activated receptor couples to its effector is crucial for the efficacy of the agonist. Considerable progress in this area has been facilitated by the tools provided by the techniques of molecular biology and modeling. Current drug design considers not only the receptor selectivity and affinity of the agonist but also postreceptor conformation changes produced by the agonist.

The pharmacologic action of antagonists is also governed by their selectivity and affinity of binding for the two receptor subtypes, with the same caveats that applied to the agonists. The potency of an antagonist is often expressed by its pA_2 value, which reflects the molar concentration of antagonist required to produce the same agonist effect when the concentration of the agonist is doubled. At this point, the efficacy of antagonists does not appear to be related to postreceptor events.

THE OPIOID SYSTEM IN THE CENTRAL NERVOUS SYSTEM

The opioid system has been spatially characterized by autoradiographic studies.[8] Opioid receptors are highly concentrated in areas known to be associated with pain perception. For instance, clusters of opioid receptors form a dense and narrow band in the substantia gelatinosa in the spinal cord. It is at this level that incoming sensory fibers synapse and initial integration of nociception occurs. The periaqueductal gray is a small circular zone in the brain stem where electrical stimulation produces analgesia, which can be antagonized with naloxone. The localization of opioid receptors in the limbic system has been implicated in the euphoria that is produced by certain opioids. It is noteworthy that one of the densest concentrations of opioid receptors exists in the locus ceruleus, the source of the major ascending and descending noradrenergic tracts in the brain. High concentrations of opioid receptors also exist in the nucleus tractus solitarius, which may be involved in opioid-induced respiratory depression. Pupillary diameter is regulated by a group of brain stem nuclei within the superior colliculus and the pretectal nuclei. These same areas are rich in opioid receptors, which may account for opioid-induced miosis.

Immunohistochemical stains have mapped out the enkephalin-containing neurons in the mammalian brain. The enkephalins are released by depolarization in a calcium-dependent manner and can thus be considered to be the major opioidlike neurotransmitter in the mammalian brain. High densities of enkephalin neurons occur in the dorsal part of the spinal cord, limbic nuclei (including the amygdala), the vagal nuclei, and the locus ceruleus.

Receptor Subtypes

Several lines of evidence support the existence of multiple opioid receptors. Different classes of opioid drugs produce distinct behavioral syndromes, and tolerance to one group of opioids does not result in cross-tolerance to another class of opioid drug.[9] While Martin and his colleagues proposed the existence of three distinct subtypes—μ for morphinelike compounds, κ for ketocyclazocinelike drugs, and σ for drugs such as SKF-10,047—the last is nonopioid in nature. It has been replaced by the δ receptor, initially named for the mouse vas deferens bioassay, where enkephalin peptides are particularly potent. The δ opioid receptors are more limited in their distribution and appear densest in olfactory-related neural areas, neocortex, caudate-putamen, nucleus accumbens, and amygdala. The function of these opioid receptor sites is not clear, but they may play a role in motor integration, olfaction, and cognitive functioning. μ opioid receptors are widely distributed throughout the forebrain, midbrain, and hind brain and correspond well with their putative role in pain regulation and sensorimotor integration. κ opioid receptors are localized in an intermediate number of brain areas, with the densest areas of binding observed in the caudate-putamen, nucleus accumbens, amygdala, hypothalamus, neural lobe of the pituitary, median eminence, and nucleus tractus solitarius. The distribution of κ opioid receptors is consistent with their probable role in regulating water balance, food intake, pain perception, and neuroendocrine functioning.

Signal Transduction and Function of the Different Subtypes

Since their discovery, opioid receptor subtypes have been implicated in negative coupling to adenylate cyclase in certain cell culture and brain areas. However, in general, it has been difficult to demonstrate an important second messenger response of any functional consequence. In common with adrenergic receptor subtypes, the opioid receptor classes are associated with the specific G-protein called G_i, which accomplishes the first stage of receptor signal transduction through the hydrolysis of GTP. Thus, especially for the μ and δ receptor subtypes, there is some evidence from biochemical, pharmacologic, and neurophysiologic studies that all the biological responses to opioid receptor activation depend on a pertussis-toxin-sensitive G-protein. For example, the antinociceptive effects of intrathecally administered enkephalins can be attenuated by pretreatment with pertussis toxin.[10]

Since activation of all types of opioid receptors both inhibits transmitter release and slows cell firing, it was assumed that the signal transduction mechanisms would be similar. But there is more than one way to change the membrane properties of a cell so that it will release less transmitter, and there are several distinct ion conductances that could be responsible for slowing the rate of spike discharge. Activation of the μ opioid receptor in the locus ceruleus appears to increase potassium conductance through a similar G-protein-coupled process as has been found for the α_2-adrenergic agonist.[11] The properties of the potassium conductance coupled to the μ receptors have been well characterized at the whole-cell level in the locus ceruleus, where the conductance is in the order of 5 nS, is voltage-independent in the range -50 mV to -120 mV, and is insensitive to tetra-ethylammonium or 4-aminopyridine. In dorsal root ganglion cells, activation of μ receptors also results in an increase in potassium conductance but is not associated with membrane hyperpolarization. The increase in potassium has the effect of accelerating the repolarization phase of an action potential. Activation of the δ receptor in the guinea pig submucous plexus increases the conductance of an inwardly rectifying potassium conductance that strongly hyperpolarizes the membrane in much the same manner as occurs for the μ receptor in the locus ceruleus.[12] Similarly, a guanine nucleotide binding protein is involved in the direct coupling between the δ opioid receptor and the potassium channel, with no evidence for activation of either cAMP-dependent protein kinase or protein kinase C. Activation of the κ opioid receptor results in a reduction in calcium entry[13] in dorsal root ganglion cells, whereas the μ and δ receptors on this cell type do not directly reduce calcium currents in these neurons. Possibly it is this action that directly inhibits neurotransmitter and substance P release.

Pharmacology of the Opioid Receptor Subtypes

At the μ receptor subtype the most selective agonists are DAGO (Tyr-D-Ala-Gly-MePhe-Gly-ol) and morphiceptin (Tyr-Pro-Phe-Pro-

NH_2), while the most potent antagonist is naloxone and the most selective are the cypridime series of compounds. At the δ receptor subtype the most selective agonists are DPDPE (Tyr-D-Pen-Gly-Phe-D-Pen) and DPLPE (Tyr-D-Pen-Gly-Phe-L-Pen), with ICI 174864 being quite potent as an antagonist at this receptor. Recently a new family of naltrexone-derived antagonists have been synthesized, of which naltrindole shows the best combination of potency and selectivity for the δ receptor. For the κ receptor subtype, the most selective agonists appear to be dynorphin and U-50,488H, while the most potent antagonist appears to be naloxone, although the newer bimorphinan compounds appear to be even more selective. It appears that each opioid receptor subtype can inhibit neurotransmitter release but appears to be located on different neurotransmitter pathways. Thus, μ receptors inhibit norepinephrine release, δ receptors inhibit acetylcholine release, and κ receptors inhibit dopamine release.[14]

INTERACTIONS BETWEEN OPIOID AND α-ADRENERGIC MECHANISMS

From the foregoing it appears that the α_2-adrenergic and opioid receptor types are analogous and that these receptors often coexist in the same cell. In fact, neurons containing both a catecholamine and an opioid transmitter have been proposed by Okamura et al.[15] One might ask the teleologic reason for such a set of circumstances. Their similar actions include both analgesia and sedation, which may be based on their ability to inhibit neurotransmitter release (e.g., substance P for the analgesic response) or decrease neuronal firing (e.g., in the locus ceruleus for the sedative property). It is noteworthy that some of the opioid subtypes, e.g., the κ, are more prone to produce sedation than others, for example, the μ opioid subtype, which may produce excitation at low doses and a catatonic state at high doses.[16] Furthermore, the α_2-adrenergic and opioid classes of receptor agonists also

differ in a number of important categories. First, α_2 agonists do not appear to have any important respiratory depressant effects.[17] Second, muscle flaccidity is a feature of α_2 agonists rather than the muscle rigidity produced by the potent μ opioid agonists.[18] Finally, the euphoria that is such a prominent feature of certain opioids, and that may be a factor in opioid abuse in primates, is not seen with the α_2-adrenergic agonists. It must also be considered that some α_2 actions may resemble certain opioid subtype specific actions, such as the diuretic effect of the α_2 agonist[19] and of the κ agonist[20], while differing from others, like the antidiuretic effect of μ agonists.[21]

Of particular interest to anesthesiologists is the use of a combination of drugs to produce a quality of analgesia or anesthesia, in association with hemodynamic stability, that holds great promise for the future in the clinical paradigm. The following discussion concerns preclinical studies that may provide insight into the appropriate use of such a combination of drugs.

Analgesic Effects

An increasing number of reports now suggest that α_2-adrenergic and opioid agonists, acting either at different levels in the nociceptive pathways or by different mechanisms at the same locus, may enhance the analgesic properties of each agent. Tamsen and Gordh[22] showed that the combination of epidurally administered clonidine and morphine produced longer duration of analgesia than either did alone without the onset of tolerance when used in combination for as long as two weeks. In another case report, the intrathecal analgesic doses of hydromorphone could be dramatically reduced by coadministration of intrathecal clonidine.[23] Clonidine has been added to intrathecal morphine in intractable cancer pain after the patient had become tolerant to morphine alone. The patient was maintained three months without pain.[24] In a series of reports concerning the efficacy of clonidine versus morphine for the control of deafferentation pain, clonidine appeared to be superior to narcotics in the majority of the patients studied.[25] In another case report, a patient with spinal deafferentation pain was successfully weaned off a combination of systemic and epidural diamorphine by substituting oral and epidurally administered clonidine.[26] In a randomized double-blind study of 20 patients with chronic pain, epidural morphine and clonidine were found to be similar in efficacy.[27] Thus, such a combination may have important clinical uses:

1. To limit the side effects present when a higher dose of the single agent is used.
2. To delay the onset of tolerance to the analgesic properties of either agent.
3. To substitute one agent for another when tolerance does occur.
4. To treat withdrawal syndromes from one agent with the other class of agent.

Up to this point most of these issues have not been rigorously tested in the clinical setting. While some of the data suggest that these attributes are attainable, other, conflicting reports place the realization of these clinical goals further away.

What is the evidence that the α_2-adrenergic and opioidergic systems differ in their nociceptive actions? The analgesic and behavioral properties of intrathecally administered α_2-adrenergic and opioid agonists appear to be quite similar,[28] although their mechanisms of action may differ. For example, morphine, but not α_2-adrenergic agonists, are capable of releasing adenosine from synaptosomes prepared from the dorsal columns of the spinal cord in a rat.[29] Since adenosine is capable of exerting an antinociceptive action,[30] this suggests at least one clear difference in the antinociceptive actions of these two classes of analgesics. α_2-adrenergic agonists have also recently been reported to increase the release of dynorphin from the spinal cord of rats, and antiserum to dynorphin will block the analgesic action of clonidine intrathecally.[31] Interestingly, intrathecal naloxone has been shown to result in a dose-dependent inhibition of intrathecal norepinephrine-induced antinociception in the rat.[32]

Electrical stimulation of the periaqueductal gray or microinjection of opioids into this region will significantly increase the nociceptive threshold. This effect can be blocked by the intrathecal administration of an α_2-adrenergic antagonist.[33] Additionally, analgesics tend to increase the amount of norepinephrine in the spinal cord.[34] This would suggest that opioids acting supraspinally activate α_2-adrenergic receptors in the spinal cord by facilitating the release of norepinephrine, the endogenous neurotransmitter for this receptor. However, this is seemingly at variance with the ability of opioid receptors to decrease firing rates in the noradrenergic pathways. Perhaps part of this paradox can be addressed by the likelihood that the α_1-agonist action of norepinephrine may be excitatory and functionally antagonize the inhibitory α_2-adrenergic receptor.[35]

Intrathecal clonidine potentiates the inhibitory effects of intrathecal morphine on electrically evoked C fiber activity in dorsal horn neurons of the rat.[36] Activity in C fibers has been associated with release of substance P in nociceptive pathways.[37,38] The involvement of α_2 adrenoceptors in potentiating the antinociceptive effects of morphine has been reported in the primate[39] and in the rat[40], in which the intrathecal agonist ST-91, selective for α_2 adrenoceptors, increased the antinociceptive action of intrathecal morphine, with a sevenfold decrease in the ED_{50} for the opiate in the rat studies. This was recently confirmed in studies with a combination of oxymetazoline and morphine administered intrathecally.[41]

Potentiation of morphine by clonidine has also been reported when both are given systemically.[42–44] Recently Drasner and Fields[45] demonstrated that systemically administered morphine potentiated the analgesic action of intrathecally administered clonidine.

It is notable that in certain species the interaction between α_2-agonists and opioids does not potentiate the analgesic action of one or the other. Eisenach and colleagues[46] demonstrated that in the pregnant ewe, morphine does not potentiate the antinociceptive action of clonidine.

Cross-Tolerance

There are conflicting data on the issue of cross-tolerance in different species and from different analgesic paradigms. Repeated intrathecal administration of ST-91 (a selective α_2-adrenergic agonist) to rats produced a significant tolerance to ST-91's ability to block the attenuate hot-plate and tail-flick responses. Once tolerance to ST-91 was obtained, the injection of morphine was observed to produce an effect that was indistinguishable from saline (i.e., cross-tolerance to morphine).[47] Yaksh and Reddy[39] have demonstrated that combined intrathecal administration of morphine and an α_2-adrenergic agonist delays the development of tolerance to either drug. They speculated that tolerance was avoided because the synergistic interaction allowed for a lesser degree of activation of each of the independent receptor systems. If this hypothesis is correct, then developing techniques that will produce adequate analgesia with the lowest possible receptor activation are essential.

In an analgesic paradigm in which the electric shock necessary to produce vocalization was determined, a previously analgesic dose of morphine was no longer effective following chronic administration of clonidine systemically, suggesting cross-tolerance.[48] Cross-tolerance to clonidine and morphine has been demonstrated in rats by measuring tail-flick latency response. An analgesic dose of clonidine was ineffective following induced morphine tolerance.[49] In rats made tolerant by a continuous intrathecal morphine infusion, the antinociceptive effect of intrathecal norepinephrine was significantly attenuated.[32]

Since the possibility of cross-tolerance exists, investigators have questioned whether naloxone will reverse the reported analgesic effects of α_2-adrenergic agonists. Tchakarov et al.[50] have reported that naloxone reverses the antinociceptive action of clonidine in hyper-

tensive rats. Analgesia produced by intracerebral administration of clonidine was effectively antagonized by both naloxone and yohimbine (an α_2-adrenergic antagonist) in the monkey.[51] Mohrland and Von-Voigtlander[52] have failed to show any reversal by naloxone of analgesia produced by a clonidine analogue. Thus, this issue is also clouded.

Cardiovascular Effects

The epinephrine-containing $C1^2$ cell group in the rostral ventrolateral medulla oblongata forms a monosynaptic connection to preganglionic sympathetic cell bodies in the intramedial lateral columns. These cells are tonically active and are sympathoexcitatory.[53] Stimulation of the C1 area electrically or by the excitatory amino acid L-glutamate results in elevated blood pressure.[54,55] Inhibition of these cells by α_2-adrenergic agonists,[50] opioid agonists,[56] H2 histamine agonists,[57] and imidazole agonists[57] results in sympathoinhibition. The C1 cell group receives innervation from many brain stem nuclei that control cardiovascular function (including the nucleus tractus solitarius, vagal motor center, reticular areas, locus ceruleus, and the amygdala) and is the efferent limb of the baroreceptor reflex arc. This connection with the baroreceptor system tonically links the sympathetic system to the cardiac cycle.[53] The C1 area gates the outflow from these higher brain centers to the preganglionic sympathetic neurons, thus controlling "sympathetic tone."

As stated, several neurotransmitters act to modulate the tonic activity of this area and therefore exert control on the sympathetic preganglionic cells. This common anatomical juncture affords a theoretical explanation for the similarity in some of the hemodynamic effects of clonidinelike and opioid drugs. During anesthesia and surgery both types of drugs have been shown to attenuate hemodynamic responses to noxious stimuli (see the following section "Clinical Uses of a Combination of α_2-Adrenergic Agonist and Opioids during General Anesthesia").

A pressor effect has also been noted following microinjections of an opioid μ agonist. μ receptors in the nucleus tractus solitarius elicit increased sympathetic nerve activity and, surprisingly, attenuation of the baroreceptor reflex following microinjection of DAGO (a selective μ antagonist).[58] In addition to the C1 area, where L-glutamate is sympathoexcitatory, there has been a depressor area reported that when stimulated by L-glutamate is sympathoinhibitory. Microinjection of opioid agonists on this site results in increased blood pressure and heart rate via the sympathetic nervous system,[56] i.e., opioids applied in this location inhibit this inhibitory center. This duality could explain some of the reported disparities and also why the narcotics could have different effects (or little to no effect) depending on the relative dominance of either the pressor or depressor area under different experimental conditions.

Other clinical reminders of the opiate adrenergic connection include the occasional catastrophic sympathetic discharges following naloxone reversal.[59–65] Clonidine has been found to attenuate the adrenergic response that occurs when naloxone is used to reverse fentanyl in dogs.[66]

Conflicting results have been reported regarding the ability of naloxone to partly reverse clonidine-induced hemodynamic effects. Naloxone alone, in normotensive humans[67] and hypertensive animals, does not cause significant changes in blood pressure or heart rate. This suggests that tonic opioidergic tone probably does not contribute to the normal or pathophysiological control of blood pressure. Farsang et al.[68] have found, in spontaneously hypertensive rats, that naloxone prevents and reverses the antihypertensive effects of clonidine. In hypertensive humans, naloxone has been reported to partially reverse the antihypertensive effects of clonidine in 50% of the individuals studied.[69]

Since the clonidine and opioid receptors are distinct and there is no cross-reaction at the receptor, for naloxone to have an effect on clonidine's hemodynamic effects one might predict the release of an opioidlike substance.

Several investigators have, in fact, reported the release of a β-endorphine immunoreactive material.[70,71]

Treatment of Addiction and Narcotic Withdrawal

Since the late 1970s clonidine has been used to manage the withdrawal syndrome associated with the detoxification of narcotic addicts.[72] The mechanism for this interaction is slowly being outlined. During withdrawal, release from the chronic narcotic inhibition (disinhibition) is thought to result in a hyperadrenergic state. These effects could presumably be mediated at the C1 area. Clonidine has been postulated, acting through either the α_2-adrenergic or imidazole receptor, to inhibit C1 neuronal traffic, attenuating the hyperadrenergic state. Consistent with this concept, the α_2-adrenergic antagonist yohimbine exacerbates morphine withdrawal in rats.[73]

Secondary to clonidine's effect on the hyperadrenergic sequelae during narcotic withdrawal, clonidine also causes some sedation. This too is probably beneficial during the early phases of withdrawal. Clonidine has been found equal but not superior to methadone treatment; however, it may be beneficial when coupled to the long-acting narcotic antagonist naltrexone.[74] In this way, the abstinence syndrome is minimized, and the temptation of returning to narcotic abuses is lessened.

Clinical Uses of a Combination of α_2-Adrenergic Agonist and Opioids during General Anesthesia

Slogoff and Keats[75] demonstrated a relationship between anesthetic or surgical events known to produce intense sympathetic stimulation and the occurrence of perioperative myocardial ischemia and postoperative myocardial infarction. Very high doses of narcotics have been used in an attempt to provide stable hemodynamic parameters without myocardial depression. Even at these doses, hypertension and tachycardia have been reported.[76,77] Secondary to these high narcotic doses, prolonged respiratory depression occurs.

For many of the foregoing reasons, several investigators have used clonidine as an adjunct medication in a balanced narcotic anesthetic technique during surgery. In general, all investigations have found improved hemodynamic stability and reduced narcotic anesthetic requirement. Flacke et al.,[78] utilizing hemodynamic determinants, found that 3.5 µg/kg clonidine given 90 minutes preoperatively and again 5 hours later in patients undergoing coronary artery bypass surgery (CABG) reduced sufentanil requirements by 41%. Even with this considerable reduction in narcotic requirement the hemodynamic responses by the patient during the stressful periods of the surgery were significantly reduced. In a similar study that also examined the effects of adding clonidine to anesthetic regimen during CABG surgery where EEG was used as the determinant of adequate anesthesia, Ghignone et al.[79] reported that clonidine reduced the fentanyl requirement at induction and intubation by 50% and 45%, respectively, with improved cardiovascular stability. Also, in hypertensive patients undergoing elective surgery, Ghignone et al. have reported that acutely administered clonidine resulted in a reduced hemodynamic lability, despite a 50% reduction in the number of pharmacological interventions required to maintain blood pressure in a predetermined normal range. Clonidine also resulted in a 75% decrease in the amount of fentanyl needed during the anesthesia.[80] Other studies have also reported improved hemodynamic stability during surgery under a balanced narcotic anesthesia when clonidine has been added.[81-84] Besides reducing the narcotic requirement, clonidine use also results in reduced ventilatory depression postoperatively.[78]

CONCLUSION

The adrenergic and opioid systems seem to interact at many different levels. These two systems are known to have receptors on the same cells, have transmitters located in the same cell, and when mapped histochemically, show a remarkable similarity in location in the brain. Their likeness also extends to a point of redundancy in function. Both the opioid and the α_2-adrenergic systems cause profound analgesia and sedation, and modulate sympathetic outflow. One major difference is that the α_2-adrenergic agonists do not seem to cause respiratory depression. Combining the two drug classes may optimize the beneficial effects of both while minimizing the unwanted side effects and delaying the onset of tolerance, especially to analgesic effects of narcotics. Clonidine has proved effective in treatment of narcotic addiction and has been shown to be especially valuable in combination with narcotics during surgical anesthesia.

Much has yet to be learned about the α_2-adrenergic class of drugs and the corresponding central (and peripheral) systems. Determining the extent to which the interdependence between the α_2-adrenergic and opioid systems can be manipulated for clinical gain will require more experience with newer and more selective α_2-adrenergic agonists and antagonists. Herein lie many fruitful years of potentially exciting developments.

REFERENCES

1. Moore RY, Bloom FE. Central catecholamine neuron systems: anatomy and physiology of the norepinephrine and epinephrine systems. Annu Rev Neurosci 1979;2:113–168.
2. Hokfelt T, Johansson O, Goldstein M. Chemical anatomy of the brain. Science 1984; 225:1326–1334.
3. Starke K, Montel H, Gayk W, et al. Comparison of the effects of clonidine on pre- and post-synaptic adrenoceptors in the rabbit pulmonary artery. Naunyn Schmiedebergs Arch Pharmacol 1974;285:133–150.
4. U'Pritchard DC, Greenberg DA, Snyder SH. Binding characteristics of a radio-labeled agonist and antagonist at central nervous system receptors. Mol Pharmacol 1977;13:454–473.
5. Unnerstall JR, Kopajtic TA, Kuhar MJ. Dis-

tribution of α_2 agonist binding sites in the rat and human central nervous system. Brain Res 1984;7:69–101.

6. Neer EJ, Clapham DE. Roles of G-protein subunits in transmembrane signalling. Nature 1988;333:129–134.

7. Yatani A, Codina J, Imoto Y, et al. A G-protein directly regulates mammalian cardiac calcium channels. Science 1987;238:1288–1292.

8. Young WS, Kuhar MJ. A new method for receptor autoradiography: $_3$H-opioid receptors in rat brain. Brain Res 1979;179:255–270.

9. Martin WR, Eades CG, Thompson JA, et al. The effects of morphine- and nalorphine-like drugs in the nondependent and morphine-dependent chronic spinal dog. J Pharmacol Exp Ther 1976;197:517–532.

10. Przewlocki R, Costa T, Lang J, et al. Pertussis toxin abolishes the antinicoception mediated by opioid receptors in rat spinal cord. Eur J Pharmacol 1987;144:91–95.

11. North RA, Williams JT. On the potassium conductance increased by opioids in rat locus coeruleus neurones. J Physiol (Lond) 1985;364:265–280.

12. North RA, Williams JT, Surprenant A, et al. μ and δ receptors belong to a family of receptors that are coupled to potassium channels. Proc Natl Acad Sci USA 1987;84:5487–5491.

13. Werz MA, McDonald RL. Dynorphin and neoendorphin peptides decrease dorsal root ganglion neuron calcium-dependent action potential duration. J Pharmacol Exp Ther 1985;234:49–56.

14. Schoffelmeer ANM, Rice KR, Jacobson AE, et al. μ, δ, and κ opioid receptor-mediated inhibition of neurotransmitter release and adenylate cyclase activity in rat brain slices: studies with fentanylisothiocyanate. Eur J Pharmacol 1988;154:169–178.

15. Okamura H, Murakami S, Yanaihara N, et al. Coexistence of catecholamine and methionine enkephalin-Arg[6]-Gly[7]-Leu[8] in neurons of the rat ventrolateral medulla oblongata: application of combined peptide immunocytochemistry and histofluorescence method in the same vibratome section. Histochemistry 1989;91:31–34.

16. Iwamoto ET. Locomotor activity and antinociception after putative μ, κ, and sigmoid opioid receptor agonists in the rat. J Pharmacol Exp Ther 1981;217:451.

17. Bloor BC, Abdul-Rasool I, Temp J, et al. The effects of medetomidine, an α_2-adrenergic agonist, on ventilatory drive in the dog. Acta Vet Scand 1989;85:65–70.

18. Weinger MB, Segal IS, Maze M. Dexmedetomidine, acting through central α_2 adrenoceptors, prevents opiate-induced muscle rigidity in the rat. Anesthesiology (in press).

19. Gellai M, Edwards RM. Mechanism of α_2-adrenoceptor agonists induced diuresis. Am J Physiol 1988;255:F317–F323.

20. Leander JD. A κ opioid effect: increased urination in rat. J Pharmacol Exp Ther 1983;224:89–94.

21. Huidobro F. Antidiuretic effect of morphine in the rat: tolerance and physical dependence. Br J Pharmacol 1978;64:167–171.

22. Tamsen A, Gordh T. Epidural clonidine produces analgesia. Lancet 1984;1:231–232.

23. Coombs DW, Saunders RL, Fratkin JD, et al. Continuous intrathecal hydromorphone and clonidine for intractable cancer pain. J Neurosurg 1986;64:890–894.

24. van Essen EJ, Bovill JG, Ploeger EJ, et al. Intrathecal morphine and clonidine for control of intractable cancer pain: a case report. Acta Anaesthesiol Belg 1988;39:109–112.

25. Glynn CJ, Jamous MA, Teddy PJ, et al. Role of spinal noradrenergic system in transmission of pain in patients with spinal cord injury. Lancet 1986;2:1249–1250.

26. Petros AJ, Bowen-Wright RM. Epidural and oral clonidine: domiciliary control of deafferentation pain. Lancet 1987;1:1034.

27. Glynn C, Dawson D, Sanders R. A double-blind comparison between epidural morphine and epidural clonidine in patients with chronic noncancer pain. Pain 1988;34:123–128.

28. Ossipov MH, Suarez LJ, Spaulding TC. A comparison of the antinociceptive and behavioral effects of intrathecally administered opiates, α_2-adrenergic agonists, and local anesthetics in mice and rats. Anesth Analg 1988;67:616–624.

29. Sweeney MI, White TD, Sawynok J. Involvement of adenosine in the spinal antinociceptive effects of morphine and noradrenaline. J Pharmacol Exp Ther 1987;243:657–665.

30. Ahlijanian MJ, Takemori AE. Effects of (-)-N[6]-(R-phenylisopropyl)-adenosine PIA and caffeine on nociception and morphine-induced analgesia, tolerance, and dependence in mice. Eur J Pharmacol 1985;112:171–179.

31. Xie CW, Tang J, Han JS. Clonidine stimulated

the release of dynorphinin in the spinal cord of the rat. Neurosci Lett 1986;65:224–228.

32. Loomis CW, Jhamandas K, Milne B, et al. Monoamine and opioid interactions in spinal analgesia and tolerance. Pharmacol Biochem Behav 1987;26:445–451.

33. Yaksh TL. Direct evidence that spinal serotonin and noradrenaline terminals mediate the spinal antinociceptive effects of morphine in the periaqueductal gray. Brain Res 1979; 160:180–185.

34. Shiomi H, Takagi H. Morphine analgesia and the bulbospinal noradrenergic system: increase in the concentration of normetanephrine in the spinal cord caused by analgesics. Br J Pharmacol 1974;52:519–526.

35. Kawaski K, Takesue H, Matsushita A. Modulation of spinal reflex activities in acute spinal rats with α-adrenergic agonists and antagonists. Jpn J Pharmacol 1978;28:165–168.

36. Sullivan AF, Dashwood MR, Dickenson AH. α₂ adrenoceptor modulation of nociception in rat spinal cord: location, effects, and interactions with morphine. Eur J Pharmacol 1987; 138:169–177.

37. Kuraishi Y, Hirota N, Sato Y, et al. Noradrenergic inhibition of the release of substance P from the primary afferents in the rabbit spinal dorsal horn. Brain Res 1985;359:177–182.

38. Jessell TM, Iversen LL. Opiate analgesics inhibit substance P release from rat trigeminal nucleus. Nature 1977;268:549–551.

39. Yaksh TL, Reddy SVR. Studies in the primate on the analgesic effects associated with intrathecal actions of opiate, α-adrenergic agonists, and baclofen. Anesthesiology 1981; 54:451–467.

40. Wang JY, Yasouka S, Yaksh TL. Studies on the analgesic effect of intrathecal ST-91 (2-[2,6-diethyl-phenylamino]-2-imidazoline): antagonism tolerance and interaction with morphine. Pharmacologist 1980;22:302.

41. Sherman SE, Loomis CW, Milne B, et al. Intrathecal oxymetazoline produces analgesia via spinal α adrenoceptors and potentiates spinal morphine. Eur J Pharmacol 1988; 148:371–380.

42. Konno F, Takayanagi I. Effects of morphine, clonidine, and papaverine on synaptosomal ⁴⁵Ca uptake in antinociceptive action in rats. Jpn J Pharmacol 1984;34:101–107.

43. Spaulding TC, Fielding S, Venafro JJ, et al. Antinociceptive activity of clonidine and its potentiation of morphine analgesia. Eur J Pharmacol 1979;58:19–25.

44. Wilcox GL, Carlsson KH, Jochim A. Mutual potentiation of antinociceptive effects of morphine and clonidine on motor and sensory responses in rat spinal cord. Brain Res 1987; 405:84–93.

45. Drasner K, Fields HL. Synergy between the antinociceptive effects of intrathecal clonidine and systemic morphine in the rat. Pain 1988; 32:309–312.

46. Eisenach JC, Dewan DM, Rose JC, et al. Epidural clonidine produces antinociception but not hypotension in sheep. Anesthesiology 1987;66:496–501.

47. Yaksh TL. Pharmacology of spinal adrenergic systems which modulate spinal nociceptive processing. Pharmacol Biochem Behav 1985; 22:845–858.

48. Paalzow G. Development of tolerance to the analgesic effect of clonidine in rats' cross-tolerance to morphine. Naunyn Schmiedebergs Arch Pharmacol 1978;304:1–4.

49. Post C, Archer T, Minor BG. Evidence for cross-tolerance to the analgesic effects between morphine and selective α₂ adrenoceptor agonists. J Neural Transm 1988;72:1–9.

50. Tchakarov L, Abbott F, Ramirez-Gonzalez MD, et al. Naloxone reverses the antinociceptive actions of clonidine in spontaneously hypertensive rats. Brain Res 1985;328:33–40.

51. Wang YC, Su CF, Lin MT. The site and the mode of analgesic actions exerted by clonidine in monkeys. Exp Neurol 1985;90:479–488.

52. Mohrland JS, Von Voigtlander PF. The analgesic activity of a clonidine analog: the formamidine, U-47,476A. Neuropharmacology 1985;24:1207–1210.

53. Reis DJ, Morrison S, Ruggiero DA. The C1 area of the brainstem in tonic and reflex control of blood pressure. Hypertension 1988; 11:I8–I13.

54. Reis DJ, Ross CA, Ruggiero DA, et al. Role of adrenaline neurons of ventrolateral medulla (the C1 group) in the tonic and phasic control of arterial pressure. Clin Exp Hypertens 1984;6:221–241.

55. Ward-Routledge C, Marshall P, Marsden CA. Involvement of central α and β adrenoceptors in the pressor response to electrical stimula-

tion of the rostral ventrolateral medulla in rats. Br J Pharmacol 1988;94:609–619.

56. Punnen S, Sapru HN. Cardiovascular responses to medullary microinjections of opiate agonists in urethane-anesthetized rats. J Cardiovasc Pharmacol 1986;8:950–956.

57. Granata AR, Reis DJ. Hypotension and bradycardia elicited by histamine into the C1 area of the rostral ventrolateral medulla. Eur J Pharmacol 1987;136:157–162.

58. Hassen AH, Feuerstein G. μ opioid receptors in NTS elicit pressor responses via sympathetic pathways. Am J Physiol 1987;252:156–162.

59. Tanaka GY. Hypertensive reaction to naloxone. JAMA 1974;228:25–26.

60. Michaelis LL, Hickey PR, Clark TA, et al. Ventricular irritability associated with the use of naloxone hydrochloride. Ann Thorac Surg 1974;18:608–614.

61. Flacke JW, Flacke WE, Williams GD. Acute pulmonary edema following naloxone reversal of high-dose anesthesia. Anesthesiology 1977;47:376–378.

62. Azar I, Turndorf H. Severe hypertension and multiple atrial premature contractions following naloxone administration. Anesth Analg (Cleve) 1979;58:524–525.

63. Andree RA. Sudden death following naloxone administration. Anesth Analg (Cleve) 1980; 59:782–784.

64. Pallasch TJ, Gill CJ. Naloxone-associated morbidity and mortality. Oral Surg 1981; 52:602–603.

65. Ward S, Corall IM. Hypertension after naloxone. Anaesthesia 1983;38:1000–1001.

66. Flacke JW, Flacke WE, Bloor BC, et al. Effects of fentanyl, naloxone, and clonidine on hemodynamics and plasma catecholamine levels in dog. Anesth Analg 1983;62:305–313.

67. Pedrinelli R, Bernini GP, Salvetti A. Naloxone does not modify the hemodynamic and neuroendocrine effects of clonidine in normal humans. J Cardiovasc Pharmacol 1985;7:953–957.

68. Farsang C, Kunos G. Naloxone reverses the antihypertensive effect of clonidine. Br J Pharmacol 1979;67:161–164.

69. Farsang C, Kapocsi J, Juhasz I, et al. Possible involvement of an endogenous opioid in the antihypertensive effect of clonidine in patients with essential hypertension. Circulation 1982; 66:1268–1272.

70. Kunos G, Farsang C. β-endorphin: possible involvement in the antihypertensive effect of central α receptor activation. Science 1981; 211:82–84.

71. Mastrianni JA, Ingenito AJ. On the relationship between clonidine hypotension and brain β-endorphin in the spontaneously hypertensive rat: studies with α-adrenergic and opiate blockers. J Pharmacol Exp Ther 1987;242:378–387.

72. Gold MS, Potash ALC, Extein I. Clonidine in acute opiate withdrawal. N Engl J Med 1980;302:1421–1422.

73. Dwoskin LP, Neal BS, Sparber SB. Yohimbine exacerbates and clonidine attenuates acute morphine withdrawal in rats. Eur J Pharmacol 1983;90:269–273.

74. Gossop M. Clonidine and the treatment of opiate withdrawal syndrome. Drug Alcohol Depend 1988;21:253–259.

75. Slogoff S, Keats AS. Does perioperative myocardial ischemia lead to postoperative myocardial infarction? Anesthesiology 1985;62:107–114.

76. Wynands JE, Townsend GE, Ong P, et al. Blood pressure response and plasma fentanyl concentrations during high- and very-high-dose fentanyl anesthesia for coronary artery surgery. Anesth Analg 1983;62:661–665.

77. Wynands JE, Wong P, Whalley DG, et al. Oxygen-fentanyl anesthesia in patients with poor left ventricular function: hemodynamics and plasma fentanyl concentrations. Anesth Analg 1983;62:476–482.

78. Flacke JW, Bloor BC, Flacke WE, et al. Reduced narcotic requirement by clonidine with improved hemodynamic and adrenergic stability in patients undergoing coronary bypass surgery. Anesthesiology 1987;67:11–19.

79. Ghignone M, Quintin L, Duke PC, et al. Effects of clonidine on narcotic requirements and hemodynamic response during induction of fentanyl anesthesia and endotracheal intubation. Anesthesiology 1986;64:36–42.

80. Ghignone M, Calvillo O, Quintin L. Anesthesia and hypertension: the effect of clonidine on perioperative hemodynamics and isoflurane requirements. Anesthesiology 1987; 66:3–10.

81. Woodcock TE, Millard RK, Dixon J, et al. Clonidine premedication for isoflurane-induced hypotension: sympathoadrenal responses and

a computer-controlled assessment of the vapour requirement. Br J Anaesth 1988;60:388–394.

82. Helbo-Hansen S, Fletcher R, Lundberg D, et al. Clonidine and the sympatico-adrenal response to coronary artery bypass surgery. Acta Anaesthesiol Scand 1986;30:235–242.

83. Ghignone M, Noe C, Calvillo O, et al. Anesthesia for ophthalmic surgery in the elderly: the effects of clonidine on intraocular pressure, perioperative hemodynamics, and anesthetic requirement. Anesthesiology 1988; 68:707–716.

84. Pouttu J, Scheinin B, Rosenberg PH, et al. Oral premedication with clonidine: effects on stress responses during general anesthesia. Acta Anaesthesiol Scand 1987;31:730–734.

Chapter 3 Discussion

EZZAT AMIN: In this chapter, the authors have presented a detailed discussion of the anatomy, physiology, and pharmacology of the noradrenergic and opioid systems. It appears that there are remarkable similarities between the two systems regarding their locations in the brain, their receptors on the same cell, and the functional coupling between their receptors and effectors. This can allow possible interactions between the two systems at different levels of the central nervous system.

Attention has been focused on the α-adrenergic receptors. Clonidine (an α_2 agonist) produces analgesia and sedation, but it differs from the classical opiate drugs (e.g., morphine) in not bringing about respiratory depression and euphoria. When clonidine and morphine are given together by the systemic, intrathecal, or epidural routes, the analgesic effect of either drug is enhanced. It seems possible that the α_2 agonist and the opioid agonist may act at different levels in the nociceptive pathway, or by different mechanisms at the same locus.

It is claimed that combinations of the two drug classes may provide optimal analgesia with fewer side effects and delayed onset of tolerance. This may prove useful in some clinical situations like management of chronic pain, treatment of narcotic addiction, and production of balanced general anesthesia.

WERNER E. FLACKE: The chapters in Part I, especially the chapter by Bloor et al., concerning the interaction between the opioid system and α_2-adrenergic agonists, represent the gap between detailed information about ligands, receptors, and events beyond the ligand-receptor interaction on the one hand, and observations in intact animals and humans on the other. It seems to me that we urgently need more information bridging this gap.

I know that this is the standard situation in biology, especially the biology of the central nervous system (CNS), and it is a platitude to say that we need to understand normal functioning better before we can set out to alter this functioning. Of course, if we wait for full comprehension of the vertebrate CNS, we will have to wait a very long time, perhaps forever. However, we must start to emphasize research directed not at further dissection but at integration. Although such research is being done today, it is very difficult work, and yet work considered by many not to be at the "cutting edge." Bloom,[1] commenting recently upon central neurotransmission, expressed the hope that the present emphasis on molecular mechanistic insight evaluated in in vitro preparations would lead to future studies "in such a way as to restore the data to the concepts of how the intact brain operates."

This is indeed necessary. Even full knowledge of the single pieces of the puzzle will not enable us to put together the functioning whole. Some time ago, McGrath,[2] speaking of difficulties in understanding α_1- versus α_2-adrenergic functions, said, "If the interaction of drug and receptor can modify performance of cellular elements, e.g., opening of ion channels, then it must be possible that, conversely, such elements can modify the conformation of the receptor." He reasoned that transition from in vitro to in vivo would bring about other changes in the environment that might modify the properties of receptors. Some factors he listed are pH, temperature, the ionic composition of the extracellular fluid, and the presence of blood-borne factors, including hormones. One complexity that can only be seen under physiological conditions is cotransmission, which was postulated for enkephalinergic fibers some time ago. Today, the coexistence of amino acid and aminergic transmitter with peptides is accepted as a new principle in synaptic transmission.[3]

The authors of these chapters have presented a large amount of detailed information about opioid peptides, their precursors, storage, patterns of release, metabolic alteration, and inactivation. They have discussed the receptors involved, and their classification and biochemical structure, including the cloning of different receptors. Yet, as Simon stated in Chapter 1, "In no case has the endogenous ligand-receptor relationship been proved." We know much about the nature of the linkages between the activated transmitter detector and the ion channels, enzyme activation, and other manifestations of receptor occupancy. However, most of this information has been obtained with biochemical and molecular methodology, or through in vitro preparations. What is lacking is knowledge linking this information to the functioning of the intact brain in the intact organism.

This is a surprising fact, given that so much detail is known, and especially surprising in that it is true even for the effects most studied, i.e., the role of opioid peptides and receptors in pain perception and modulation and in respiratory depression. If this is so in cases where no one doubts that such relationships exist, how much more so in the case of opioids and functions less firmly linked to them! How about the link to control of cardiovascular function, control of appetites, such as hunger, thirst, sexual drives? What about the physiologic role of opioid peptides in endocrine functions, of which we know little more than that hormonal changes occur when agonists are given and that antagonists can block these changes. When we go farther afield to effects on mood and role in mental illness, the postulated cross-talk between the opioid system and the immune system is based upon nothing more than the similarity of molecules shared by the immune system and the nervous system. On the other hand, knowledge about cellular and subcellular mechanisms may help in better understanding of tolerance and dependence.

As much as we relish our increasingly detailed knowledge, we have to fill the gap between this knowledge and physiologic, pathophysiologic, and pharmacologic function. Nowhere is this more apparent than in the interaction between opioid peptides and the α_2-adrenergic system. There, we have accumulated a certain amount of whole-animal and clinical experience, whereas the basis of the interaction at the cellular level is meager. It is not surprising that there are apparent contradictions between results obtained by different investigators and under different circumstances. Not until we have a much better understanding of the physiology underlying the events in functioning intact animals and humans will we be able to resolve these contradictions.

Of course, this is not an unusual situation. In fact, when it comes to the CNS, clinical, so-called serendipitous observations have often provided critical impetus for detailed study. Increasingly, I hope, we will see the opposite: that laboratory observations provide the rationale for clinical trials. However, we should not be too optimistic. Where the CNS is concerned, the sheer complexity of neurophysiologic functioning is likely to prevent successful deductive reasoning for some time to come. More realistically, we may anticipate that the laboratory results will provide us retrospectively with a basis for the clinical observations. Heuristically and with caution we may then make tentative predictions that may prove useful.

Research in the field of endogenous opioid peptides and receptors has not been very productive in terms of clinically useful results. This is not unexpected. The enormous complexity of the opioid peptide system at every level means that useful application may turn out to be equally complex. Let me illustrate by contrast what I mean. Impulse transmission across the neuromuscular junction is fairly straightforward: a single transmitter acting upon a single type of postjunctional receptor. The functioning of this system is simple impulse transmission without modulation. In consequence, we have been able to develop drugs that are satisfactorily selective. Present-day neuromuscular blocking drugs do what they are designed to do with no or minimal side effects. The situation in the opioid system is quite different. Apart from the complication on the postsynaptic side, transmitter release may generate "mosaics of opioid peptides." Carr et al. emphasize in their chapter that "the constellation of enzymes acting to metabolize opioid peptides at a particular tissue site is very sensitive to local biochemical changes." This implies that it will be difficult or impossible to influence such function by single-entity drugs. Perhaps we should look not so much for synthetic agonists or antagonists as for agents that may affect the constellation of factors at certain sites and conditions. It means that we may have to pay close attention to the exact circumstances in which such drugs act. We should not, perhaps, look for the "magic bullet," but for bullets or combination of bullets that will produce the desired effects under specific conditions. Such agents may not be highly selective in terms of specific targets, but they may be sufficiently selective to achieve a desired result.

Pharmacologists know that often therapeutic value lies not in selective agonists and antagonists but rather in agents that alter functioning in more indirect ways. For example, anesthesiologists use anticholinesterase agents every day to reverse neuromuscular block. Everybody will agree that anticholinesterase drugs are "dirty" drugs because their target enzyme is so widely distributed. However, if used appropriately, these dirty drugs do their job well.

This type of thinking may also be useful in considering the clinical use of α_2-adrenergic agonists in conjunction with opioids. We have heard that the combination of opioids and α_2 adrenoceptor agonists has been used to clinical advantage. The interaction between α_2 agonists and opioids has been traced to anatomical structures and cellular events where the two ligands show a surprising degree of similarity of postreceptor functioning. Not only do the two types of agents produce the same electrophysiological effects in the same cells; even the postreceptor mechanisms show great similarity. Pertussis toxin blocks the electrophysiological events evoked by both opioids and α_2 agonists, in the same cells.[4] Now we will have to see how this synergism can be used most advantageously. We will hear more about cross-tolerance between the two types of agonists and about buildup of tolerance. We have to explore what other synergism and, perhaps, antagonism may be present that we can exploit for therapeutic purposes. When I say "therapeutic purposes," I don't mean to restrict our area of interest to the anesthetic period alone. Anesthesiologists are very much concerned with postanesthesia care, and one of the important parts of that is analgesia. In fact, pain control is the province of anesthesiologists in all patients, not just those who come to surgery. α_2 agonists are agents that convey potent analgesia without respiratory depression. There may be more to the interaction between opioids and α_2 agonists than their synergism as analgesics. There is some indication that the combination is more effective in alleviating one of the consequences of pain: stress. The same seems to be true of the stress that is a major component of withdrawal reactions. However, before we adopt uncritical generalizations, we have to look carefully at all pharmacologic interactions between these agents. The past gives reason for optimism, yet optimism tempered by caution. We know more about the mechanism of action of opioids and α_2 adrenoceptor agonists than even the greatest optimist had reason to expect a few years ago. And we have only just started to explore their therapeutic potential.

REFERENCES

1. Bloom FE. Neurotransmitters: past, present, and future. FASEB J 1988;2:32–41.
2. McGrath JC. Evidence for more than one type of postjunctional alpha adrenoceptor. Biochem Pharmacol 1982;31:467–484.
3. Hokfelt T, Fuxe K, Pernow B. Coexistence of neuronal messengers: a new principle in chemical transmission. Progr Brain Res 1987;68:1–411.
4. Aghajanian GK, Wang Y-Y. Pertussis toxin blocks the outward current evoked by opiate and alpha$_2$ agonists in locus coeruleus neurons. Brain Res 1986;371:390–394.

4 FUNCTIONAL COUPLING AMONG OPIOID RECEPTOR TYPES

John W. Holaday, Frank Porreca, and Richard B. Rothman

The clinical utility of opioids in anesthesia is complicated by their many well-known side effects, including constipation, urinary retention, respiratory depression, alteration of body temperature, immunosuppression, and addictive liability.[1] For more than a century, medicinal chemists and pharmacologists have synthesized opioid ligands in attempts to develop opioid analgesic molecules devoid of these side effects. It was the hope of opioid pharmacologists that the characterization of the multiple opioid receptor types (e.g., μ, δ, and κ; see Chapter 2) and the availability of receptor-selective ligands would allow for a dissociation of desirable and undesirable actions of opioids, ultimately resulting in an ideal opioid analgesic. Unfortunately, this has not happened.

Ever since the first description of heroin as a nonaddictive analgesic in the mid-1800s, each newly discovered opioid has ultimately been demonstrated to share many of the known undesirable side effects. Although each new opioid compound is initially heralded as being pure and selective, as its pharmacologic profile becomes more thoroughly characterized, these adjectives become meaningless; biochemical and pharmacologic data establish that the li-

gands cross-react with μ, δ, or κ receptors, or function as mixed agonist/antagonist molecules.

What can account for these confusing opioid responses? Consider for the moment that these diverse pharmacologic profiles of opioids do not always reflect the different chemical faces presented by the various opioid ligands to the receptor but may instead reflect conformational changes brought about by the ligand's binding to different sites on a large, flexible opioid receptor complex. In this light, it may be helpful to re-examine opioid receptor systems by reviewing extensive data to indicate that a functional coupling among μ, δ, and κ binding sites may explain the repeating patterns of pharmacologic and biochemical responses that typify opioid pharmacology.

FUNDAMENTAL CONCEPTS OF LIGAND-RECEPTOR INTERACTIONS

When a flexible ligand molecule binds to its receptor, both the ligand and receptor will slightly modify their shapes to accommodate each other. For agonist interactions, this conformational change evoked by the receptor is important in conveying information to transmembrane-signaling mechanisms and second messenger systems, ultimately coupling receptor occupancy with intracellular events. Because of the myriad binding sites offered by large, flexible receptor molecules, it is not surprising that complex pharmacologic and biochemical profiles may be a consequence of conformational changes produced by allosteric interactions among binding sites on a common receptor macromolecule.

Allosterism, a term borrowed from enzymology, refers to binding of a ligand at a site other than the active "receptor" site. This form of receptor plasticity has been known to pharmacologists for some time. For example, allosteric coupling among the α, β, δ, and γ subunits of the acetylcholine receptor has been recognized for over 20 years.[2] More recently, unique pharmacologic, electrophysiologic, and biochemical profiles of ligand interactions with the GABA-benzodiazepine-chloride ion channel complex have become widely accepted as evidence for allosteric coupling in that system.[3] Current thinking about the N-methyl-D-aspartate (NMDA) receptor complex, including the potentiating effects of glycine and zinc on the agonist glutamate, as well as the characterization of phencyclidine-σ binding sites, unnatural ($+$) opioid (dextromethorphan), and magnesium interactions, are also compatible with allosteric mechanisms.[4,5]

This review will provide evidence that combinations of so-called selective opioid agonists and antagonist ligands result in repeating patterns of pharmacologic responses that may indicate involvement of allosteric receptor mechanisms. The characterization of these pharmacologic profiles requires the simultaneous assessment of responses to at least two ligands, including combinations of agonists and antagonists. We shall emphasize our collaborative studies using combinations of agonist/antagonist opioid ligands in the rat endotoxic shock model, the rat flurothyl seizure model, production of antinociception, urinary bladder motility, measurements of changes in striatal cyclic adenosine monophosphate (cAMP), and receptor binding.

These interactions are not as confusing as they may seem at first glance, since they describe a very consistent pattern of responses. Germinal to this concept is the observation that antagonist molecules may antagonize the actions of other antagonists. Specifically, these experimental paradigms provide evidence that compounds with μ antagonist actions block the effect of δ antagonists. Furthermore, many of these μ antagonists also function as κ agonists, and vice versa. Data indicate that these interactions occur among the low-affinity binding sites and that allosteric modulation of these sites may play a role in opioid tolerance mechanisms. These patterns of μ, δ, and κ interactions not only have predictive value in defining the pharmacologic profiles of opioid ligands but also indicate that the use of μ, δ, or κ agonists for the treatment of pain may have predictable consequences for the clinical anesthesiologist.

EVIDENCE FOR SEPARATE OPIOID RECEPTORS

Many laboratories have provided evidence that μ, δ, and κ receptors exist as separate macromolecular species with anatomically distinct localizations and unique pharmacologic profiles.[6] In fact, the concept that opioid receptor types only exist as unique and separate entities reflected the prevailing opinion expressed in the earlier literature. Evidence to support this concept includes data obtained using sequential combinations of opioid agonist ligands to indicate a lack of cross-tolerance among "selective" agonists when given over time.[7,8] Cross-protection studies using selective reversible ligands to block nonselective receptor alkylation have provided further evidence to distinguish multiple opioid receptor types as separate entities.[9,10] These observations may be considered strong evidence for the individuality of multiple opioid receptors.

Indeed, evidence to support the concept that opioid receptor types may not be physically or functionally independent is not entirely inconsistent with our allosteric hy-

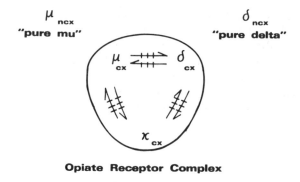

Opiate Receptor Complex

χ_{ncx}
"pure kappa"

FIGURE 4.1 A schematic model of the opioid receptors.

pothesis. We propose that there are separate μ, δ, and κ sites that may have different anatomical distributions and functions than those of the interacting μ, δ, and κ allosteric sites[11] (Figure 4.1).

EVIDENCE FOR INTERACTING (ALLOSTERIC) OPIOID RECEPTORS

Over the past decade, several investigators have performed in vivo and in vitro experiments to indicate that μ and δ receptor sites may functionally interconvert[12] or interact through noncompetitive molecular mechanisms.[13–15] Consistent with these observations, evidence from our laboratories also indicates that noncompetitive interactions among μ and δ binding sites may occur in vivo and in vitro. We have extended earlier observations by demonstrating that interactions among multiple opioid binding sites are not restricted to μ and δ receptors but may also involve an important functional role for κ receptors.[16–22]

To demonstrate interactions among all three opioid binding sites, it is necessary to evaluate responses following administration of combinations of agonist and antagonist ligands. Using this strategy, it has been shown that many (if not all) opioid ligands classified as κ ago-

nists also function as μ antagonists in certain preparations. These include the alkaloidlike ligands such as ketazocine, ethylketazocine, tifluadom, bremazocine, and U-50,488H as well as the peptide analogs of dynorphin (1-17).[23–26] Another opioid ligand, β-funaltrexamine (β-FNA), widely accepted as an irreversible μ antagonist, was originally described as having κ agonist effects.[27] Thus, all these opioid ligands may be classified as having both κ agonist and μ antagonist properties.

Antagonists of Antagonists

We have also observed that many of these κ agonists (μ antagonists) prevent the ability of δ antagonists to block or reverse δ agonist effects. In other words, they function as antagonists of antagonists. This concept, first mentioned by Villarreal and colleagues[28] for opioid systems, has also been described for ligand interactions at the GABA-benzodiazepine-chloride ion receptor complex.[29] In those studies, it was demonstrated that β-carbolines, the inverse agonist at this receptor, when administered at doses that do not show intrinsic activity, block the antagonistic actions of the antagonist Ro 15-1788 against benzodiazepines. Similarly, from our studies with opioid ligands summarized in the following sections, we observe a consistent pharmacologic profile to indicate that certain μ antagonists also block the antagonistic actions of δ antagonists.

Endotoxic Shock and Cardiovascular Function

Septic shock is a common problem facing anesthesiologists who practice critical care medicine. Endotoxin is the lipopolysaccharide component of the cell wall of gram-negative organisms, and release of endotoxin during sepsis is believed to account for many of the pathophysiologic events that typify septic shock. Over the past several years, we have demonstrated that high doses of opioid antagonists such as naloxone (Narcan) reverse many of the pathophysiologic events produced by the administration of endotoxin in various animal models of endotoxic shock.[1,30,31] Naloxone, which is generally accepted as a pure opioid antagonist, lacks adequate selectivity for the different opioid receptor types.

In our initial investigations into the type(s) of opioid receptors responsible for shock hypotension, we used a variety of ligands with reported receptor selectivity. The μ-selective antagonists, including naloxazone (now known to be active as naloxonazine), β-FNA, and dynorphin (1-13), failed to improve endotoxic hypotension.[17,18,32] However, high doses of naloxone or the δ-selective antagonists ICI 154129 or ICI 174864 were quite effective.[16–18,32] From these results, it appeared that endogenous opioids released in endotoxic shock act upon δ (not μ) receptors to produce their pathophysiologic effects.

These studies in endotoxemic rats, however, also revealed unexpected findings when combinations of antagonist ligands were administered. Curiously, pretreatment with any of the μ antagonists naloxazone, β-FNA, or dynorphin (1-13), which were inactive in this model, when administered prior to high-dose naloxone or the δ antagonists ICI 154129 or ICI 174864 rendered the latter substances ineffective in reversing endotoxic shock hypotension.[16,17,32] From these studies of endotoxic shock in rats, we concluded (1) that endogenous opioids contribute to endotoxic hypotension by acting on δ opiate receptors, and (2) that μ antagonists like naloxazone, β-FNA, and dynorphin also antagonize the actions of δ antagonists.

In other studies addressing direct cardiovascular responses, it was revealed that the μ antagonist effects of dynorphin were time-dependent. Morphine-induced bradycardia, believed to be mediated at peripheral μ receptors, was antagonized by dynorphin 8 hours following intracerebroventricular (icv) injection but potentiated by icv dynorphin pretreatment 4 hours before intravenous morphine injections.[22] Garcia and Kunos[33] demonstrated that the δ receptor antagonist ICI 174864 antagonized clonidine hypotension in spontaneously hyper-

tensive rats but was ineffective in normotensive rats. Conversely, the μ antagonist β-FNA antagonized clonidine hypotension in normotensive rats but not in hypertensive rats. Taken together, these studies demonstrate that such factors as time of injection, site of injection, and hypertension can further modify apparent interpretations of opioid receptor interactions.

Seizures

To confirm the pattern of opioid interactions initially observed in the endotoxic shock model, we investigated the same interactions using these selective opioid ligands in a model of flurothyl-induced seizures in rats.[19] Flurothyl is a volatile convulsant, and rats exposed to a defined titration of flurothyl vapors experience tonic-clonic convulsions within approximately 360 sec.[34,35] Unlike the endotoxic shock model, where endogenous opioids are physiologically released to act upon δ receptors, in the flurothyl seizure studies opioid agonists and antagonists are pharmacologically administered. Using this approach, it has been shown that several classes of opioid agonist ligands may act upon separate receptor sites to elevate seizure thresholds.[34,45] For example, the anticonvulsant effects of etorphine were completely blocked by the μ antagonist β-FNA, whereas β-FNA only partly antagonized the effects of the δ agonist D-Ala^2-D-Leu^5-enkephalin (DADL).[20] Similarly, the δ antagonist ICI 154129 completely blocked the anticonvulsant effects of DADL but was without effect on the anticonvulsant actions of etorphine.[20,35,36]

Consistent with the pattern of interactions observed in the endotoxic shock model, β-FNA pretreatment prevented naloxone or ICI 154129 from blocking the anticonvulsant response to DADL.[20]

More recent evidence provided additional support for these unique interactions. After the initial anticonvulsant effects of dynorphin (1-13) pretreatment had ended—2 hours following dynorphin (1-13) pretreatment (unpublished observations)—subsequent treatment with the μ agonist DAGO (Tyr-D-Ala^2-MePhe^4

DADL binds to a μ site, and morphine binds to δ opioid receptors.

At a functional level, in vivo studies described previously indicated that β-FNA could serve as an antagonist of an antagonist. Rothman et al.[63] demonstrated this phenomenon using receptor binding studies to indicate that β-FNA pretreatment, either in vivo or in vitro, significantly increased the amount of naloxone required to displace radio-labeled DADL from its low-affinity binding site in rat brain membranes. More recent evidence from their laboratory indicates that this low-affinity opioid receptor complex is significantly up-regulated by chronic morphine and naltrexone.[65,66] These data indicate the possible involvement of the opioid receptor complex in tolerance mechanisms.

Electrophysiologically, both μ and δ receptors have been shown to be coupled to potassium channels.[67] Zieglegansberger and colleagues (personal communication) have demonstrated using brain slices that both μ and δ receptors are located on the same neurons. Similar findings have been reported by Shen and Crain[68] using cultured spinal cords. From these observations, at least μ and δ receptors have been shown to coexist in a manner consonant with their colocalization as part of a receptor complex.

Evidence that μ and δ receptors are differentially distributed within the brain[69] is consistent with the hypothesis of a μ-δ complex, since published anatomical studies are optimized to label the δ site not associated with the receptor complex. Moreover, biochemical evidence for a μ-δ complex was recently published.[70] Additionally, it has been demonstrated using the radiation inactivation technique that κ, μ, and δ "receptors" are all about the same molecular weight.[71] Recent work by Lee and colleagues (personal communication) indicates that antibodies directed against an isolated and purified opioid binding protein equally inhibit the binding of "selective" μ, δ, and κ agonists. Thus, anatomical, biochemical, behavioral, and physiologic evidence is available to indicate that multiple opioid "recep-

tors" may instead be multiple opioid binding sites that may interact as part of the same macromolecular cluster or complex.

HYPOTHESES FOR LIGAND INTERACTIONS

The pattern of ligand interactions described in these three separate models of opioid responses may appear hopelessly complex. However, the pattern of responses across these studies consistently demonstrates that many compounds described as κ agonists are also μ antagonists that further antagonize the actions of δ antagonists (Table 4.1). Thus, several different lines of evidence indicate that simultaneous interactions among all three binding sites have a precise pattern that is only revealed by experiments using combinations of opioid agonist and antagonist ligands.

In an attempt to define the reasons for these sometimes confusing and interdependent phenomena, several working hypotheses may be proposed:

1. One ligand may display several moieties that account for cross-reactivity among receptor types.
2. In vivo studies or tissue preparation stud-

TABLE 4.1 Selected opioid ligands demonstrating κ, μ, and δ interactions

κ-agonists	μ-antagonists	Antagonists of δ-antagonists
?	Naloxazone (Naloxonazine)	Yes
Yes	β-funaltrexamine	Yes
Dynorphin (1-13)	Yes	Yes
U-50,488H, tifluadom Nalbuphine Bremazocine Ethylketazocine	Yes	?

ies in vitro must be interpreted with caution because of the existence of neuronal networks.

3. Combinations of ligands may alter the uptake or metabolism of other ligands.
4. Combinations of ligands may result in alterations of receptor coupling to second messengers.
5. Cooperatively or allosteric coupling may exist among multiple binding sites of a macromolecular receptor complex.

These multiple working hypotheses are not all mutually exclusive.

In response to the first of these hypotheses, it is difficult to conceive that molecules as different as the synthetic alkaloids β-FNA, U-50,488H, bremazocine, and so on, would share similar structural moieties with the peptide dynorphin (1-13) to explain their actions as κ agonists, μ antagonists, and antagonists of δ antagonists.

Concerning the second and fourth possibilities, although neuronal networks and altered neuronal uptake may still exist within the striatum, evidence obtained in studies of striatal cAMP, as well as confirming studies using opioid receptor binding, are consistent with the hypothesis that these pharmacologic profiles are mediated at receptors and expressed at a postreceptor coupling level.

On the third hypothesis, alterations of metabolism are difficult to invoke because of the similar pharmacologic profiles and different chemical structures of the many synthetic alkaloid and peptide ligands we used. Furthermore, these actions of naloxazone, β-FNA, and dynorphin occur at a time when the ligands no longer express an intrinsic activity of their own.

Finally, on the last point, although it is by no means proved from the evidence presented in this review, we are unable to rule out the possibility that a single agonist or antagonist ligand may affect the binding of other agonist or antagonist ligands at other opioid binding sites through noncompetitive allosteric interactions.

CONCLUSION

The experimental evidence we have reviewed may ultimately have direct consequences in the practice of clinical anesthesiology. For example, the concurrent use of κ agonists like bremazocine, nalbuphine, and others, or the δ agonists, may modify the analgesic effects of other opioid agonists such as morphine or fentanyl that act primarily upon μ receptors. Opiate antagonists such as naloxone, compounds that may ultimately be used for the treatment of shock and trauma,[30] would have limited efficacy if κ agonists were used as anesthetics. The future development of opioid agonists and antagonists must take into account the pharmacologic consequences of receptor interactions. Perhaps these concepts will lead to a more enlightened approach to the biochemical characterization of opioid receptors and to the development of novel opioid ligands.

REFERENCES

1. Holaday JW. Endogenous opioids and their receptors. In: Current concepts. Kalamazoo, Mich.: Upjohn Company, 1985.
2. Changeaux J-P. The acetylcholine receptor: an "allosteric" membrane protein. Harvey Lect 1981;75:85–254.
3. Braestrup C, Nielsen M. Benzodiazepine receptor binding in vivo and efficacy. New York: Alan R. Liss, 1986;167–184.
4. Kushner L, Lerma J, Zukin RS, et al. Coexpression of N-methyl-D-aspartate and phencyclidine receptors in Xenopus oocytes injected with rat brain mRNA. Proc Natl Acad Sci USA 1988;85:3250–3254.
5. Musacchio JM, Klein M, Santiago LJ. Allosteric modulation of dextromethorphan binding sites. Neuropharmacology 1987;26(7B): 997–1001.
6. Paterson SJ, Robson LE, Kosterlitz HW. Classification of opioid receptors. Br Med Bull 1983;39:31–36.
7. Schulz R, Wuster M, Kreuss H, et al. Selective development of tolerance without dependence in multiple opiate receptors of mouse vas deferens. Nature 1980;285:242–243.

studies with fentanyl isothiocyanate. Eur J Pharmacol 1988;154:169–178.

57. Schoffelmeer ANM, Rice KC, Heijna MH, et al. Fentanyl isothiocyanate reveals the existence of physically associated μ and δ opioid receptors mediating inhibition of adenylate cyclase in rat neostriatum. Eur J Pharmacol 1988;149:179–182.

58. Chang KJ, Cuatrecacas P. Multiple opiate receptors: enkephalins and morphine bind to receptors of different specificity. J Biol Chem 1979;254:2610–2618.

59. Rothman RB, Bowen WD, Herkenham M, et al. A quantitative study of [³H]-D-Ala²-D-Leu⁵-enkephalin binding to rat brain membranes: evidence that oxymorphone is a noncompetitive inhibitor of the lower-affinity δ binding site. Mol Pharmacol 1985;27:399–408.

60. Rothman RB, Bowen WD, Bykov V, et al. Preparation of rat brain membranes greatly enriched with either type-I-δ or type-II-δ opiate binding sites using site directed alkylating agents: evidence for a two-site allosteric model. Neuropeptides 1985;4:201–215.

61. Rothman RB, Danks JA, Herkenham M, et al. Evidence that the δ-selective alkylating agent, FIT, alters the μ-noncompetitive opiate δ binding site. Neuropeptides 1985;6:227–237.

62. Rothman RB, Danks JA, Jacobson AE, et al. Leucine enkephalin noncompetitively inhibits the binding of ³H-naloxone to the opiate μ-recognition site: evidence for δ-μ binding site interactions in vitro. Neuropeptides 1985; 6:351–363.

63. Rothman RB, Long JB, Bykov V, et al. β-FNA binds irreversibly to the opiate receptor complex: in vivo and in vitro evidence. J Pharmacol Exp Ther 1988;247:405–416.

64. Sarne Y, Kenner A. Biphasic competition between opiates and enkephalins: does it indicate the existence of a common high-affinity ("μ-1") binding site? Life Sci 1987;41:555–562.

65. Rothman RB, Bykov V, Long JB, et al. Chronic administration of morphine and naltrexone up-regulate opioid binding sites labeled by ³H-(D-Ala²-MePhe⁴-Gly-ol⁵) enkephalin: evidence for two μ binding sites. Eur J Pharmacol 1989;160:71–82.

66. Rothman RB, Danks JA, Jacobson AE, et al. Morphine tolerance increases μ-noncompetitive δ binding sites. Eur J Pharmacol 1986; 124:113–119.

67. North RA, Williams JT, Surprenant A, et al. μ and δ receptors belong to a family of receptors that are coupled to potassium channels. Proc Natl Acad Sci USA 1987;84:5487–5491.

68. Shen KF, Crain SM. Dual opioid modulation of the action potential duration of mouse dorsal root ganglion neurons in culture. Brain Res 1989;491:227–242.

69. Goodman RR, Snyder SH, Kuhar MJ, et al. III Differentiation of δ and μ opiate receptor localization by light microscopic autoradiography. Proc Natl Acad Sci USA 1980;77:6239–6243.

70. Schoffelmeer A, Yao Y-H, Simon EJ. Cross-linking of human ¹²⁵I-β-endorphin to a μ-δ opioid receptor complex in rat striatum. Eur J Pharmacol 1989;166:357–358.

71. Ott S, Costa T, Hietel B, et al. The molecular size of multiple opiate receptors. Naunyn Schmiedebergs Arch Pharmacol 1983;324:60.

5 CELLULAR AND SUBCELLULAR ACTIONS OF OPIOIDS IN THE HEART

Jack K. Pruett, John R. Blair, and Robert J. Adams

The purpose of this chapter is to discuss our limited current knowledge about the cardiac effects of opioids and the subcellular mechanisms by which these agents affect ion fluxes involved in mediating excitation-contraction in the heart. Although the opioids have been, and continue to be, used primarily as analgesics and general anesthetics, their myocardial actions have not received the attention of investigators to the same extent as have agents like propranolol that are used specifically for treatment of heart ailments. This statement is easily verified, as illustrated in Figures 5.1 and 5.2. These computer-generated data are shown only to illustrate the limited number of studies concerning the influence of opioids on the heart.

In whole-animal and patient studies, the general impression is that therapeutic doses of opioids have little or no major effect on cardiac rate, rhythm, or contractility. Most cardiovascular effects of morphine and related opioids have been attributed to histamine release or central nervous system mediated alterations in autonomic control,[1] although there are reports of positive or negative inotropic and chronotropic actions of opioid agonists and antagonists in the heart.[2]

ELECTROPHYSIOLOGIC EFFECTS

Our initial studies of opioid effects on cardiac tissues were based on a simple question: Does the synthetic opioid fentanyl affect the electrical activity of isolated canine cardiac Purkinje fibers? Our initial experiments revealed that 0.19 μM (100 ng/ml) fentanyl produced a significant prolongation of action potential duration.[3,4] Very quickly we confirmed our suspicion that the more potent congener sufentanil also would produce a similar effect[3,4] (see Figure 5.3). The results of these pilot studies led us to extend the electrophysiologic examination of these agents in an attempt to answer more specific questions regarding potential membrane sites of actions of these popular drugs.

Opioid Receptors

Early in these studies we questioned the possibility that the prolongation of action potential duration was mediated via opioid receptors. We speculated that the observed actions of fentanyl and sufentanil might act through these or similar receptors. The existence of opioid

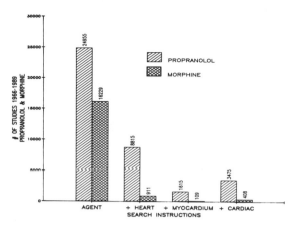

FIGURE 5.1 The number of published studies involving propranolol and morphine between 1966 and 1989. The numbers shown in this figure were obtained using a computer program called Crosstalk. The computer was instructed to search for the key words *propranolol* and *morphine*. The total number of studies for each drug between 1966 and 1989, regardless of the type of study, are shown above AGENT. More specific instructions for the type of study of each agent resulted in reduced numbers for each category, HEART, MYOCARDIUM, and CARDIAC.

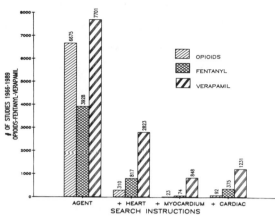

FIGURE 5.2 The number of studies listed under the key words *opioids, fentanyl,* and *verapamil.* The computer was instructed to perform the same search as before (Figure 5.1), but the agents were changed.

receptors in the heart was somewhat controversial. Laurent et al.[5] had shown that enkephalins induce a direct positive inotropic response in cultured avian myocytes via a specific opiate receptor interaction, and others[6,7] have provided additional convincing evidence that indicates the presence of specific opioid receptors in the heart. Dashwood and Spyer,[8] however, were unable to detect opioid receptors in rat and cat hearts using rather uncritical autoradiographic techniques. We knew from a report by Frame and Argentieri[9] that high concentrations of naloxone would produce prolongation of action potential duration and depression of the maximum rate of rise of the depolarization phase (V_{max}), effects that resembled the actions of Class I antiarrhythmic agents and effects that would, in part, resemble those of fentanyl and sufentanil. We found that lower concentrations of naloxone, be-

tween 2.0 μM and 10.0 μM (1.0 and 3.5 mg/L), produced little or no effect on action potential characteristics when administered alone. Regardless of whether naloxone was administered before or after the agonists, it failed to prevent or reverse action potential prolongation produced by the agonists. These concentrations of naloxone were much greater than clinically useful doses but were used in an attempt to prevent or reverse action potential prolongation caused by fentanyl and sufentanil. Despite the failure of naloxone to prevent or reverse the effects of the opioids, the possibility still exists that the effect to prolong action potential duration is mediated by specific receptors insensitive to naloxone.

Ionic Currents

With the failure of naloxone to prevent or reverse the effects of fentanyl and sufentanil on action potential duration, we began to explore possible ionic channel actions that would alter duration. Three principal ionic currents, or combinations of these currents, control action potential duration: (1) a slow inward current (I_{si}), carried by calcium ions during phase

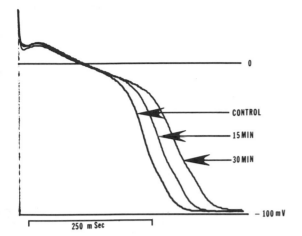

FIGURE 5.3 Superimposed action potentials recorded from canine cardiac Purkinje fibers during control and after 15 and 30 minutes' exposure to 0.17 μM sufentanil. In most cases, the maximum increase in duration occurred within 30 minutes. Changes in duration shown in this figure are typical of changes caused by both fentanyl and sufentanil. Phase 0 has been retouched for clarity.

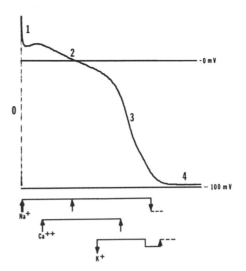

FIGURE 5.4 Action potential phases and ionic currents that generate action potentials. Phase 0 is the rapid depolarization of the membrane caused by a fast inward current carried by sodium ions (indicated by Na+, heavy arrow). Phase 1 is rapid repolarization. Phase 2 is the plateau that results from three ionic currents: an inward background sodium "window" current (second small arrow on the Na+ scale), a second inward current carried by calcium (Ca++ arrow), and an outward current carried by potassium (K+ arrow). These currents control action potential duration. Phase 3 is terminal repolarization that results when the inward Ca++ and Na+ ("window") currents are inactivated, leaving the outward K+ current to repolarize the membrane. Phase 4 is the resting or diastolic potential of the membrane. Notice that the Na+ and K+ currents are reversed at the end of phase 3 and the beginning of phase 4. The channels that regulate the ionic currents are voltage- and time-dependent, e.g., the fast sodium current is inactivated at membrane potentials positive to -60 mV, and the calcium current is activated at membrane potentials positive to -40 mV.

2, that tends to maintain the plateau at or near zero potential (I_{si} is slow relative to the fast sodium current, I_{Na}, responsible for the maximum rate of depolarization, V_{max}); (2) a sodium background current (sodium "window" current) that tends to maintain the plateau; and (3) an outward potassium current (I_K) that repolarizes the cell back to its resting or maximum diastolic potential (see Figure 5.4). Action potential duration could be prolonged by enhancing or delaying the inactivation of I_{si}, inhibiting the inactivation of the sodium "window" current, inhibiting or delaying the activation of I_K, or a combination of these actions.

Sodium Currents

Although we had not observed an effect of fentanyl on V_{max}, we considered the possibility that the effect of fentanyl on these fast sodium channels might be rate- or voltage-dependent or both. In a series of membrane responsiveness determinations, where stimulation rate was varied between 1.0 and 3.0 Hz, fentanyl was without an effect on the fast sodium channels. We then focused our attention on action potential duration.

It is well established that 1.0 μM tetrodotoxin (TTX) abolishes the sodium "window" current in Purkinje fibers.[10] In fibers with the sodium "window" current blocked by TTX, 0.26 μM sufentanil prolonged action potential duration in a manner similar to that observed in fibers not pretreated with TTX.[11] On the basis of these experiments, it appeared that the increase in action potential duration caused by the opioids was not mediated via an effect on the sodium "window" current.

Calcium Current

We next turned our attention to the possible involvement of the slow inward calcium current, I_{si}, in the prolongation of action potential duration caused by sufentanil. In these experiments, Purkinje fibers partly depolarized with 20.0 mM potassium in the bathing solution were utilized. Depolarizing the membranes to approximately -50 mV effectively inactivated the fast sodium channels, and the slow action potentials then elicited by stimulation were generated primarily by calcium entering the cell. Sufentanil enhanced V_{max}, increased overshoot, and prolonged the duration of these slow action potentials[12] and TTX pretreatment did not prevent the increase in duration.[11] These results suggested to us that sufentanil either enhanced I_{si} or delayed the inactivation of I_{si} or both. Thus it appeared that an alteration in the calcium current was involved in the action potential prolongation caused by sufentanil.

Potassium Current

Our initial attempts to examine the possible role of potassium in the sufentanil effect on action potential duration consisted of two simple maneuvers. In the first experiment, stimulus rate was increased from 1.0 Hz to 2.0 Hz. This action has at least two effects on I_K: I_K is still partly activated, and extracellular potassium ($[K^+]_o$) is elevated. Both of these actions are known to increase the outward potassium current, I_K.[13] The change produced by sufen-

tanil in duration was approximately 25% less at the higher stimulus rate than at the lower stimulus rate. In the second experiment, the potassium concentration in the bathing solution was increased from 2.7 mM to 5.4 mM and, as noted, this action is known to increase I_K.[13] The change produced in action potential duration of fibers exposed to 5.4 mM K^+ and 0.26 μM sufentanil was approximately 30% less than the changes produced in fibers exposed to 2.7 mM K^+ and the same concentration of sufentanil.[14] The results of these experiments suggest that sufentanil may also act through the outward potassium current to prolong action potential duration.

To summarize, our experiments indicate that fentanyl and sufentanil have little or no effect on the fast sodium current and the sodium "window" current. They may enhance the calcium current that occurs during the plateau and depress the outward potassium current that is responsible for terminal repolarization. Either of these actions or a combination of the two would prolong action potential duration. Additional voltage or patch clamp studies are needed to quantify the alterations in these membrane ionic currents.

QT Prolongation

In some experiments, we observed large changes in action potential duration at concentrations of fentanyl and sufentanil only slightly greater than those reported in patients. We reasoned that if changes of similar magnitude occurred in heart cells of patients receiving high doses of the opioids, these changes would be reflected in the electrocardiograms of these patients. An examination of the electrocardiograms revealed a prolongation of the QT interval, which we subsequently reported.[15,16] In a small group of patients who received sufentanil for induction and maintenance of anesthesia, we observed that 10 minutes after the start of induction, the QTc (QT corrected for heart rate[17]) was significantly longer than recorded before the start of induction.[18] The QTc remained prolonged throughout the 90-minute study period and at some points exceeded the upper limit of normal (0.44 second[19]). Although prolongation of the QTc was not directly related to serum levels of sufentanil, the effect may be related to redistribution and uptake of sufentanil into cardiac tissue.

Opioid Antiarrhythmic Actions

Electrophysiologic changes caused by fentanyl and sufentanil in isolated canine cardiac Purkinje fibers[14] and in patients' electrocardiograms[18] resembled changes one would expect with class III antiarrhythmic agents,[20] an observation that led us to consider the possibility that the opioids might exhibit antiarrhythmic activity.

Opioid agonists and antagonists had been shown to be effective against a variety of experimental arrhythmias in isolated tissue and intact animal studies and to produce electrophysiologic changes consistent with those seen with antiarrhythmic agents.[9,21-24] Meptazinol, a partial opioid agonist, was reported to reduce the incidence of ventricular extrasystoles as well as of ventricular fibrillation and mortality that resulted from acute coronary occlusion in rats.[21] In addition, meptazinol significantly prolonged action potential duration and depressed V_{max} in papillary muscles isolated from rats.[21] These actions were dose-dependent. Helgesen and Refsum[22] have shown that meperidine increased the effective refractory period in isolated rat atrial preparations without increasing electrical threshold. They suggested that the effect on the effective refractory period was a result of an increase in action potential duration caused by meperidine. In the same study, piritramide and morphine had no significant effect on refractoriness. In another study, methadone prolonged the functional refractory period in isolated atria obtained from guinea pig hearts, an effect that was naloxone-insensitive.[23] In isolated sheep cardiac Purkinje fibers, methadone depressed V_{max} and increased action potential duration in a concentration-dependent manner.[23] Brasch[24] compared the effects of morphine to those of

naloxone. While changes in action potential characteristics recorded from guinea pig papillary muscles exposed to morphine were not as large as those seen with naloxone, morphine caused a lengthening of action potential duration, increased the functional refractory period, and depressed V_{max}.[24] In general, the concentrations of agents used in all the preceding studies were much greater than blood levels one would anticipate from clinical use of these agents. Furthermore, it is unlikely that these high concentrations would be required to produce an effect solely mediated via opioid receptors.

Naloxone

The cardiac effects of the opioid antagonist naloxone have been the subject of several investigations.[9,24-29] In guinea pig papillary muscles[24] and canine cardiac Purkinje fibers,[9] naloxone caused a lengthening of action potential duration and depression of V_{max}, actions that the investigators considered to be potentially antiarrhythmic. Naloxone has been effective against arrhythmias resulting from coronary artery ligation and reperfusion in isolated rat hearts and intact rats and dogs.[25-28] The usefulness of naloxone to protect against digitalis-induced arrhythmias is in question. While Lee et al.[29] observed a protective effect with naloxone against ouabain-induced ventricular fibrillation, Rabkin and Roob,[30] using a similar guinea pig model, found that naloxone hastened the onset of ventricular fibrillation produced by digoxin. The results of naloxone arrhythmia experiments in our laboratories agree with those of Rabkin and Roob: we found that naloxone hastened the onset of ventricular fibrillation produced by ouabain in guinea pigs.[31]

Sufentanil

We conducted experiments designed to test the effectiveness of sufentanil against ouabain-induced ventricular fibrillation in guinea pigs anesthetized with pentobarbital.[31] Sufentanil doses ranged from 3.75 μg/kg to 50.0 μg/kg. In control animals, the average time to ventricular fibrillation was approximately 15 minutes after the start of the ouabain infusion. In animals pretreated with 7.5 μg/kg sufentanil, the average time to ventricular fibrillation was approximately 20 minutes and significantly different from control. Other doses of sufentanil, both higher and lower than 7.5 μg/kg, did not change the time to fibrillation significantly. In fact, at 50 μg/kg, sufentanil hastened the onset of fibrillation. While sufentanil appeared to provide protection against ouabain-induced ventricular fibrillation, it did so over a very narrow dose range, for which we have no explanation. It is well known from isolated tissue studies that cardiac glycosides produce several changes in action potentials associated with arrhythmias. Among these changes are enhanced automaticity, shortened duration, and delayed afterdepolarizations. Sufentanil may delay the onset of ouabain arrhythmias by preventing the shortening of action potential duration caused by ouabain. Such an action could have a dual effect: first, the effective refractory period of the tissue would be maintained, and second, development of delayed afterpotentials might be inhibited. The influence of sufentanil on automaticity has not been examined.

INOTROPIC EFFECTS

Opioid Agonists

The influence of opioid agonists and antagonists on cardiac muscle contractile force has been examined in a variety of preparations with a variety of results, including positive, negative, and biphasic (both positive and negative) inotropic effects. In most studies involving isolated myocardium, negative inotropic effects are the predominantly observed action of opioids such as morphine,[22,32–34] pentazocine,[32] fentanyl,[33–36] piritramide,[22,34] and meperidine.[35] Most reported changes in contractile force appear to have occurred only at relatively high concentrations (greater than 1 μM) and there have been no consistently deter-

mined 50% effective concentrations (EC^{50}) for any given agent in any given species of animal studied. A minor positive inotropic effect of fentanyl and meperidine (between 10 nM and 10 μM) was reported by Rendig et al.[32] in isolated cat papillary muscle. Higher concentrations of both drugs caused a marked depression of contractile force, which was not prevented by pretreatment with naloxone (0.1 mM).

Because of the high concentrations of opioids required to elicit any of the preceding effects, one might conclude that no specific interaction with classic opioid receptors is involved. However, evidence of cardiac opioid receptors has been presented by Laurent et al.,[5] who reported that several different enkephalins caused directly mediated, concentration-dependent positive inotropic effects. The enkephalin-induced increase in contractile force of embryonic avian myocytes was unaffected by α and β adrenoceptor blockade or histamine receptor antagonism but could be antagonized by naloxone.[5] Consistent with this observation are reports that opioid receptors, as well as endogenous opioids, exist in cardiac tissue.[7]

Opioid Antagonists

Naloxone effects on myocardial contractility also appear to be quite variable. Sagy et al.[37] reported that both the *d*- and *l*- isomers of naloxone (40 μM) produced positive inotropic effects in intact rat heart, isolated rat atria, and human atrial strips (effects not influenced by either α or β adrenoceptor blockade). In contrast, Brasch[24] found that neither isomer (30 to 120 μM) had an effect on contractile force of isolated left guinea pig atria. It is interesting, however, that in the same study Brasch found that both naloxone isomers had potent negative chronotropic effects in spontaneously beating right atria.

Fentanyl and Sufentanil

In our hands, the opioid agonists fentanyl and sufentanil also produced variable contractile responses in isolated cardiac tissues. Despite the variability, statistically significant groups of inotropic responses have been observed for isolated tissues of two species (Figure 5.5). Initial studies of guinea pig left atria revealed that fentanyl caused a concentration-dependent biphasic change in contractility; decreases in contractile force at low concentrations (1 to 50 nM) were followed by increased contractile force after cumulative addition of fentanyl up to 1 μM. Of 24 dog papillary muscles studied to date, 2 have responded in a manner similar to that of the guinea pig atria, 15 have displayed only a negative inotropic response, and

7 have responded to only a positive inotropic effect of the drug. Single administrations of fentanyl variably elicit negative or positive inotropic effects or no effect, depending on the concentration. The onset of action, duration, and washout time of single-dose effects on contractile force are similar to those observed for electrophysiologic changes in Purkinje fibers. Because of the unpredictable nature of fentanyl's action on contractile force, the potential blocking actions of naloxone or histamine and adrenergic receptor antagonists have not been well defined. In preliminary experiments, sufentanil has been observed to have the same qualitative effects as fentanyl but over a slightly lower concentration range.

BIOCHEMICAL EFFECTS

Because of the possibility that the electrophysiologic and inotropic effects of fentanyl or sufentanil were mechanistically related, biochemical experiments have been performed in an attempt to identify possible subcellular sites that may be involved. These experiments, utilizing sarcolemmal membranes isolated from canine ventricular myocardium, focused on the opioid effects at sites of subcellular regulation of sodium, potassium, and calcium.[38] It was found that the activity of the sodium pump enzyme (Na^+,K^+-ATPase), which regulates a large number of cellular functions including transmembrane potentials, was unaffected by any concentration of fentanyl, sufentanil, or naloxone studied (1 nM to 100 μM). These data are consistent with the lack of effect of fentanyl and sufentanil on the maximal diastolic potential of isolated Purkinje fibers. Another site studied, the sarcolemmal Na^+/Ca^{2+} exchange antiporter, was found to be inhibited by fentanyl (Figure 5.6) but in an inconsistent manner. This antiporter, which is electrogenic and thus dependent on membrane potential, acts in concert with the sodium pump to regulate cellular sodium and calcium, and therefore can modulate the contractile and electrophysiologic state of cardiac cells.[41] It is interesting to speculate that the inconsistent effects of fentanyl on this site may somehow be related to

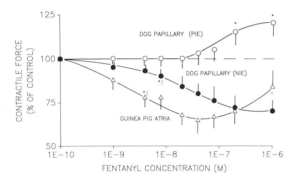

FIGURE 5.5 Concentration-dependent effects of fentanyl on isometric contractile force of canine papillary muscles and guinea pig left atria. Isolated tissues were attached to a calibrated force transducer and mounted in a tissue chamber containing aerated (97% O_2, 3% CO_2) Krebs solution maintained at pH 7.4, 37°C. A preload of 9 mN was maintained on papillary muscles and atria throughout each experiment, and both tissues were electrically paced to contract under physiologic conditions. After tissue equilibration (90 minutes), cumulative administration of the opioid resulted in low concentration negative (NIE) or biphasic inotropic effects or high concentration positive inotropic effects (PIE), expressed as percent change of contractile force from the predrug control level. Statistical significance for data compared to control level is denoted by * for $p < 0.05$; *I indicates $p < 0.05$ for data obtained at all successive higher concentrations except where + denotes not significant compared to control.

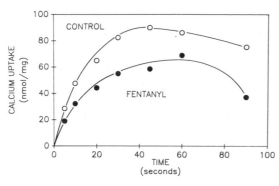

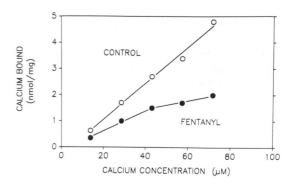

FIGURE 5.6   Effect of 0.2 μM fentanyl on cardiac sarcolemma Na$^+$/Ca^{2+} exchange. Sarcolemma vesicles were prepared according to the procedure of Van Alstyne et al.[39] and loaded internally with 160 mM NaCl, 20 mM MOPS/Tris buffer, pH 7.4. Sodium-dependent uptake of ^{45}Ca, assayed by the method of Reeves and Sutko,[40] was initiated by transferring 10 μg/ml Na$^+$ loaded sarcolemma to a 37°C medium containing 160 mM KCl, 20 mM MOPS/Tris, pH 7.4, and 30 μM ^{45}CaCl^2 in the absence (control) or presence of 0.2 μM fentanyl citrate. At the indicated times, calcium uptake was terminated by dilution of the reaction medium with cold 200 mM KCl, 20 mM MOPS/Tris and 0.1 mM EGTA followed by vacuum filtration to wash away free or loosely bound ^{45}Ca. Sarcolemma vesicle content of ^{45}Ca was then determined by liquid scintillation spectrometry. The maximum net calcium uptake (determined by subtracting sodium-independent calcium binding/uptake (see Figure 5.7) from total uptake at the 55 to 60-second uptake point) was found to be inhibited by fentanyl (65% of control uptake) in 12 out of 17 experiments; fentanyl had no significant effect in 5 experiments.

FIGURE 5.7   Effect of fentanyl (0.95 μM) on high-affinity calcium binding (or passive uptake) to sarcolemma, which was independent of a transmembrane sodium gradient. Sodium-gradient-independent binding/uptake was determined as described in Figure 5.6, except the uptake medium contained 160 mM NaCl instead of KCl and the ^{45}CaCl^2 concentration was varied between 15 and 70 μM. Under these conditions, fentanyl reduced calcium binding to the membranes by 50 to 60% at any given calcium concentration.

the variable inotropic response elicited by the opioid.

One absolutely consistent action of fentanyl, observed in the Na$^+$/Ca^{2+} exchange experiments, was inhibition of calcium binding to the sarcolemma (Figure 5.7). Because sarcolemma preparation is composed of naturally oriented (right-side-out) as well as inside-out vesicles, it cannot be determined from these data whether this inhibition occurs at the intracellular or extracellular face of the membrane. Consequently, little can be said for the potential role of this effect in intact tissue.

CONCLUSION

It is unknown at this time whether any of the effects of fentanyl or sufentanil observed in cardiac tissues or subcellular preparations are due to an interaction with opioid receptors. The failure of naloxone to prevent or reverse (but in some cases mimic) the effects of these opioids suggests at least two possibilities. The first is that drug-induced changes in function were mediated by nonreceptor but perhaps membrane-specific actions[42,43] that altered ionic fluxes normally involved in the cardiac excitation-contraction-relaxation cycle. The second possibility is that the changes were, in fact, mediated by specific opioid receptors not blocked by naloxone. The findings that (1) cardiac opioid receptors may not include the naloxone-sensitive μ subtype, (2) other subtypes (κ and γ) may exist as high- and low-affinity forms, and (3) the number of these receptor subtypes may be quite different for atrial and ventricular myocardium, should be considered in light of the variety as well as the variability of responses observed.[7]

Several of the effects observed in cardiac tissue should not be regarded as merely non-specific, since, as in the case of increased action potential duration, other action potential parameters were not indiscriminately altered. It has been demonstrated that specific membrane effects of the highly lipophilic opioids (like other anesthetic agents) can be exerted by interactions with specific phospholipids (boundary or annular) surrounding specific ion channels and thus alter protein function.[44,45] Alternatively, direct opioid effects could be exerted by interactions with hydrophobic domains of affected proteins within the region of a membrane bilayer.

Opioids produce interesting actions in cardiac tissues. Our understanding of these actions will require future studies in the areas of biochemistry, ion channels, and membrane function.

REFERENCES

1. Jaffe JH, Martin WR. Opioid analgesics and antagonists. In: Gilman AG, Goodman LS, Rall TW, Murad F, eds. The pharmacologic basis of therapeutics. 7th ed. New York: Macmillan, 1985;491–531.

2. Rosow CE. Cardiovascular effects of narcotics. In: Covino B, Covino BG, Fozzard HA, Rehder K, Strichartz G, eds. Effects of anesthesia. Bethesda, Md.: American Physiological Society, 1985;195–204.

3. Blair JR, Pruett JK, Adams RJ, et al. The electrophysiologic effects of opiates in canine cardiac Purkinje fibers. Anesthesiology 1986; 65:A406. (Abstr.)

4. Pruett JK, Blair JR, Adams RJ, et al. The influence of fentanyl on canine cardiac Purkinje fiber action potentials. Fed Proc 1987; 46:1437. (Abstr.)

5. Laurent S, Marsh JK, Smith TW. Enkephalins have a direct positive inotropic effect on cul-

6. tured cardiac myocytes. Proc Natl Acad Sci USA 1985;82:5930–5934.

6. Gautret B, Schmitt H. Cardiac slowing induced by peripheral κ opiate receptor in rats. Eur J Pharmacol 1984;102:159–163.

7. Krumins SA, Faden AI, Feuerstein G. Opiate binding in rat hearts: modulation of binding after hemorrhagic shock. Biochem Biophys Res Commun 1985;127:120–128.

8. Dashwood MR, Spyer KM. Autoradiographic localization of α adrenoceptors, muscarinic acetylcholine receptors, and opiate receptors in the heart. Eur J Pharmacol 1986;127:279–282.

9. Frame LH, Argentieri TM. Naloxone has local anesthetic effects on canine cardiac Purkinje fibers. Circulation 1985;72 (suppl 3):234. (Abstr.)

10. Atwell D, Cohen I, Eisner D, et al. The steady state TTX-sensitive ("window") sodium current in cardiac Purkinje fibers. Pfluegers Arch 1979;379:137–142.

11. Pruett JK, Blair JR, Adams RJ, et al. Tetrodotoxin does not prevent prolongation of slow action potential duration by sufentanil. FASEB J 1989;3:A1171. (Abstr.)

12. Blair JR, Pruett JK, Introna RPS, et al. Enhancement of slow response action potentials by sufentanil. Anesthesiology 1988;69:A63. (Abstr.)

13. Noble D. The initiation of the heartbeat. Oxford: Clarendon Press, 1975;62–68, 122–125.

14. Blair JR, Pruett JK, Introna RPS, et al. Cardiac electrophysiologic effects of fentanyl and sufentanil in canine cardiac Purkinje fibers. Anesthesiology 1989;71:565–570.

15. Blair JR, Pruett JK, Crumrine RS. Prolongation of QT interval associated with the administration of large doses of opiates. Anesthesiology 1987;67:442–443.

16. Blair JR, Pruett JK, Adams RJ, et al. Prolongation of QT intervals in patients receiving high-dose sufentanil. Fed Proc 1987;46:545. (Abstr.)

17. Bazett HC. An analysis of the time relationships of electrocardiograms. Heart 1920;7:353–370.

18. Blair JR, Pruett JK, Introna RPS, et al. Prolongation of QTc interval in association with the administration of sufentanil in high dose. Unpublished.

19. Surawicz B, Knoegel S. Long QT: good, bad or indifferent? J Am Coll Cardiol 1984;4:398–413.

20. Singh BN, Opie LH, Harrison DC, et al. Anti-arrhythmic agents. In: Opie LH, ed. Drugs for the heart. 2d ed. Orlando, Fla.: Grune & Stratton, 1987;74–78.

21. Fagbemi O, Kane KA, Lepran I, et al. Anti-arrhythmic actions of meptazinol, a partial agonist at opiate receptors, in acute myocardial ischaemia. Br J Pharmacol 1983;78:455–460.

22. Helgesen KG, Refsum H. Arrhythmogenic, antiarrhythmic, and inotropic properties of opioids. Pharmacology 1987;35:121–129.

23. Mantelli L, Corti V, Bini R, et al. Effects of dl-methadone on the response to physiological transmitters and on several functional parameters of the isolated guinea pig heart. Arch Int Pharmacodyn Ther 1986;282:289–313.

24. Brasch H. Influence of the optical isomers (+)- and (−)-naloxone on beating frequency, contractile force, and action potentials of guinea pig isolated cardiac preparations. Br J Pharmacol 1986;88:733–740.

25. Zhan ZY, Lee AYS, Wong TM. Naloxone blocks the cardiac effects of myocardial ischaemia and reperfusion in the rat isolated heart. Clin Exp Pharmacol Physiol 1985; 12:373–378.

26. Lee AYS, Wong TM. Antiarrhythmic potency of naloxone determined by a screening test using the isolated ischaemic perfused rat heart preparation. Arch Int Pharmacodyn Ther 1986;286:212–215.

27. Fagbemi O, Lepran I, Parratt JR, et al. Naloxone inhibits early arrhythmias resulting from acute coronary ligation. Br J Pharmacol 1982;76:504–506.

28. Huang XD, Lee AYS, Wong TM, et al. Naloxone inhibits arrhythmias induced by coronary artery occlusion and reperfusion in anaesthetized dogs. Br J Pharmacol 1986; 87:475–477.

29. Lee AYS, Unang TWK, Wong TM. Prevention and reversal of ouabain-induced cardiotoxicity by naloxone in the guinea pig. Clin Exp Pharmacol Physiol 1986;13:55–58.

30. Rabkin SW, Roob O. Effect of the opiate antagonist naloxone on digitalis-induced cardiac arrhythmias. Eur J Pharmacol 1986; 130:47–55.

31. Blair JR, Pruett JK, Adams RJ, et al. The influence of sufentanil on cardiac glycoside toxicity. Washington, D.C.: World Congress of Anaesthesiologists, 1988. (Abstr.)

32. Rendig SV, Amsterdam EA, Henderson GL, et al. Comparative cardiac contractile actions of six narcotic analgesics: morphine, meperidine, pentazocine, fentanyl, methadone, and L- α-acetylmethadol (LAAM). J Pharmacol Exp Ther 1980;215:259–265.

33. Goldberg AH, Padget CH. Comparative effects of morphine and fentanyl on isolated heart muscle. Anesth Analg (Cleve) 1969; 48:978–982.

34. Strauer BE. Contractile responses to morphine, piritramide, meperidine and fentanyl. Anesthesiology 1972;37:304–310.

35. Motomura S, Kissin I, Aultman DF, et al. Effects of fentanyl and nitrous oxide on contractility of blood-perfused papillary muscle of the dog. Anesth Analg 1984;63:47–50.

36. Reves JG, Kissin I, Fournier SE, et al. Additive negative inotropic effect of a combination of diazepam and fentanyl. Anesth Analg 1984;63:97–100.

37. Sagy M, Shavit G, Oron Y, et al. Nonopiate effect of naloxone on cardiac muscle contractility. J Cardiovasc Pharmacol 1987;9:682–685.

38. Adams RJ, Pruett JK, Blair JR, et al. Subcellular effects of fentanyl which relate to actions in intact myocardium. Anesthesiology 1987;67:A62. (Abstr.)

39. Van Alstyne E, Burch RM, Knickelbein RG, et al. Isolation of sealed vesicles highly enriched with sarcolemma from canine left ventricle. Biochim Biophys Acta 1980;602:131–143.

40. Reeves JP, Sutko JL. Competitive interactions of sodium and calcium with the sodium-calcium exchange system of cardiac sarcolemmal vesicles. J Biol Chem 1983;258:3178–3182.

41. Reeves JP. The sarcolemma sodium-calcium exchange system. Curr Top Membranes Transport 1985;25:77–127.

42. Dodson BA, Miller KW. Evidence for a dual mechanism in the anesthetic action of an opioid peptide. Anesthesiology 1985;62:615–620.

43. Stone DJ, DiFazio CA. Anesthetic action of opiates: correlation of lipid solubility and spectral edge. Anesth Analg 1988;67:663–666.

44. Loh HH, Law PV. The role of membrane lipids in receptor mechanisms. Annu Rev Pharmacol Toxicol 1980;20:201–234.

45. Koblin DD, Eger IE II. How do inhaled anesthetics work? In: Miller RD, ed. Anesthesia. 2d ed. New York: Churchill Livingstone, 1986;1:581–623.

Chapter 5 Discussion

STEVEN SHAFER: The authors have succinctly reviewed the actions of opioids on cardiac tissue. The data presented, although substantial, yield inconsistent conclusions. For example, do opioids affect the fast sodium channel? Fentanyl and sufentanil have no effect on V_{max}, while morphine, methadone, and naloxone all decrease V_{max}. Do opioids affect inotropy? Rendig et al.[1] reported that low concentrations of fentanyl increase inotropy, while high concentrations decrease inotropy. The authors' research produced the opposite result.

These results are difficult to understand in the absence of data on the molecular mechanisms of opioid effects on cardiac tissue. Once these mechanisms are understood, then consistent explanations should emerge from the apparently conflicting data. In the interim, research in clinically relevant domains, such as the inotropic effects of opioid on the failing myocardium, may yield results that directly affect clinical practice.

REFERENCE

1. Rendig, SV, Amsterdam EA, Henderson GL, et al. Comparative cardiac contractile actions of six narcotic analgesics: morphine, meperidine, pentazocine, fentanyl, methadone, and L-α-acetylmethadol (LAAM). J Pharmacol Exp Ther 1980;215:259–265.

PETER S.A. GLASS: One of the major advantages of the fentanyl group of piperidine derivatives is their marked lack of cardiovascular effects. The most significant action of these potent opioids on vascular function is slowing of heart rate. The exact mechanism of this effect is poorly understood. However, several effects of the opioids on cellular and subcellular function that may account for this opioid function have been described by Pruett et al. They have shown that the prolongation of the action potential duration occurring after opioid administration appears unrelated to opioid receptor occupancy but is rather due to a direct effect of the opioids on ion channels. More specifically, Pruett et al. have demonstrated that calcium and outward potassium current are altered in a way that would prolong the duration of the action potential. That these mechanisms are important within the dosage range of opioids used clinically is supported by the fact that the QT interval is prolonged during opioid-based anesthesia.

The effect of opioids on myocardial contractility is far less clear. Certainly, in the clinical setting, these are minimal. The variable action of opioids on contractility in isolated preparations may well result from the fact that opioids have a very limited action and thus variability may be due to differences in the model or differences in the preparations rather than due to the drug. A still unanswered question is whether there are opioid receptors in the heart, and if so, for which actions they are responsible. The data presented by Pruett et al. in this chapter favor the absence of opioid receptor-mediated actions in the heart. They do, however, suggest the possibility of non-naloxone reversible opioid receptors being present. A nonspecific action of opioids on the heart remains a more likely explanation.

Although opioids alone may have limited effects on hemodynamics, drug combinations (most notably opioids plus benzodiazepines) may produce profound hemodynamic changes. Although it appears that these drug interactions may result from actions within the nervous system, a direct effect on cellular function may be possible. It is therefore important that the actions of anesthetic drugs either alone or in combination on cellular and subcellular function continue to be defined.

6 SPINAL OPIOID ANALGESIA: CHARACTERIZATION OF ACUTE TOLERANCE IN AN ANIMAL MODEL

Tony L. Yaksh and Maurice Sosnowski

MECHANISMS OF OPIOID ANALGESIA

Morphine administered systemically will yield a powerful and relatively selective obtundation of the pain behavior otherwise evoked by high threshold visceral and somatic stimuli. This effect is mediated by an action at specific brain stem and spinal loci. Thus, stereotaxic micro-injection studies have shown that morphine administered into circumscribed regions of the brain, notably the mesencephalic periaqueductal gray and the medial medulla, will yield a behaviorally defined analgesia. This effect reflects several mechanisms, including activation of bulbospinal monoamine pathways, that inhibit spinal sensory processing and direct local changes in the afferent input into the bulbar core.[1] In addition, the local administration of opioids into the spinal space will yield a powerful and selective analgesia. This effect is mediated by an action on small primary afferent terminals that blocks the release of the respective excitatory neurotransmitters and by a postsynaptic effect that inhibits the firing of dorsal horn nociceptors.[2]

In both brain and spinal cord, the effects observed with opioids reflect an action mediated by local opioid receptors. By systematic pharmacologic analysis, it can be shown based on agonist structure-activity relationships and antagonism by selective antagonists that in the periaqueductal gray and medulla, the effects are largely mediated by μ and μ-δ classes of receptors, respectively.[1] In the spinal cord, strong evidence exists to suggest the role of μ, δ, and κ subclasses of sites.[3]

Mechanistically, it is known that the μ and δ receptor types exert their effects by altering ion fluxes. Thus, in dorsal root ganglia in culture, these receptors are known to diminish Ca^{++} flux through voltage-sensitive Ca channels.[4] This likely accounts in part for the ability of these agents to block neurotransmitter release. In addition, agonist occupation of the μ and δ sites has been shown to be positively coupled through Gi/Go protein to K^+ channels.[5] Increase in K^+ conductance leads to membrane hyperpolarization and subsequent depression of cellular excitability.

This linkage of an agonist to its effect (e.g., increased K$^+$ conductance, inhibition of adenylate cyclase) by receptor occupancy and subsequent activation of a second messenger system has been shown to be subject to a significant degree of regulation.[6] One important manifestation of such regulation may be observed with continued exposure of the system to its agonist. This will frequently lead to a time-dependent diminution of the effect otherwise produced by a given dose of the drug. This phenomenon is often referred to as tolerance. In animal studies, efforts to produce long-term elevations in the nociceptive threshold by chronic administration of systemic morphine will reliably lead to large incrementations in the necessary dose over surprisingly short periods of time (hours to days).[7]

In rats and primates, the repeated intrathecal administration of opioids over 5 to 7 days results in a dramatic reduction in the antinociceptive effect normally produced by an otherwise maximally effective dose of morphine, metkephamid, β-endorphin and D-Ala^2-D-Leu^5-enkephalin.[8-10] As the drug was administered into the central nervous system (CNS), the possibility of changes in the blood-brain barrier could be excluded. Given the role of the opioid receptor in mediating these effects, it appears likely that changes in response to chronic drug exposure should occur with characteristics defined by the underlying pharmacodynamic properties of the receptor systems. In the following sections, we briefly summarize recent work from our laboratory[11-13] that characterizes some of the pharmacodynamic aspects of these changes in opioid-induced analgesia that are observed after chronic intrathecal administration in a well-defined rat model.

ANIMAL STUDIES ON THE PHARMACOLOGIC CHARACTERISTICS OF SPINAL OPIOID TOLERANCE

In the experiments to be described, rats are prepared with chronic indwelling spinal catheters inserted to the level of the lumbar enlargement through the cisternal membrane. To deliver drug, the catheter is connected to an osmotic infusion pump (Alzet), which delivers 1 μl/hr for 7 to 8 days. A loop of the catheter is externalized to permit access to the spinal catheter without having to do a cutdown to disconnect the pump.[14] To assess nociception, animals are tested on the 52.5°C hot plate. Failure to respond by 60 seconds is cause to terminate the test, and that number is assigned as the score.

Time Course of Tolerance Development

As shown in Figure 6.1A, rats receiving continuous infusion of morphine and tested on a daily basis displayed a concentration-dependent increase in the nociceptive threshold, with the maximum effect observed on day 1. Over the ensuing 7-day infusion period, the hot-plate response latency fell to preinfusion levels. Inspection of the curves suggests that the rate at which the effect disappeared was the same for all doses. To demonstrate that, the area under the 7-day analgesia curve was plotted versus the peak effect observed on day 1 (which is directly proportional to the infusion concentration). Had lower doses shown a slower or faster time course for development of tolerance, the distribution of the points would have been nonlinear. As shown in Figure 6.1B, the best-fit line appears linear with an intersect at the origin. Thus, the rate of tolerance development in this model is independent of infusion concentration over the range of doses employed.

Experiments similar to those described for morphine were carried out using the anilinopiperidines sufentanil and alfentanil. These agents also displayed an infusion concentration-dependent increase in the hot-plate response latency, which was maximal on day 1. Comparison of their relative potency as measured by their respective effects on day 1 during chronic intrathecal infusion, with potency as measured after bolus intrathecal administration, reveals them to be similar (Table 6.1).

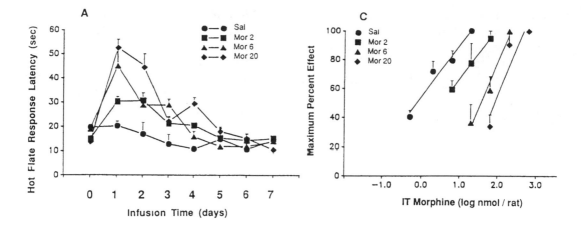

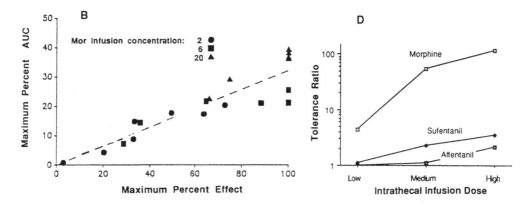

FIGURE 6.1 (A) Time course of analgesic effect (hot-plate: test: percent of maximum percent effect) observed over a 7-day period of infusion of morphine at doses of 20, 6, or 2 nmol/μl/hr or saline vehicle. Each curve presents the mean and standard error for six rats. (B) Percentage of the maximum possible area under the analgesia time course curve (AUC) plotted versus the maximum percent effect observed on the hot-plate test on day 1 of the infusion. (Data derived from those presented in A.) Each point presents the results for a single animal. (C) Intrathecal dose-response curves carried out in different groups of rats 7 days after the initiation of the infusion of vehicle or morphine at 2, 6, or 20 nmol/μl/hr. Each point presents the mean for four to six rats. (D) Tolerance ratio (ED_{50} in drug-infused animals ÷ ED_{50} in vehicle-infused animal) derived from data similar to those presented in C, plotted versus the infusion dose of morphine, sufentanil, or alfentanil. (Adapted from data presented in Stevens CW and Yaksh TL. Time course characteristics of tolerance development to continuously infused antinociceptive agents. J Pharmacol Exp Ther 1989; 251:216–223; Sosnowski M, Stevens CW, Yaksh TL. Comparison of tolerance development after continuous spinal intrathecal infusions in rats. Reg Anesth 1989; 14S:76.)

TABLE 6.1 Potency of morphine, sufentanil, and alfentanil as determined by bolus administration or by chronic infusion at 1 day after initiation of infusion

Drug	Intrathecal Bolus ED$_{50}$ (nmol)	Intrathecal Infusion ED$_{50}$ (nmol/µl/hr)
Morphine	12.6	3.0
Sufentanil	0.3	0.3
Alfentanil	10.2	32.0

Source: From Stevens CW, Yaksh TL. Time course characteristics of tolerance development to continuously infused antinociceptive agents. J Pharmacol Exp Ther 1989;251:216–223; Yaksh TL, Noueihed RY, Durant PAC. Studies of the pharmacology and pathology of intrathecally administered 4-anilinopeperidine analogues and morphine in rat and cat. Anesthesiology 1986;64:54–66; Sosnowski M, Yaksh TL. Differential tolerance between the spinal µ opioid agonists morphine and sufentanil, correlation with drug efficacy. Proc Meet Soc Neurosci, Phoenix, Arizona, 1989. (Abstr.).

Interestingly, given that the infusion represents a steady-state drug level, it would appear that the relative potency of morphine is underestimated and alfentanil overestimated after bolus injection. As with morphine, the analgesia observed after 7 days of chronic infusion showed a decline to baseline. Calculation of the area under the maximum possible time course curve (AUC) at 7 days versus the maximum effect observed on day 1 revealed a relationship that was superimposable over that demonstrated with morphine in Fig 6.1B. Thus, when these agents are matched for their peak drug effect on day 1, the rate of tolerance development during continuous infusion is the same for all agents in this model.

Magnitude of Tolerance Development

After 7 days of infusion with either vehicle or one of the several doses of morphine, the question of the magnitude of tolerance that had been induced was addressed. In separate groups, animals were prepared for infusion with the same concentrations of morphine (2, 6, or 20 nmol/µl/hr) or vehicle. These animals were not tested until the end of 7 days. At this time, it was observed, as in the animals that had been tested daily, that test latencies were not different from saline-infused controls. In these animals, dose-response studies were then carried out in which a given bolus dose of morphine, the probe drug, was given through the external arm of the intrathecal catheter and the effect on the hot-plate response latency was assessed. As shown in Figure 6.1C, these dose-response curves for bolus morphine carried out in animals that had received 7 days of infusion of vehicle or one of the three doses of morphine revealed an infusion concentration-dependent rightward shift. This is emphasized by plotting the degree of shift as a function of infusion concentration. Thus, calculating the tolerance ratio (ED$_{50}$ of test drug in drug-infused animals ÷ ED$_{50}$ of test drug in saline-infused animals) reveals that the magnitude of the shift was proportional to the log of the infusion concentration (Fig 6.1D).

Experiments similar to the preceding one were carried out with sufentanil and alfentanil. As with morphine, there was a parallel rightward shift in the probe dose-response curves. To our surprise, the magnitude of the shift was considerably less than that observed with morphine. Note that the 7-day AUC values for the low, medium, and high infusion concentrations of morphine (2, 6, and 20 nmol/µl/hr), sufentanil (0.06, 0.2, and 0.6 nmol/µl/hr), and alfentanil (6, 20, and 60 nmol/µl/hr) could be matched for effect, as shown in Figure 6.1D. At these respective infusion concentrations, the degree of shift was reliably greater with morphine than with the anilinopiperidines.

Cross-Tolerance between Drugs

Given that morphine and sufentanil act largely upon the µ opioid receptor,[15] we sought to address the characteristics of the cross-tolerance between these drugs in animals that had been exposed for 7 days to equieffective concentration of either drug. Table 6.2 presents the intrathecal ED_{50} values on the hot-plate test for morphine or sufentanil in animals that had received 7 days of infusion of morphine (20 nmol/μl/hr), sufentanil (0.6 nmol/μl/hr), or saline (vehicle).

As indicated, the magnitude of the shift of the probe drug ED_{50} for both morphine and sufentanil as a function of the infusion regimen was morphine > sufentanil > saline. In other words, given the similarity of the peak analgesia curve and the area under the drug analgesia curve, there was clear asymmetry in the tolerance induced by these two agents in that the degree of shift for morphine and sufentanil was always greater after morphine than after sufentanil.

Reversibility of Intrathecal Tolerance

To assess the reversibility of tolerance induced by intrathecally infused morphine, rats received intrathecal infusion of the highest dose of morphine (20 nmol/μl/hr) for 7 days. The animals were then tested at 3 hours or 9 days for their sensitivity to intrathecal morphine. As indicated in Table 6.3, the intrathecal ED_{50} of morphine displayed a reduction over the ensuing days in which the animals were not exposed to morphine, such that the ED_{50} displayed an approximate 60% recovery by 9 days.

MECHANISMS OF INTRATHECAL TOLERANCE

In the preceding sections, experiments detailing the characteristics of the change in drug sensitivity observed after spinal infusion in a rodent model for three agents known to act at the μ subclass of opioid receptors were reviewed. In the following section, the implications of these results for the interpretation of the tolerance phenomena is briefly discussed.

The mechanisms whereby apparent changes in drug-effect coupling can occur following chronic exposure may be broadly classed in four categories: learning, change in the effective stimulus, pharmacokinetics, and pharmacodynamics.

Learning

There is evidence to suggest that repeated pairing of a drug and a stimulus can give rise to conditioned events that are antagonistic to the effect otherwise produced by the drug.[16,17] While this phenomenon may be relevant in certain precise behavioral paradigms, in the present class of studies the loss of effect (elevated hot-plate response latency) could be demonstrated even in animals in which the drug (spinal opioid)–stimulus (hot-plate) pairing never occurred until the end of 7 days.

TABLE 6.2 Intrathecal ED_{50} values for morphine and sufentanil measured in animals after chronic intrathecal infusion of morphine (20 nmol/μl/hr), sufentanil (0.6 nmol/μl/hr) or vehicle

Infusion Drug	Test Drug			
	Morphine (ED_{50} (nmol) tol. ratio)		Sufentanil (ED_{50} (nmol) tol. ratio)	
Vehicle	0.6	—	0.07	—
Morphine	30.0	45.0	0.68	9.7
Sufentanil	6.1	9.5	0.2	3.0

Tolerance ratio = ED_{50} of drug ÷ ED_{50} of vehicle.

TABLE 6.3 ED_{50} values (nmol) for intrathecal morphine assessed at times after chronic spinal infusions for 7 days in rats

Infusion Agent	ED_{50} of Intrathecal Morphine (nmol) (Days Posttermination of Infusion)	
	0	9
Vehicle	0.6	—
Morphine	30.0[a]	10.0[a,b]

[a] $p < 0.05$ as compared to vehicle animal.
[b] $p < 0.05$ as compared to morphine-infused rats tested 0 days posttermination.

Change in Effective Stimulus

It is clear that as the nociceptive stimulus intensity rises, the dose of spinal drug required to block the effect also rises.[18] It is also clear that different stimulus modalities may result in CNS effects that are differentially sensitive to opioid modulation. Thus, in studies examining the ability to block the allodynia induced by spinally administered strychnine, opioids displayed a clearly diminished activity as compared to other classes of spinally administered agents, such as N-methyl-D-aspartate receptor antagonists or adenosine agonists.[19,20] While the use of the fixed thermal stimulus in the present study precludes such variability, it is probable that changes in the nature of the effective pain stimulus may affect the activity of opioids in terminal cancer patients. In such a situation, the pain report in the later stages often reveals an increasing incidence of dysesthetic pain,[21] a condition that may involve central substrates not influenced by opioids.[22,23]

Pharmacokinetics

In the present model, plasma and spinal cord levels of morphine, sufentanil, and alfentanil were assessed at times after the initiation of their intrathecal infusion. These levels were routinely maximal at 1 day after the initiation of infusion and did not change between 1 and 7 days (Sosnowski, Hill, and Yaksh, unpublished observations). Moreover, the loss of ef-

fect observed with morphine, sufentanil, and alfentanil is limited to the μ opioids. Thus, following the development of tolerance to morphine, there is no loss of effect to either δ opioid agonists[11] or to α_2 agonists.[24] While these data indicate that the change in response observed in this intrathecal model was not due to changes in spinal drug levels, it should be noted that following epidural placement in a variety of animal models, there may be a local aseptic inflammatory reaction that prevents free distribution of the drug.[25,26] In humans the distribution of drug into the cerebrospinal fluid after administration through epidural catheters that have been in place for some period may in fact be considerably altered.[27] In such cases, incrementations in dose in a terminal patient might be anticipated to reflect such incomplete redistribution.

Pharmacodynamics

Aside from the preceding variables, the change in drug effects observed after chronic exposure of the preparation to an agonist may be largely predicted on the theoretical assumption that the total number of receptors or the number of receptors coupled to the second messenger may be reduced. Such pharmacodynamic explanations of the loss of drug effect with continuous agonist exposure have been shown relevant in well-defined in vitro neuronal models for a number of receptor systems, including those for the opioid receptor.[28,29]

Appreciation of the significance of receptor down-regulation to opioid analgesia requires the following consideration. In classical pharmacology, it was believed that a maximum effect was achieved when all receptors were occupied.[30] Since Stephenson,[31] it has been widely appreciated that a receptor agonist may yield a complete effect by occupying a given, subtotal, number of the receptor population. Thus, it is possible to express the efficacy of a drug in terms of the fraction of the total receptor population that an agonist must occupy (fractional receptor occupancy: FRO) to yield a given effect in a specific physiological

Psychopathology in animals. New York: Academic Press, 1985;143–168.

17. Kalant H. Tolerance, learning, and neurochemical adaptation. Can J Physiol Pharmacol 1985;63:1485–1494.

18. Yaksh TL. Tolerance: factors involved in changes in the dose effect relationship with chronic drug exposure. Dahlem Konferenzen, Berlin (West), 30 Nov 1989 (in press).

19. Yaksh TL. Behavioral and autonomic correlates of the tactile evoked allodynia produced by spinal glycine inhibition: effects of modulatory receptor systems and excitatory amino acid antagonists. Pain 1989;37:111–123.

20. Sosnowski M, Yaksh TL. The role of spinal adenosine receptors in modulating the hyperesthesia produced by spinal glycine receptor antagonism. Anesth Analg 1989;69:587–592.

21. Foley KM. Pharmacologic approaches to cancer pain management. Ad Pain Res Ther 1985;9:629–653.

22. Arner S, Arner B. Differential effects of epidural morphine in the treatment of cancer-related pain. Acta Anaesthesiol Scand 1985;29:32–36.

23. Arner S, Meyerson BA. Lack of analgesic effect of opioids on neuropathic and idiopathic forms of pain. Pain 1988;33:11–23.

24. Stevens CW, Monasky MS, Yaksh TL. Spinal infusion of opiate and α_2 agonists in rats: tolerance and cross-tolerance studies. J Pharmacol Exp Ther 1988;244:63–70.

25. Durant PAC, Yaksh TL. Epidural injections of bupivacaine, morphine, fentanyl, lofentanil, and DADL in chronically implanted rats: a pharmacologic and pathologic study. Anesthesiology 1986;64:43–53.

26. Sabbe M, Mjanger E, Sosnowski M, et al. Study on tolerance development after daily epidural injection of sufentanil in dogs. Anesthesiology 1988;69(suppl 3A):A392.

27. Samuelsson H, Nordberg G. CSF and plasma morphine concentrations in cancer patients during chronic epidural morphine therapy and its relation to pain relief. Pain 1987;30:303–310.

28. Zukin RS, Temple A. Neurochemical correlates of opiate receptor regulation. Biochem Pharmacol 1986;35:1623–1627.

29. Christie MJ, Williams JT, North RA. Cellular mechanisms of opioid tolerance: studies in single brain neurons. Mol Pharmacol 1987;32:633–638.

30. Goldstein A, Aronow L, Kalman SM. Principles of drug action. New York: Wiley, 1974:82–87.

31. Stephenson RP. A modification of receptor therapy. Br J Pharmacol 1956;11:379–393.

32. Mjanger E, Yaksh TL. Funaltrexamine (β-FNA) versus opioid receptors in the spinal cord. Proc Meet Soc Neurosci, Toronto, 1988. (Abstr.)

33. Twycross RG, Lack SA. Symptom control in far advanced cancer: pain relief. London: Pitman, 1983.

34. Yaksh TL, Onofrio BM. Retrospective consideration of the doses of morphine given intrathecally by chronic infusion in 163 patients by 19 physicians. Pain 1987;31:211–223.

35. Onofrio BM, Yaksh TL. Long-term pain relief produced by intrathecal morphine infusion in 53 patients. J Neurosurg 1990;72:200–209.

36. Shetter AG, Hadley MN, Wilkinson E. Administration of intraspinal morphine sulfate for the treatment of intractable cancer pain. Neurosurgery 1986;18:740–747.

37. Krames ES, Gershow J, Glassberg A. Continuous infusion of spinally administered narcotics for the relief of pain due to malignant disorders. Cancer 1985;56:696–702.

38. Coombs DW, Saunders RL, Gaylor MS. Relief of continuous chronic pain by intraspinal narcotics infusion via an implanted reservoir. JAMA 1983;250:2336–2339.

39. Russell RD, Leslie JB, Su YF, et al. Continuous intrathecal opioid analgesia: tolerance and cross-tolerance of μ and δ spinal opioid receptors. J Pharmacol Exp Ther 1987;240:150–158.

40. Moulin DE, Max MB, Kaiko RF, et al. The analgesic efficacy of intrathecal D-Ala²-D-Leu⁵-enkephalin in cancer patients with chronic pain. Pain 1985;23:213–221.

41. Tamsen A, Gordh T. Epidural clonidine produces analgesia. Lancet 1984;1:231–232.

42. Yaksh TL, Noueihed RY, Durant PAC. Studies of the pharmacology and pathology of intrathecally administered 4-anilinopeperidine analogues and morphine in rat and cat. Anesthesiology 1986;64:54–66.

43. Sosnowski M, Yaksh TL. Differential tolerance between the spinal μ opioid agonists morphine and sufentanil, correlation with drug efficacy. Proc Meet Soc Neurosci, Phoenix, Arizona, 1989. (Abstr.)

Chapter 6 Discussion

STEVEN SHAFER: Dr. Yaksh offers very compelling data that low-efficacy drugs like morphine will produce tolerance at a faster rate than high-efficacy drugs like sufentanil. These conclusions appear to conflict with those of Dr. Farley, who observes faster addiction and acceleration of drug dosing with fentanyl and sufentanil than with morphine. Perhaps the resolution of this apparent contradiction is that tolerance in the spinal cord of the rat is very different from clinical addiction in humans, for whom opioid effects on mood and behavior, rather than spinal-mediated analgesia, dominate the physical effects of dependence.

Dr. Yaksh's data show that the magnitude of tolerance following equipotent infusions of morphine and sufentanil is far greater with morphine, and this is explained by the experimentally verified observation that morphine is a low-efficacy drug with a higher FRO requirement than sufentanil. Why is the rate of onset of tolerance, when adjusted for peak effect, the same for morphine and sufentanil in this animal model, when the differences of FRO requirement imply that the rate for morphine should be greater? Perhaps the low-resolution data collection (1 point/animal/day), high interanimal variability, and nonparametric rate estimation (AUC/peak effect) contributed to the inability to discern a difference in the rate of tolerance onset. I obtained reasonably good fits with a parametric analysis of the rate of the onset of tolerance to morphine by fitting the reported effect data (Figure 6.1A) to the model:

$$\text{Effect } (t) = \text{peak effect } * e^{-kt}$$

where

Effect   = observed effect − baseline effect
Peak effect = effect on day 1 − baseline effect
k = rate constant of effect
              onset (in days^{-1})
t = time (days)
e = base of natural
              logarithms

The half-life of tolerance development to intrathecal morphine with the preceding model was 1.3, 1.1, and 1.1 days for the 2, 4, and 20 nmol/hr doses, respectively. Perhaps a similar parametric analysis of the onset of sufentanil tolerance, combined with higher resolution sampling, would demonstrate a slower onset of tolerance for sufentanil, as Dr. Yaksh's conclusions suggest should be observed.

PETER S.A. GLASS: Acute tolerance is a fascinating phenomena easily demonstrated in animal models but as yet not well defined in humans. Dr. Yaksh has presented data to answer three questions important to the development of tolerance: (1) Does the rate of tolerance depend on the concentration of drug presented to the opioid receptor? Dr. Yaksh ensured a constant concentration by utilizing a continuous infusion. His data tend to indicate that the rate at which tolerance occurred is independent of concentration. (2) Does the degree of tolerance produced differ according to the concentration to which the opioid receptor is exposed? Using a second probe drug to provide dose response curves in tolerant animals, Dr. Yaksh has clearly shown that the degree of tolerance varies according to the concentration. The higher the concentration, the greater the degree of tolerance. (3) Is the degree of tolerance that occurs different between different opioid agonists given at equipotent doses? When sufentanil is compared to morphine, it appears the degree of tolerance induced is greater with morphine than sufentanil. This latter phenomenon, Dr. Yaksh speculates, is due to the lower fractional receptor occupancy of sufentanil (being a more potent drug) than morphine.

How do these results relate to the development of tolerance in humans, and what are their clinical implications? The model used by Dr. Yaksh isolated opioid exposure to receptors in the spinal cord. Thus these data may only be applicable to spinal opioid administration, as tolerance to systemic opioids may be influenced by a multitude of neurosensory regulatory mechanisms present in the brain and not at the level of the spinal cord. Also, tolerance was tested by the intermittent application of a painful stimulus. In the clinical setting, opioids are administered for continuous pain. The inability to clearly define tolerance in patients with acute or chronic pain may be the result of complex interaction of neuroreceptor activation and opioid receptor occupancy.

Several groups are at present developing pharmacokinetic model-driven drug delivery systems enabling patients to be maintained at constant plasma concentrations.[1-4] Equipotent analgesic concentrations are also being defined in humans. The use of pharmacokinetic model-driven drug delivery systems, combined with the knowledge of relative drug potency, will enable studies similar to those performed by Dr. Yaksh to be done in humans. This will allow us to obtain a greater understanding of tolerance in humans and its significance to acute and chronic administration of opioids.

REFERENCES

1. Ausems ME, Vuyk J, Hug CC Jr, et al. Comparison of a computer-assisted infusion versus intermittent bolus administration of alfentanil as a supplement to nitrous oxide for lower abdominal surgery. Anesthesiology 1988;68:851–861.
2. Martin RW, Hill HF, Yee HC, et al. An open-loop computer-based drug infusion system. IEEE Trans Biomed Eng 1987;BME34:642–649.
3. Shafer SL, Martin GM, Stanski DR, et al. Pharmacokinetic analysis of fentanyl administered by a computer-controlled infusion pump. Anesthesiology 1987;67:A666. (Abstr.)
4. Glass P, Jacobs JR, Hawkins ED, et al. Accuracy and efficacy of a pharmacokinetic model driven device to infuse fentanyl for anesthesia during general surgery. Anesthesiology 69:A290. (Abstr.)

Part I Discussion

DR. THEODORE H. STANLEY: I'm interested in the interaction between not only the α_2 agonists in the opioids but other classes of drugs. Is there any evidence that the interaction may be precipatory at the receptor level or at the subcellular level rather than simply additive by different receptors? Is it possible that one class of drugs, like the α_2 agonists, actually potentiates opioid action by facilitating the interaction at the opioid receptor?

DR. BYRON C. BLOOR: If you define receptor as a binding site, the answer is clearly no. We have done experiments to see whether there is either an inhibitory or facilitory action of these other drugs on opioid binding, and there is not, until huge concentrations. On the other hand, if you define receptor as the binding site plus the G-protein plus ion channel or cyclase, then I think there is much more likelihood of a common pathway at that level.

DR. DANIEL B. CARR: What about the motor dysfunctions seen with peptides? A number of different mechanisms have been proposed that may actually be acting to a greater or lesser degree simultaneously. The degree of toxicity through N-methyl-D-aspartate seems to be a true finding. Other mechanisms that have been posited include mechanisms dependent on vasospasm; on alterations in calcium flux; in release of free radicals; and so on. So you could say several things are known to cause neurotoxicity in the setting of other drug administration. All of these may play a role to one or another degree. On the other hand, there are many examples of opioid peptides or analogues that are safe to give. The problem at this point seems to arise from the particular sequence of individual amino acids that are liberated upon metabolism.

SPEAKER FROM THE FLOOR: Is there any evidence that species differences between opioid receptor actions are based on receptors or on any kind of blood mechanism?

DR. ERIC J. SIMON: Well, one very clear difference is the distribution of these receptors. The species differences are difficult to understand. For instance, the cerebellum of some species, like the rat, has almost no perceptible receptors. The cerebellum of the guinea pig has a huge level of cab κ receptors. The cerebellum of the rabbit has almost all μ receptors. There are many other cases like this. The rat in general has a very low level of κ receptors. What does it mean about the importance of these receptors when a species can get along with a low level in an important area of the brain? That is one area where there are clear species differences. In terms of identifying the differences between molecular entities of particular receptors, or actions of receptors, we are not yet able to tell. I have some evidence that in lower species, like the frog and the toad, receptors may be different from their mammalian counterparts.

DR. STANLEY: Which animal species usually studied is closest to humans? This is some work that Dr. Labkowski Silver and I did, and this rather chaotic pattern is indicative of what clinicians face. To explain the slide, these little sets are percentages of maximum possible effect on analgesic testing from administration of selective agonists that were directed either against δ, μ, or κ receptors, and you see little clusters. Each cluster is one individual animal. Clinicians are often bewildered as to why there seems to be such variability among individual animals. In fact, a large body of statistical techniques is used by pharmacologists to smooth out individual differences. The whole question of individual differences has been perceived as a bothersome and vexing thing that we want to brush aside and smooth out. But if one specifically focuses on individual animals that are genetically identical—Sprague Dawley rats, for instance—that are all the same sex and prepared in the same way, it is impressive how much individual variability there is. It is difficult to predict the responses to one agonist even in the same animal. How is that animal going to respond to another agonist of different type? It is a chaotic situation; even if you take into account interspecies variability, there seems to be a nondeterministic aspect to opioid receptor effects, such as for analgesia.

DR. CARL C. HUG, JR.: There is another aspect to this. With due regard to the differences in receptors, some of the apparent differences in species may be related to experimental techniques. These drugs have multiple actions, and when those actions are not appropriately controlled for, I think you can find experimental differences. Let me give you a hypothesis I had concerning one of the differences that has been emphasized between dog and human. In dogs, you can give huge doses of opioids, for example, 30 mg/kg, and the dog will survive. If one gave 30 mg/kg to a human, I doubt the human would survive. One of the differences, of course, is respiratory function. The dog has two functions for respiration: the exchange of oxygen and carbon dioxide, and control of body temperature. When you give an opioid to a dog, the body temperature will tend to fall, and the dog, unlike the human, ventilates. So if you compare dog and human, just as individuals unsupported any other way, you might find this difference. But if you intubate the dog and the human, and you control ventilation, and you look not only at doses but at concentration-effect relations, you find that the dog and the human (for example, in terms of anesthetic component contribution of the opioids) are almost identical. If you combine, for example, alfentanil–nitrous oxide in the human so that there is no response to a typical stimulus, for example, a skin incision, you will find that the concentration of alfentanil matches exactly the concentration of alfentanil required as supplement to enflurane to reduce MAC by the tail-clamp method in the dog. Thus, there are not only very important receptor differences in distribution but also important differences in experimental techniques.

DR. SIMON: These receptor differences may be important but, on the other hand, there may be no correlation between mass of receptor distribution and function. In other words, it may take a tiny amount to do the job, and so when we say this has a very high or low level, it may not mean very much. In terms of which species to work with, it depends a lot on what aspect of the whole domain you are studying. In terms of distribution, the guinea pig happens to be a little closer to humans than the rat or some of the others. But I think there is much more to pain and to pain modulation than that.

Maybe I can add a historical vignette showing that I am a Stone Age pharmacologist. I trained with Dr. John C. Crantz. He maintained 30 years ago that there were differences between dogs and cats in their reactions to morphine: dogs get sedated and sleep, and cats get excited and doped up like horses. And the next step—I can prove this; I have notes—is that there are gender differences in human responses. The human male reacts like a dog whereas the human female reacts like a cat.

SPEAKER FROM THE FLOOR: They have proposed μ_1, μ_2 receptor sites and also different actions in terms of analgesia.

DR. SIMON: I have no trouble with subtypes, and we may very well find a μ_1, μ_2, and maybe μ_3. The μ_1 postulated by Pasternak has the curious characteristic that it's the favorite receptor for all the different ligands, μ, δ, κ, and just heliologically, I have some trouble with that. I think it's still an open question whether that particular μ is real and does what Dr. Pasternak says it does. If it does, it is clearly a very important and exciting story.

DR. STANLEY: Is there any perceived relation between the percent of opioid centers of varying subtypes in given species and the abilities of those species to perceive different types of pain? For example, many wild-life biologists believe that wild animals do not seem to be receptive to normal pain as they would be in a laboratory environment due, perhaps, to the interaction of the α or the synthetic nervous system. Is there any relation between the percent of receptors of one species and that species' ability to perceive a standard stimulus like the tail-flick test?

DR. SIMON: I can't claim any special lab knowledge about different species, but I would add a cautionary note, because in studies of human disorders that appear dependent on receptor abnormalities, a whole host of abnormalities have been identified (for example, in insulin resistance) that do not depend upon an abnormality of the binding site but instead on some abnormal post-binding-site affector mechanism. So, considering all the different post-binding-site affector mechanisms involved—coupling to other proteins, and so on—and considering that such abnormalities have been identified in human disorders like diabetes, there may be much more to it than just a percentage distribution of receptors that methodologically are actually just binding sites.

SPEAKER: Just another cautionary note. Binding does not necessarily imply function, so if you just look at the amount of binding in trying to infer back to function, it doesn't always work. It would be very hard to make that kind of speculation.

DR. SIMON: There is some evidence perhaps in terms of sensitivity to opioids and opioid receptor levels. But in terms of pain and pain perception, there is no evidence I know about. My own opinion is that in some of the things mentioned with regard to wild animals, the set under which pain occurs is far more important than any distribution of receptors.

DR. EZZAT AMIN: Dr. Simon presented evidence that the three types or subtypes of pure receptor are distinct in each species. Are they coded by separate genes or some modification?

DR. SIMON: We don't know. I would say they might very well be coded by separate genes. The reason I say that is simply in analogy to the neuroadrenergic field, where there have been about five or six different subtypes, α_1, α_2, α_3, and so on.

DR. AMIN: Is the amino acid sequence of these receptor genes well established?

DR. STANLEY: We do not have amino acid sequences for any of them.

DR. HORACE LOH: I want to comment on a few points. First, on opioid binding and pain relief, an additional point should be made regarding spare receptors. Certain systems, such as the neuroblastoma cell, have only δ receptors. The function of this receptor is measured by measuring its adenylcyclase activity. Scientists have shown that the adenylcyclase activity can still be calculated after 90% of the receptors have been destroyed. If there is no adenylcyclase activity to measure, there is no way to correlate opioid binding to the receptor activity. In a complicated system like the brain or any analgesic system or the nervous system, there are many levels of control in addition to the binding sites; therefore, it is hard to correlate binding to its effect.

Another comment I would like to make concerns ε receptors. To the best of my recollection, Professor Albert Herz of Germany originally proposed their existence to show that endorphin has its own opioid receptor. Thus, more than 10 years ago his research showed that binding sites correlate with the characteristics of opioids, just as receptors do. There is also evidence in the literature showing that ε receptors, which specifically bind to β-endorphin, can be displaced by μ or δ receptors, together or separately.

Many analogues of β-endorphin have been made simply by deleting one, two, or three amino acids in various places. Thus, researchers were able to identify that the β-endorphin receptor may be called an ε receptor, since the C terminal (the N terminal which is enkephalin) naturally binds the μ receptor. That is the site where morphine binds. Based on this data, I believe ε β-endorphin receptors probably consist of 2 sites, the so-called classical μ and δ site.

DR. FAWZY G. ESTAFANOUS: I have two questions for Dr. Carr. Exogenous opioids are addictive, while endogenous opioids are not. First, why? And second, can we prepare analogues of the endogenous opioids and use them as nonaddictive opioids?

DR. CARR: The question is predicated on the hypothesis that exogenous opioids are addictive and endogenous opioids are not. But it is not clear that exogenous opioids are more addictive than endogenous opioids. Exogenous opioid alkaloids are simply more stable, hence less easily degraded, and hence more popularly used as a means of addiction. But at the receptor level it is not clear that one couldn't become addicted to anything that occupied one or another opioid receptor. This issue of being able to understand and treat addiction to opioids, which is a major societal problem, by generating more sophisticated molecules is still elusive. People claim that they are addicted to their own endorphins released in exercise. It is a very elusive issue, and whether we can make nonaddictive opioid analogues is unknown.

DR. HUG: When I went through pharmacology, we had to learn a long list of compounds and their effects. That has all shifted. Now we have to learn a long list of opioid receptors.

It might be interesting to reflect on where we have come to over the last 50 or 60 years. Lyndon Small, of the University of Virginia, was an organic chemist. Himmelsbach was at the addiction research center in Lexington. And Nathan Eddy was at the University of Michigan. They started in the 1930s to synthesize a whole series of compounds and test them for ability to produce analgesia without respiratory depression or physical dependence. And here we are 50 years later, still without a compound that produces potent analgesia without respiratory depression and physical dependence. But we keep working at it.

7 CLINICAL PERSPECTIVES ON OPIOID ANESTHESIA

Edward Lowenstein

Although I first published a perspective on morphine "anesthesia" in an editorial almost two decades ago,[1] I believe it is useful to take stock periodically. Perhaps the most impressive evidence of the magnitude of the current role of narcotics in the practice of anesthesia is the existence of this volume, and the broad base of clinical anesthesia specialties represented in it. In this chapter, I first discuss several specific issues from my earlier experience that remain topical; next I take note of issues that have faded or been resolved; and then I paint a few broad brush strokes about the future.

ISSUES OF THE PAST

Morphine anesthesia was born of the need to anesthetize safely for cardiac surgery, patients with the combination of severely impaired heart muscle and a requirement for supernormal cardiac performance due to abnormalities of the heart valves. Besides the empirical observation that morphine was not only well tolerated but also beneficial for patients with acute myocardial infarction or pulmonary edema, a convincing body of experimental work suggested that morphine caused little or no myocardial depression in molar concentrations that ex-

ceeded any likely to be achieved clinically.[2] In fact, enhanced myocardial contractility was demonstrated in neurally intact animals, and this was shown to depend upon an intact autonomic nervous system.[3] A similar lack of myocardial depression has been demonstrated for most of the currently available synthetic narcotics.

From the early days of narcotic anesthesia, we recognized that the properties of narcotics that represented their greatest advantages under some circumstances could also, under other circumstances, be so detrimental as to contraindicate their use. Neutrality of narcotic effect upon myocardial contractility is one example of this. Provision of profound analgesia, circulatory stability, and conditions suitable for operation were achieved by morphine and oxygen with some reliability in patients with cardiac cachexia associated with valvular heart disease, probably because of lack of myocardial depression.[4] These patients often required little or no supplementation with an inhalation anesthetic to avoid apparent circulatory responses to surgical stimulation. However, this lack of circulatory depression turned out to be a major and limiting disadvantage in robust patients. This became quickly evident soon after coronary artery surgery was initiated.[5]

Whether a narcotic by itself can provide protection from the circulatory responses associated with anesthetic and surgical stimulation as typified by hypertension and tachycardia is, remarkably, still a subject of investigation and controversy. For instance, Stanley and de Lange[6] recently published an unblinded though randomized study in which one-third of patients undergoing myocardial revascularization under fentanyl (113 μg/kg) oxygen anesthesia required treatment for hypertension prior to cardiopulmonary bypass, compared to none receiving a sufentanil (9 μg/kg) anesthetic. In contrast, Philbin (personal communication) has been unable in a double-blind study to differentiate fentanyl (100 μg/kg) from sufentanil (up to 40 μg/kg). The incidence of requirement for treatment of hypertension (> 115% of control) was high in this study (about 80% of patients) and not different between the opioids or among the doses studied. He confirmed for sufentanil the observations of Wynands et al.[7] in patients anesthetized with fentanyl, that no blood level achieved invariably prevented circulatory responses to stimulation. We are left with a hypothesis that I believe is proved, that profound narcotic-associated analgesia does not prevent "breakthrough" and that simply giving more is not the answer. Whether it is preferable to prevent end organ reactivity directly (vasodilators, β-adrenergic blockers) or to administer a volatile anesthetic to achieve the same endpoint is not known. Both appear to be effective. However, it is unlikely that a so-called "better" narcotic will prevent this problem.

A second advantage of narcotics as anesthetics, which is often perceived as a disadvantage, is respiratory depression. Morphine anesthesia was developed directly from the observation that high doses of morphine administered following anesthesia and operation would permit retention of an oral or nasal endotracheal tube and elective, prophylactic mechanical ventilation. The alternatives were often acute respiratory failure and secondary circulatory decompensation, or prophylactic tracheostomy. In 1966, 30% of the cardiac surgical patients at the Massachusetts General Hospital underwent tracheostomy.[8] At present many groups would like to achieve early extubation safely, as they now consider routine prolonged postoperative endotracheal intubation and mechanical ventilation costly and hazardous.[9] In fact, halving the time until the patient met criteria for extubation was considered an advantage of sufentanil relative to fentanyl by Stanley and de Lange.[6] Flacke and associates[10] also observed a shorter duration of respiratory depression in patients receiving small doses of sufentanil compared with similar doses of fentanyl.

In our postoperative cardiac surgical unit, several factors cause us to consider more rapid awakening and extubation undesirable in many cardiac surgical patients. These include hypothermia, excessive chest tube drainage, residual neuromuscular blockade, and circulatory instability. Particularly vexing is the phenomenon of sudden, abrupt arousal from a completely anesthetized state. Often supplementary narcotics, benzodiazepines, and muscle relaxants are administered in order to continue the period of assured ventilation while these various issues are resolved. If early extubation is a priority, should we be using an ultrashort-acting narcotic like alfentanil, or should we revert and advocate primarily inhalation techniques, using intravenous drugs as supplements rather than primary drugs?

This brings us to the third topic, that of postoperative hypertension. Clearly, the incidence in many units remains high. Is the incidence obligatorily higher with shorter-acting than with longer-acting narcotics (e.g., fentanyl, sufentanil versus morphine, methadone)? Is it primarily a response to endotracheal intubation in a poorly sedated, painful patient? Is it a manifestation of acute narcotic withdrawal? Is it due to recurrence of rigidity, as recently suggested?

Two of the most difficult periods in narcotic anesthesia may be during slow induction, when narcosis and neuromuscular blockade are both incomplete, and during recovery, when the criteria for respiratory competence have not been achieved but the patient is uncomfortable with the endotracheal tube. Both produce their anxious moments for patient and anesthetist alike.

While these are seemingly mundane questions, they remain important, and cry out for definitive answers. Other topics raised in previous perspectives include permanent neurological damage, excessively increased requirement for blood volume replacement, effects on renal blood flow and liberation of antidiuretic hormone, histamine release, change in the quality of the circulatory response by anesthetic adjuvants, and recall.[1] The first three have proved not to be real problems. The last three are now widely recognized, and are dealt with effectively. These have been resolved and are no longer issues of concern.

ISSUES OF THE PRESENT AND FUTURE

Since the initial development of narcotic anesthesia, the understanding of how narcotics work has exploded. The demonstration of narcotic receptors has represented perhaps the most important discovery.[11] The definition of different kinds of narcotic receptors, each having a different spectrum of properties, even holds the eventual promise of narcosis without respiratory depression.

The ceiling effect of systemically administered opioids has led to a search for more effective methods of delivery. The knowledge of the presence of narcotic receptors in the spinal cord has led to local deposition of narcotics, producing more profound blockade of nociceptive information.[12] This has raised the possibility of dramatically altering the postoperative course of patients undergoing major surgery and perhaps improving outcome. Surely all anesthesiologists are now aware of the study of Yaeger et al.[13] demonstrating lower morbidity with postoperative epidural narcosis than with parenteral analgesics. Yet Anand and Hickey's data (personal communication), revealing a superior outcome with extremely high doses of parenteral sufentanil in infants undergoing surgery for complex congenital heart dis-

ease, suggest that narcotics may produce their beneficial effects in more than one way.

The consequences of avoiding pain after surgery have only begun to be defined and present one of the most important and exciting avenues for clinical research potentially leading to major changes in practice. Local (spinal and intracerebral) deposition of narcotics for cancer pain is another example of the application of the discovery of narcotic receptors, and one in which anesthesiologists are increasingly more involved.[14]

Opioids have emerged (or re-emerged) as integral to the clinical practice of anesthesia. This volume bears evidence that all the fields within anesthesiology use opioids as an important part of their practice. This is not what anyone would have predicted a generation ago, when the documented circulatory and respiratory depression made elimination of narcotics one of the goals of then-current anesthetic thought.

We now have drugs that act at different narcotic receptors and that have dramatically different durations of action. The role of the α_2 component of the autonomic nervous system in anesthetic practice is just beginning to be defined. We know narcotic agonists are potentiated by α_2-adrenergic agonists.[15] Active, central α_2 adrenergically mediated vasodilation by sufentanil has been demonstrated in the innervated vascularly isolated, separately perfused canine gracilis muscle, reinforcing the possibility that opioids and α_2 agonists bind to the same or similar receptors.[16] I believe we are practicing during an era when our use of opioids will continue to expand, based upon the rational application of basic scientific research. It promises to be a stimulating and rewarding period.

REFERENCES

1. Lowenstein E. Morphine "anesthesia"—a perspective. Anesthesiology 1971;35:563–565.
2. Goldberg AH, Padget CH. Comparative effects of morphine and fentanyl on isolated

heart muscle. Anesth Analg (Cleve) 1969;48: 978–982.

3. Vasko JS, Henney RP, Brawley RK, et al. Effects of morphine on ventricular function and myocardial contractile force. Am J Physiol 1966;210:329–334.

4. Lowenstein E, Hallowell P, Levine FH, et al. Cardiovascular response to large doses of intravenous morphine in man. N Engl J Med 1969;281:1389–1393.

5. Lowenstein E, Philbin DM. Narcotic "anesthesia" in the eighties. Anesthesiology 1981; 55:195–197.

6. Stanley TH, de Lange S. Comparison of sufentanil-oxygen and fentanyl-oxygen anesthesia for mitral and aortic valvular surgery. J Cardiothorac Anesth 1988;2:6–11.

7. Wynands JE, Townsend GE, Wong P, et al. Blood pressure response and plasma fentanyl concentrations during high- and very high-dose fentanyl anesthesia for coronary artery surgery. Anesth Analg 1983;62:661–665.

8. Lowenstein E. Pulmonary consequences of cardiopulmonary bypass. In: Thirty years of extracorporeal circulation: proceedings of the symposium, Munich: Deutsches Herzzentrum, 1984.

9. Lichtenthal PR, Wade LD, Niemyski PR, et al. Respiratory management after cardiac surgery with inhalation anesthesia. Crit Care Med 1983;11:603–605.

10. Flacke JW, Bloor BC, Kripke BK, et al. Comparison of morphine, meperidine, fentanyl, and sufentanil in anesthesia: a double-blind study. Anesth Analg 1985;64:897–910.

11. Lord JAH, Waterfield AA, Hughes J, et al. Endogenous opioid peptides: multiple agonists and receptors. Nature 1977;267:495–499.

12. Yaksh TL, Noueihed R. The physiology and pharmacology of spinal opiates. Annu Rev Pharmacol Toxicol 1985;25:433–462.

13. Yeager MP, Glass DD, Neff RK, et al. Epidural anesthesia and analgesia in high-risk surgical patients. Anesthesiology 1987;66:729–736.

14. Combs DW. Management of chronic pain by epidural and intrathecal opioids: newer drugs and delivery systems. Int Anesthesiol Clin 1986;24:59–74.

15. Flacke JW, Bloor BC, Flacke WE, et al. Reduced narcotic requirement by clonidine with improved hemodynamic and adrenergic stability in patients undergoing coronary bypass surgery. Anesthesiology 1987;67:11–19.

16. O'Keefe RJ, Domalik-Wawrzynski L, Guerrero JL, et al. Local and neurally mediated effects of sufentanil on canine skeletal muscle vascular resistance. Pharmacol Exp Ther 1987; 242:699–706.

8 OPIOIDS AND THE CARDIAC PATIENT

Fawzy G. Estafanous and Thomas Higgins

In the last two decades, the use of opioid anesthetics for patients with cardiac disease has become well established and has far exceeded the use of any other anesthetic regimen. All agree that anesthesia management for patients with heart disease should ensure continuous myocardial protection by maintaining a positive balance between myocardial oxygen supply and demand, and by minimizing myocardial depression to maintain adequate cardiac output for vital tissue perfusion. Advantages of opioid anesthetics for patients with heart disease include decreased heart rate, lack of myocardial depressant effects, maintained perfusion pressure, attenuated responses to sympathetic stimulation, and minimum changes in heart rate (HR) and blood pressure (BP). Opioid use was most promoted by the development of the new synthetic opioids, which are much more potent than morphine and have better hemodynamic characteristics, minimal side effects, and variable durations of action.

Fentanyl anesthesia has almost replaced morphine anesthesia for open-heart surgery. Its advantages over morphine anesthesia are very clear. Sufentanil, a newer opioid, is shown to have several advantages over fentanyl, including faster induction and recovery and absence of the ceiling effect. However, early clinical experiences with the use of sufentanil were complicated by rare and unexpected events, including hypotension, bradycardia, or both. The reasons for such unexpected events were probably epidemiological rather than pharmacodynamic. Between the time sufentanil went through the initial studies for Food and Drug Administration approval and the time it was released for clinical use, multiple changes did occur in the epidemiology of patients with coronary artery disease and their preoperative medical treatment. Currently, the population undergoing coronary artery surgery is older, hypertension is better controlled, and angina is well treated. β-sympathetic blockers and calcium channel blockers have achieved widespread use, and new muscle relaxants have been developed. These developments have had a significant effect on the hemodynamic responses to sufentanil anesthesia as well as to every other anesthetic agent. All these factors must be taken into consideration when selecting the appropriate inducing agents and muscle relaxants and the adjuvant agents to accompany fentanyl and sufentanil anesthesia.

CHARACTERISTICS OF OPIOID ANESTHETICS

Morphine

Morphine is the prototype of opioid anesthetics. It was used briefly in the late nine-

93

or calcium channel blockers alone or combined were used for treatment of a large number of patients with coronary artery disease or hypertension. In our very early clinical experience with sufentanil/vecuronium, we reported three cases of severe bradycardia, even sinus arrest, complicating the induction of anesthesia (Figure 8.2).[34] Analysis of the sequence of events and the doses used showed that these three cases occurred in patients receiving both calcium channel blockers and β blockers, and that initial HR was already slow. Both sufentanil and muscle relaxant were administered over a short period of time. These incidents emphasized that preoperative drug therapy, the muscle relaxant used and its dose, and the rate of administration determine the hemodynamic changes observed during sufentanil induction. Preoperative β and calcium channel blocker therapy reduces not only the HR but also the sympathetic responses to stimulation. However, when using a muscle relaxant like vecuronium, which is free of cardiovascular effects, the negative chronotropic effects of opioids are unopposed and severe bradycardia may result.

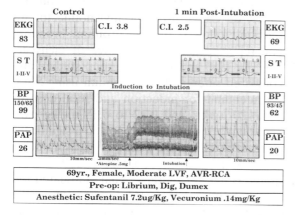

69yr., Female, Moderate LVF, AVR-RCA

Pre-op: Librium, Dig, Dumex

Anesthetic: Sufentanil 7.2ug/Kg, Vecuronium .14mg/Kg

FIGURE 8.2 Sufentanil/vecuronium induction. A drop in the HR and BP was noticed and immediately corrected by atropine administration. Notice lack of signs of ischemia as indicated by absence of change in ST segment levels. (Information gathered at the Cleveland Clinic Foundation.)

All opioid anesthetics except meperidine have negative chronotropic effects and can cause bradycardia. The exact mechanism of bradycardia is not fully known but is probably due to central vagal stimulation of the vagal nucleus in the medulla,[35] as it can be totally blocked by bilateral vagotomy.[36] Other proposed mechanisms include direct effect on the sinoatrial node[37] or depression of ventricular function.[38] Repeated doses of fentanyl produce less bradycardia than the initial dose.[39] The negative chronotropic opioids are supposed to have a protective effect on the myocardium during periods of ischemia.[40] Slowing of the HR reduces myocardial oxygen consumption unless extreme bradycardia decreases the cardiac output and perfusion pressure. Bradycardia is usually minimized by prior administration of atropine[41] or pancuronium bromide[42] and is dose-related.[5] Also, the use of nitrous oxide is known to minimize the incidence of bradycardia.

Sufentanil anesthesia in the early 1980s was reported to be complicated by hypertension.[43] However, it became evident that this hypertension was related to the use of pancuronium bromide as the muscle relaxant and occurred mainly in patients with good ventricular function who had not been treated by either β or calcium channel blockers. Unlike that linked with fentanyl, hypertension related to sufentanil anesthesia can be minimized or treated by increasing the sufentanil doses and by further supplements of sufentanil, since there is no ceiling effect.

Patients receiving small doses of sufentanil may have a higher incidence of postoperative hypertension due to early emergence from anesthesia and may require BP control by peripheral vasodilators such as sodium nitroprusside. The rise in BP is probably due to the short duration of action of sufentanil. Using large doses of sufentanil or using another opioid such as morphine sulphate at the end of the procedure minimizes this postoperative rise in BP.

Hypotension during sufentanil induction is mainly related to bradycardia, as discussed earlier. Later studies by our group, confirmed by our clinical experience, demonstrated that slow administration of sufentanil for induction, over 2 to 3 minutes, and the appropriate choice of muscle relaxant produce hemodynamic stability with sufentanil anesthesia (Figures 8.3 and 8.4). The muscle relaxant is usually chosen according to the preinduction HR as discussed earlier.

A multicenter Canadian clinical trial involving 616 patients undergoing elective, major, noncardiac surgical procedures reported an incidence of hypotension in 37 patients, but the hypotension was easily managed without adverse effects.[44] Comparison of sufentanil with inhaled agents in coronary artery bypass patients demonstrated far less hypotension with sufentanil than with any volatile anesthetic.[45] In patients anesthetized with sufentanil, nitrous oxide, and midazolam for open-heart surgery, hypotension was noted in some patients during unstimulated periods, and these episodes were associated with decreases in systemic vascular resistance.[46] These studies suggest that while use of sufentanil alone is associated with hemodynamic stability, using additional vasodilating agents makes BP support reliant on the degree of sympathetic stimulation that remains.

EPIDEMIOLOGICAL CHANGES AND THEIR INFLUENCE ON THE HEMODYNAMIC CHANGES RELATED TO OPIOID ANESTHESIA

The evaluation of opioid anesthetics and their hemodynamic effects in patients with heart disease cannot be complete without discussing the epidemiological and therapeutic changes in the last decade, particularly those related to the use of preoperative therapy and to the adjuvants of opioid anesthesia.

Muscle Relaxants and Heart Rate

The development of pancuronium bromide presented a new era in the use of muscle relaxants. Since pancuronium did not cause histamine release or hypotension, it replaced d-tubocurarine as the preferred muscle relaxant. For over a decade pancuronium bromide was the most commonly used relaxant for cardiac patients and often the sole relaxant for intu-

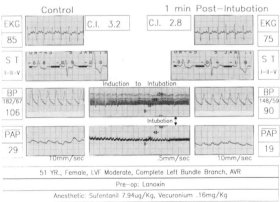

FIGURE 8.4 Sufentanil/vecuronium anesthesia for mitral valve replacement. Notice hemodynamic stability (mild decrease in HR and BP and significant decrease in PAP). Note lack of signs of ischemia as indicated by absence of change in ST segment levels. (Information gathered at the Cleveland Clinic Foundation.)

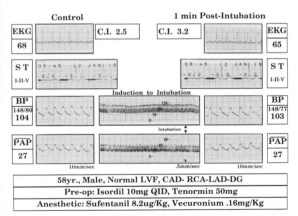

FIGURE 8.3 Sufentanil/vecuronium induction. Notice the extreme hemodynamic stability. Note lack of signs of ischemia as indicated by absence of change in ST segment levels. (Information gathered at the Cleveland Clinic Foundation.)

bation and perioperative management. Pancuronium has strong vagolytic chronotropic effects because it tends to increase the HR, cardiac output, and BP.[47-49] However, reports vary about the magnitude of tachycardia caused by pancuronium bromide. Tachycardia was less significant when succinylcholine was used to facilitate intubation and only small doses of pancuronium were used to maintain muscle relaxation.[13,50] Tachycardia was frequently reported with fentanyl/pancuronium anesthesia.[23,24] A high incidence of tachycardia was reported with the early use of sufentanil/pancuronium anesthesia.[32,33,47,51] Later it became clear that tachycardia caused by the use of pancuronium bromide with opioid anesthesia can be accompanied by ST segment changes and may well be the cause of myocardial ischemia in patients with coronary artery disease.[52] However, prevention or treatment of tachycardia can minimize the incidence of ischemia.[53]

Vecuronium, Atracurium, and Pipecuronium

Studies by our group and others using different muscle relaxants (vecuronium, atracurium, and pipecuronium) reaffirmed that they did not cause tachycardia as observed with pancuronium. Indeed, the appropriate choice of muscle relaxant, based upon the initial HR, will help in maintaining stable hemodynamics during sufentanil induction. To facilitate intubation we do not use pancuronium bromide except in patients with initial HR < 60 beats per minute. For patients with HR > 60 beats per minute, vecuronium is the preferred muscle relaxant. Initial studies have demonstrated that sufentanil/pipecuronium has the same hemodynamic effects as sufentanil/vecuronium. Changes in HR are best minimized by administering an initial dose of the muscle relaxant (25 to 50%) and monitoring the HR response. The remainder of the paralyzing dose can be the same relaxant or changed to another relaxant according to the chronotropic effect and the hemodynamic response.

β-Adrenergic Blocking Drugs

β-adrenergic blocking drugs are widely used for symptomatic treatment of angina pectoris, reduction of resting HR, and control of supraventricular arrhythmia (Table 8.1). Large-dose opiates minimize responses to stress and also impair the ability of the sympathetic nervous system to support cardiovascular homeostasis, thus enhancing the susceptibility of the cardiovascular system to depression by β-adrenergic blockade. While preoperative β-adrenergic blockade was once thought to contribute to morbidity,[54] subsequent experience with the effects of withdrawal of β blockage have resulted in the conclusion that it is advisable to continue β blockers until the morning of surgery.

Hyperdynamic responses to anesthetic induction with high-dose narcotics have been reported even in patients receiving preoperative β blockade.[55] Since potent opioids alone are insufficient to protect the myocardium adequately from autonomic sympathetic responses,[56] many anesthesiologists use β-blocking drugs during primary opioid anesthesia. Propranolol,[57] labetalol[58,59] and esmolol[60,61] have been shown effective in preventing HR increases during induction and surgical stimulation.

Differences within the β blocker family also modify opioid-adrenergic interactions. β-blocking agents can be distinguished by their degree of cardioselectivity, the presence or

TABLE 8.1 Frequency of β and calcium blocker therapy in patients undergoing coronary artery surgery

	Number of Patients	Percent
None	944	31.8
β	302	10.2
CaCh	1,191	40.1
Both	531	17.9
Total	2,968	100.0

Source: Cleveland Clinic Foundation.

absence of intrinsic sympathomimetic activity, and duration of action. In awake patients with angiographically documented coronary artery disease, left ventricular function was better maintained after intravenous β blockade with agents that had intrinsic sympathomimetic activity (such as oxprenolol) than after treatment with metoprolol or propranolol.[62] Cardioselectivity, however, offers no significant hemodynamic advantage either at rest[62] or in patients undergoing elective coronary artery bypass surgery exposed to isoproterenol challenge (i.e., sympathetic stimulation).[63] Drug interactions can contribute to observed differences in opioid response in β-blocked patients. First-pass uptake of fentanyl is decreased in those receiving propranolol, with the possibility that as much as four times the injected dose of fentanyl may enter the systemic circulation of patients on chronic propranolol therapy.[64] Higher plasma levels of propranolol not only inhibit stress-induced changes in HR but may also cause a decline in cardiac index and increased systemic vascular resistance.[65] Anesthesia with either fentanyl–nitrous oxide–oxygen or isoflurane has been shown to affect the disposition of propranolol, partly because of decreased clearance.[66]

Calcium Channel Blockers

Calcium channel blockers play an important role in muscle excitations and contraction coupling of all muscles. (During excitation, calcium moves through the slow channels, which are very selective to calcium, while sodium and potassium move through the fast channels.)[67] Calcium channel blockers inhibit the normal calcium influx into cells.[68] Cardiac muscles and vascular smooth muscles contain a relatively small amount of endoplasmin calcium. Therefore, these muscles are more dependent on calcium flux than are skeletal muscles.[69] Thus, calcium channel blockers can be potent myocardial depressants as well as peripheral vasodilators, mainly arteriolodilators, and have little effect on skeletal muscles.

Calcium channel blockers decrease SVR, MAP, and myocardial contractility. However, different calcium channel blockers affect these parameters and HR to variable degrees.

Verapamil, which is a potent local anesthetic, blocks both the fast and the slow channels, and is a potent myocardial depressant. Verapamil can cause a variable degree of AV block. Diltiazem has negative chronotropic effects and can reduce HR by up to 10%. Both verapamil and diltiazem can decrease the HR and even cause sinus arrest in patients with SA node disease. Nifedipine and, to a lesser degree, verapamil can cause reflex increase in the HR,[70] particularly with acute administration. Verapamil and diltiazem have more negative inotropic effects than nifedipine,[71] which is a potent peripheral vasodilator.[72]

These hemodynamic effects of calcium channel blockers help to explain the possible interactions between these agents and various anesthetics. The administration of verapamil to patients or animals anesthetized with halothane results in significant decreases in arterial BP, SVR, increased LVEDP, PR interval, and cardiac output,[73,74] The administration of verapamil during enflurane or isoflurane anesthesia produces the same hemodynamic changes but to a lesser extent than with halothane anesthesia.[75] Nifedipine also interacts with halothane anesthesia and causes a transient (up to 30 minutes) decrease in BP, SVR, cardiac output, and ventricular dP/dt.

We can postulate about the possible interactions between different calcium channel blockers and opioid anesthetics. Unlike inhalation agents, opioids have no direct myocardial depressant effect, and they do not directly affect cardiac conduction. However, they have definite chronotropic effects and cause bradycardia by several mechanisms. The vagotonic effect of fentanyl and, to a lesser degree, sufentanil can block or decrease the reflex tachycardia caused by nifedipine or verapamil.[76] Administration of pancuronium with fentanyl and verapamil administration did not change the HR. PR interval still increased and MAP decreased.[76]

In spite of these hemodynamic effects, our clinical experience and that of others[77] is that chronic administration of calcium channel blockers is safe in patients receiving anesthesia for open-heart surgery. Therefore, our group and others recommend the continuation of calcium channel blocker therapy until the day of surgery. However, we exercise extreme caution when using calcium channel blockers intraoperatively.

Combined β-Adrenergic and Calcium Entry Blockade Therapy

This combination has gained favor in the therapy of angina pectoris in patients who are unresponsive to a single agent alone.[78] The interaction between opioids, adrenergic receptor blockers, and calcium channel antagonists is complex and of importance, since the patient presenting for open-heart surgery is likely to be exposed to all three classes of agents. At the cellular level, enkephalins affect the level of cyclic adenosine monophosphate, calcium uptake, and contractile state.[79] Reduced mechanical activity of the heart has been experimentally demonstrated following morphine or enkephalin peptide administration.[80] Conversely, opioid antagonists have been shown to enhance myocardial response to isoproterenol.[81]

This combination therapy has been associated with severe conduction disorders (bradycardia, asystole) when anesthesia is induced with potent narcotics, both in experimental preparation[82] and in the clinical setting.[34] The reflex increase in HR in response to vasodilation produced by calcium channel blockers can increase CO and may maintain MAP. If β blockers are added, the reflex increase in the HR will be obtunded. Therefore, the β-blocked patient will also be more vulnerable to hypotension. It is expected that opioid anesthetics, when administered to patients receiving both calcium channel and β blockers, will produce slowing of HR and possible reduction of MAP. The magnitude of such changes will be influenced by the muscle relaxant used as discussed earlier.

Effective blockade of either calcium channel or β blockers in cardiac tissue may be tested by determining the degree of suppression of the cardiac rate response to the hand-grip maneuver[83] or by the vasodilation and fall in pressure induced by either isoproterenol or sodium nitroprusside (Table 8.2). In each case, the blockade of the reflex tachycardia induced by either the sympathofacilitory stimulus of isotonic contraction or the fall in BP may be used as an estimate of effective interruption of the calcium channel and β sympathetic blockade.

Clinically, the hand-grip test can be applied to most patients preoperatively and provides a reliable, although rough, guide to the degree of blockade. A modified test is to ask the patient to hold a tight fist, using only the muscles of the forearm, for a period of 1 to 3 minutes and record any changes of HR. Less than a 10% increase in HR indicates a significant degree of blockade.

These tests are not specific, since any drug that interferes with pre- or postsynaptic sympathetic transmission will produce similar effects. Nevertheless, the hand-grip test can be valuable clinically in assessing the degree of blockade prior to induction of anesthesia, thus helping appropriate selection of relaxants and vasoactive drugs.

TABLE 8.2 Tests for degree of β or calcium channel blockade (test degree of suppression of heart rate change in response to challenge)

Test	Response
Exercise (hand grip test)	Direct increase in HR
Isuprel test	Direct increase in HR
Sodium nitroprusside	Reflex increase in HR
Lab tests	Changes in plasma renin activity to above

Clonidine

Clonidine is an antihypertensive agent and a central α_2-adrenergic agonist or antagonist. It modulates efferent sympathetic vasomotor tone but preserves the sympathetic mediated reflex control of BP.[84] These central sympathetic inhibitory effects result in decreased HR, SVR, CO, and BP.[85] The reduction in BP is accompanied by vasodilation; vital organ perfusion is well preserved.[82] Besides its central sympathetic effects, clonidine has been shown in animals to have some analgesic properties[86,87] and to reduce the amount of halothane required for anesthesia.[88] Clonidine interacts centrally with opioid analgesics.[89,90] It minimizes the untoward effects of naloxone[89] and opioid withdrawal.[91] Preoperative treatment with clonidine is effective in blocking the cardiovascular reflexes to intubation, more than the combination of lidocaine and fentanyl.[92] The incidence of postintubation tachycardia in clonidine-treated patients was 15% less than the non-clonidine-treated group, where ischemic changes were additionally noticed in two patients.[92] Preoperative administration of clonidine reduces the amount of fentanyl required for intubation by 45% and the sufentanil requirement by 40%.[90] These results were confirmed by correlating both electroencephalographic (EEG) and hemodynamic changes.

Studies by Flacke et al.[92] demonstrated that clonidine reduced the opioid requirement for anesthesia by 40% and also resulted in significantly lowered HR and BP at different stages of anesthesia and surgery (pre- and postinduction and postincision). Following cardiopulmonary bypass, the rise in SVR that is frequently observed and that leads to post myocardial revascularization hypertension[93] was not observed in the clonidine-treated patients.[92] The same study also reported that the clonidine-treated patients resumed spontaneous ventilation and were extubated earlier than the non-clonidine-treated patients.[92]

Therefore, it seems that preoperative treatment with clonidine may play an important role in minimizing the hemodynamic responses as well as opioid requirements during opioid anesthesia. However, there maybe a higher incidence of bradycardia that will require treatment.[92] Also, clonidine treatment may be a risk to patients with poor ventricular function that is dependent upon a high sympathetic drive.

ADJUVANTS TO OPIOID ANESTHESIA

Nitrous Oxide

The addition of 50% nitrous oxide to the inspired gases in patients receiving fentanyl anesthesia (50 μg/kg) resulted in myocardial depression, a significant drop in Cl, and increase in SVR.[94] These effects are more pronounced in patients with impaired ventricular function[95] and in those with severe coronary artery obstruction. Similar myocardial depression also occurs in patients receiving sufentanil anesthesia.[96]

Benzodiazepines

Benzodiazepines have hypnotic, amnesic, antianxiety, anticonvulsant, and muscle-relaxing effects. Benzodiazepines are frequently used as premedicants in combination with opioids during induction and to prevent awareness during maintenance of opioid anesthesia. Different benzodiazepines have variable hemodynamic effects.

Diazepam alone as an anesthetic agent does not change HR, Cl, and filling pressures.[97–99] It provides hemodynamic stability in patients with coronary artery disease as well as in patients with heart valve disease[100,101] but occasionally can cause a decrease in MAP.

The addition of diazepam to fentanyl anesthesia has additive depressant effects on SVR and MAP as well as cardiac output.[12] This may result from a negative inotropic effect and myocardial depression attributed to reduction in plasma catecholamine levels.[102] Similarly, the combination of diazepam with sufentanil anesthesia produced significant reductions in MAP and SVR.[103] The reasons for these hemodynamic changes caused by opioid/benzodiazepine combinations are not clear. It was demonstrated that large doses of fentanyl or sufentanil can be myocardial depressants; however, these doses were up to 400 times those used in clinical practice.[104] On the contrary, recent experimental studies by our group and others indicate that clinical concentrations of fentanyl may have positive inotropic effects.[105,106] In our experiments, equal concentrations of sufentanil had similar positive inotropic responses. Moreover, propranolol blocked these positive inotropic responses, while naloxone did not.[107] Most probably the drop in BP when using the opioid/diazepam combination is due to peripheral vasodilation and decreased SVR. This may partly explain why the addition of diazepam to morphine anesthesia does not produce further reduction in MAP and Cl.[108]

Midazolam causes a significant decrease in MAP (20%) and SVR (15 to 33%) and increases HR in patients with coronary artery disease.[97,109] The drop in BP produced by midazolam is greater than that caused by diazepam, which suggests that midazolam may have a more negative inotropic effect.[109,110] Midazolam did not cause a significant change in Cl or pulmonary vascular resistance (PVR), suggesting that its main effect is on the capacitance vessels.[111]

Lorazepam when combined with fentanyl anesthesia causes a significant drop in BP but less than that observed with both diazepam and midazolam,[112,113] and this may be a safer combination.

CHARACTERISTICS OF PATIENTS

Age

In the last decade, more older patients have presented for coronary artery bypass graft surgery (Figure 8.5). The percentage of patients over the age of 70 has increased from 0.2% in

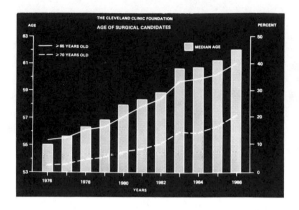

FIGURE 8.5   Increased age of patients undergoing coronary artery surgery. Cleveland Clinic—1976–1986. (Information gathered at the Cleveland Clinic Foundation.)

the early 1970s to about 10% in the early 1980s and appears to be headed to 30% or more in the 1990s.

As age increases, hepatic blood flow decreases.[114] Hepatic clearance of opioids is flow-dependent, and clearance of fentanyl approximates hepatic blood flow.[115] In the elderly, microsomal enzyme activity is also decreased.[116] Studies by Bentley et al.[117] demonstrated that following standard administration of fentanyl in two age groups (< 50 and > 60 years) higher serum fentanyl concentrations were found in the older group.

The effects of age on recovery from sufentanil anesthesia can be expected to be similar to those of fentanyl anesthesia. Plasma clearance and terminal elimination half-life of sufentanil are 935 ml/min and 164 minutes, respectively, in comparison with 956 ml/min and terminal elimination half-life of 219 minutes[118] for fentanyl. We have observed longer time to extubation in octogenarians after either fentanyl or sufentanil anesthesia. Increased age attenuates elasticity of blood vessels and baroreceptor reflex. The characteristics of the endothelial linings of the blood vessels and the vasoactive substance they secrete are changed. Therefore, it is also expected that the hemodynamics may be less stable during induction of anesthesia, as there are more BP fluctuations and a possibility of hypotension. The pharmacokinetics of sufentanil, which allow faster induction and earlier recovery, may significantly change with age. With increased age, lower doses of opioids are required to achieve similar levels of anesthesia when compared with younger age groups. The duration of recovery and return to spontaneous respiration can be prolonged.

Reoperations

The percentage of reoperations recently exceeded 20% of all coronary and heart valve surgeries at our institution and similar referral centers. These patients usually have a higher incidence of preoperative ischemia and impaired ventricular function, and are of relatively older age groups (Tables 8.3 and 8.4). The magnitude and duration of surgery is higher than first-time surgery. Such higher-risk patients with limited reserves mandate ultimate hemodynamic stability to prevent ischemia. These patients can benefit from well-planned opioid anesthesia using sufentanil or fentanyl as the main inducing agent with a properly selected muscle relaxant.

ANESTHESIA MANAGEMENT

Our anesthesia management for patients with heart disease can be summarized as follows.

All patients presenting to surgery are advised to maintain β and calcium channel blocker therapy and other antihypertensive treatment up to the day of surgery. Patients are advised on the day of surgery to have their morning dose of β blocker therapy. Preoperative medication consists of a strong analgesic, such as morphine sulphate, and an amnesic, such as scopolamine, in doses adjusted according to the age and clinical condition. Benzodiazepines are recommended by some of our staff as a substitute for scopolamine. Routinely all coronary artery patients receive transdermal nitroglycerin patches, which have effect for 12 to 24 hours. Continuation of these preoperative medications has almost eliminated preinduction anginal pain. Induction of anesthesia is usually smooth, with minimal hemodynamic changes and minimal incidence of ischemia, as detected by continuous electrocardiogram (EKG) monitoring with ST measurements.

All patients have comprehensive hemodynamic monitoring, which is initiated prior to induction of anesthesia. This includes arterial BP and all parameters that can be obtained from pulmonary artery catheters such as central venous pressure (CVP), pulmonary capillary wedge pressure, CO, SVR, and other calculated indices. Pulse oximetry and temperature changes are also continuously monitored. We continuously display two EKG leads, one of them a chest lead, preferably V5, although practically the leads may be at either V6 or V7. New EKG monitors allow measurements of ST segment changes and have the ability to store and display this information. Transesophageal echo can add some advan-

TABLE 8.3 Severity of disease in patients undergoing coronary artery surgery reoperations

	Primary (%)	Reoperations (%)
Number of patients	3,529	844
Severe LMT	8.4	15.5
Prior myocardial infarction	41	50

Source: Cleveland Clinic Foundation.

TABLE 8.4 Left ventricular asynergy for the first 1,000 cohort series

Year	LV Asynergy (%)
1967–70	41
1973	41
1976	45
1979	54
1982	55
1985	56
1987	56
1988	57

Source: Cleveland Clinic Cardiovascular Registry.

tages in early detection of ischemia, particularly in reoperations that require more dissection and manipulation of the heart.

In the last few years coronary artery patients are coming to the operating room with slow heart rates compared to a decade ago. This is because of the frequent β blocker and calcium channel blocker treatments, particularly when long-acting β blockers are used. The degree of such blockade can be relatively assessed by the hand-grip test, as described earlier. This, together with the evaluation of the ventricular function, helps to anticipate the possible hemodynamic responses to inducing agents and to design the anesthesia management accordingly. Our goal is to maintain the slowest HR that does not significantly lower CO and that will maintain BP adequate for coronary perfusion.

As a guideline to facilitate endotracheal intubation, we use vecuronium bromide, a muscle relaxant free of cardiovascular effects, for patients with HR > 60 beats per minute. For patients who are blocked and present with slow HR, < 60 beats per minute, we use pancuronium bromide. Its anticholinergic effects will balance the bradycardic effects of opioids. However, the response to the muscle relaxant can be further assessed after the administration of about a half-dose, with the option to change the relaxant according to the response. For induction of anesthesia we use 6 to 10 μg/kg sufentanil or up to 50 to 70 μg/kg fentanyl. We prefer sufentanil in hyperdynamic patients with high BP or HR (Figure 8.6). However, because of the extreme variability in ventricular function, blood volume and baroreceptor function, and the effect of β and calcium channel blockade, BP and HR fluctuations during induction and anesthesia are not uncommon. Therefore, vasoactive drugs such as vasopressors, vasodilators, and β blockers should be available for immediate use during induction and thereafter to adjust instantly any undesirable hemodynamic changes and to prevent any episodes of ischemia.

Anesthesia is supplemented by 1 to 2 μg/kg sufentanil every 30 to 45 minutes or by 5 to 10 μg/kg fentanyl every half hour and as

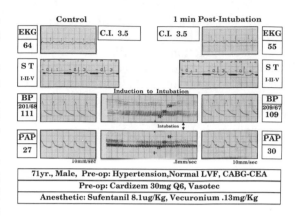

FIGURE 8.6 Sufentanil/vecuronium induction in a preoperatively hypertensive patient. Notice hemodynamic stability. Note lack of signs of ischemia as indicated by absence of change in ST segment levels. (Information gathered at the Cleveland Clinic Foundation.)

needed. Vasodilators are frequently used during surgery to control BP during dissection of the internal mammary arteries to minimize bleeding, to prevent or control the increase in SVR, and to prevent or minimize the incidence of postoperative hypertension. Nitroglycerin is used deliberately in the presence of any signs of ischemia and for control of moderate degrees of hypertension. However, sodium nitroprusside is used more to lower SVR and control hypertension, particularly at the end of surgery.

Neither muscle relaxants nor opioids are reversed at the end of surgery. Their effects are allowed to dissipate while the patient is mechanically ventilated. Over 60 to 70% of patients do not require ventilatory support after the first 12 hours postoperatively and can be extubated when they are hemodynamically stable. A similar percentage of patients are usually discharged from the intensive care unit (ICU) on the first postoperative day. A large number of patients are sufficiently comfortable from residual operating room opioids that they do not request further pain medication during their ICU stay. Occasional patients who awaken suddenly are treated with additional narcotics, if hemodynamic stability or other reasons proscribe early extubation.

Opioid anesthesia has considerably simplified the anesthesiologist's task in the operating room. Outcome after cardiac surgery continues to improve, and while it is impossible to separate out the many factors responsible (cardioplegia, anesthetic and surgical experience, advanced monitoring, better equipment, etc.), we believe opioid anesthesia has contributed to the improvement. The advantages of opioid anesthesia in the heart patient have been recognized and transferred to anesthetic care of all patients. Further work needs to be pursued into the role of continuing opioid anesthesia and analgesia in the early postoperative period to ameliorate the stress response. The future holds exciting possibilities with the advent of short-acting opioids, muscle relaxants, and sedative-hypnotics that can be administered by continuous intravenous infusion, allowing the anesthesiologist to precisely time awakening.

REFERENCES

1. Hasbrouck JD. Morphine anesthesia for open-heart surgery. Ann Thorac Surg 1970;10:364–369.
2. Lowenstein E, Hallowell P, Levine FH, et al. Cardiovascular response to large doses of intravenous morphine in man. N Engl J Med 1969;281:1389–1393.
3. Lowenstein E. Morphine "anesthesia"—a perspective. Anesthesiology 1971;35:563–565.
4. Dalton B. Anaesthesia and coronary heart disease. J Ir Coll Physicians Surgeons 1972; 2:36–40.
5. Benthuysen JL, Smith NT, Sanford TT, et al. Physiology of alfentanil-induced rigidity. Anesthesiology 1986;64:440–446.
6. Conahan TJ III, Ominsky AJ, Wollman H, et al. A prospective random comparison of halothane and morphine for open-heart anesthesia: one year's experience. Anesthesiology 1973;38:528–535.
7. Stanley TH, Gray NG, Stanford W, et al. The effects of high-dose morphine on fluid and blood requirements in open-heart operations. Anesthesiology 1973;38:536.
8. Rosow CE, Moss J, Philbin DM, et al. His-
tamine release during morphine and fentanyl anesthesia. Anesthesiology 1982;56:93–96.
9. Wong KC, Martin WE, Hornbein TF, Freund FG, Everett J. The cardiovascular effects of morphine sulfate with oxygen and with nitrous oxide in man. Anesthesiology 1973; 38:545–549.
10. Stoelting RK, Gibbs PS. Hemodynamic effects of morphine and morphine–nitrous oxide in valvular heart disease and coronary-artery disease. Anesthesiology 1973;38:45–52.
11. Lappas DG, Buckley MJ, Laver MB, et al. Left ventricular performance and pulmonary circulation following addition of nitrous oxide to morphine during coronary-artery surgery. Anesthesiology 1975;43:61–69.
12. Stanley TH, Webster LR. Anesthetic requirements and cardiovascular effects of fentanyl-oxygen and fentanyl-diazepam-oxygen anesthesia in man. Anesth Analg (Cleve) 1978;57:411–416.
13. Stanley TH, Philbin DM, Coggins CH. Fentanyl-oxygen anesthesia for coronary artery surgery: cardiovascular and antidiuretic hormone responses. Can Anaesth Soc J 1979; 26:168–171.
14. Vusse GJ, van der Belle H, van Gerven W, et al. Acute effect of fentanyl on haemodynamics and myocardial carbohydrate utilization and phosphate release during ischaemia. Br J Anaesth 1979;51:927.
15. Hall GM. Analgesia and the metabolic response to surgery. Int Cong Symp Series No 3. London: Royal Society of Medicine, 1978.
16. Barash P, Kopriva C, Giles R, et al. Global ventricular function and intubation: radionuclear profiles. Anesthesiology 1980;53: S109. (Abstr.)
17. Edde RR. Hemodynamic changes prior to and after sternotomy in patients anesthetized with high-dose fentanyl. Anesthesiology 1981;55:444.
18. Kono K, Philbin DM, Coggins CH, et al. Renal function and stress response during halothane or fentanyl anesthesia. Anesth Analg 1981;60:552.
19. Barash PG, Kopriva CJ. Narcotics and the circulation. In: Kitahata LM, Collins JG, eds. Narcotic analgesics in anesthesiology. Baltimore: Williams and Wilkins, 1982;91–132.
20. Quintin L, Whalley DG, Wynands JE, et al. Oxygen–high-dose fentanyl–droperidol anes-

of nifedipine on resistance vessels, arteries, and veins in man. Br J Clin Pharmacol 1980;10:433–438.

73. Kapur PA, Flacke WE. Epinephrine-induced arrhythmias and cardiovascular function after verapamil during halothane anesthesia in the dog. Anesthesiology 1981;55:218–225.

74. Brichard G, Zimmermann PE. Verapamil in cardiac dysrhythmias during anaesthesia. Br J Anaesth 1970;42:1005–1012.

75. Kapur PA, Flacke WE, Olewine SK. Comparison of effects of isoflurane versus enflurane on cardiovascular and catecholamine responses to verapamil in dogs. Anesth Analg 1982;61:193–194.

76. Hill DC, Chelly JE, Dlewati A, et al. Cardiovascular effects of and interaction between calcium blocking drugs and anesthetics in chronically instrumented dogs. VI Verapamil and fentanyl-pancuronium. Anesthesiology 1988;68:874–879.

77. Reves JG, Kissin I, Lell WA, et al. Calcium entry blockers: uses and implications for anesthesiologists. Anesthesiology 1982;57:504–518.

78. Packer M. Combined β-adrenergic and calcium-entry blockade in angina pectoris. N Engl J Med 1989;320:709–718.

79. Laurent S, March JD, Smith TW. Enkephalins increase cyclic adenosine monophosphate content, calcium uptake, and contractile state in cultured chick embryo heart cells. J Clin Invest 1986;77:1436–1440.

80. Clo C, Muscari C, Tantini B, et al. Reduced mechanical activity of perfused rat heart following morphine or enkephalin peptides administration. Life Sci 1985;37:1327–1333.

81. Caffrey JL, Wooldridge CB, Gaugl JF. Naloxone enhances myocardial responses to isoproterenol in dog isolated heart-lung. Am J Physiol 1986;250:H749–H754.

82. Schmeling WT, Kampine JP, Warltier DC. Negative chronotropic actions of sufentanil and vecuronium in chronically instrumented dogs pretreated with propranolol and/or diltiazem. Anesth Analg 1989;69:4–14.

83. Siegel W, Gilbert CA, Nutter DO, et al. Use of isometric handgrip for the indirect assessment of left ventricular function in patients with coronary atherosclerotic heart disease. Am J Cardiol 1972;30:48–54.

84. Kobinger W. Central α-adrenergic systems as targets for hypotensive drugs. Rev Physiol Biochem Pharmacol 1978;81:39–100.

85. Abrams WB. In summary: satellite symposium on central α-adrenergic blood pressure regulating mechanisms. Hypertension 1984;6(suppl 2):1187–1193.

86. Paalzow L. Analgesia produced by clonidine in mice and rats. J Pharm Pharmacol 1974;26:361–363.

87. Spaulding TC, Fielding S, Venafro JJ, et al. Antinociceptive activity of clonidine and its potentiation of morphine analgesia. Eur J Pharmacol 1979;58:19–25.

88. Blood BC, Flacke WE. Reduction in halothane anesthetic requirement by clonidine, an α-adrenergic agonist. Anesth Analg 1982;41:741–745.

89. Flacke JW. Flacke WE, Bloor BC, et al. Effects of fentanyl, naloxone, and clonidine on hemodynamics and plasma catecholamine levels in dogs. Anesth Analg 1983;62:305–313.

90. Ghignone M, Quintin L, Duke PC, et al. Effects of clonidine on narcotic requirements and hemodynamic response during induction of fentanyl anesthesia and endotracheal intubation. Anesthesiology 1986;64:36–42.

91. Gold, MS Redmond DE, Lkeber HD. Clonidine in opiate withdrawal. Lancet 1978:1:929–930.

92. Flacke JW, Bloor BC, Flacke WE, et al. Reduced narcotic requirement by clonidine with improved hemodynamic and adrenergic stability in patients undergoing coronary bypass surgery. Anesthesiology 1987;67:11–19.

93. Estafanous FG, Urzua J, Yared JP, et al. Pattern of hemodynamic alterations during coronary artery operations. J Thor Cardiovasc Surg 1984;87:175–182.

94. Philbin DM. Foex P, Lowenstein E, et al. Nitrous oxide causes myocardial dysfunction. Anesthesiology 1983;59:A80.

95. Meretoja OA, Takkunen O, Heikkila H, et al. Haemodynamic response to nitrous oxide during high-dose fentanyl pancuronium anaesthesia. Acta Anaesthesiol Scand 1985;29:137–141.

96. Philbin DM, Foex P, Drummond G, et al. Regional ventricular function with sufentanil anesthesia: the effect of nitrous oxide. Anesth Analg 1984:63:260.

97. Samuelson PN, Reves JG, Kouchoukos NT, et al. Hemodynamic responses to anesthetic induction with midazolam or diazepam in patients with ischemic heart disease. Anesth Analg 1981:60:802–809.

98. Rao S, Sherbaniuk RW, Prasad K, et al. Cardiopulmonary effects of diazepam. Clin Pharmacol Ther 1973;14:182–189.

99. Samuelson PN, Lell WA, Kouchoukos NT, et al. Hemodynamics during diazepam induction of anesthesia for coronary artery bypass grafting. South Med J 1980;73:332–334.

100. D'Amelio G, Volta SD, Stritoni P, et al. Acute cardiovascular effects of diazepam in patients with mitral valve disease, Eur J Clin Pharmcol 1973;6:61–63.

101. Clarke RSJ, Lyons SM. Diazepam and flunitrazepam as induction agents for cardiac surgical operations. Acta Anaesthesiol Scand 1977;21:282–292.

102. Tomicheck RC, Rosow CE, Philbin DM, et al. Diazepam-fentanyl interaction: hemodynamic and hormaonal effects in coronary artery surgery. Anesth Analg 1983;62:881–884.

103. George J, Samuelson PN, Lell WA, et al. Hemodynamic effects of diazepam-sufentanil compared to diazepam-fentanyl. Proc Annu Meet Soc Cardiovasc Anesthesiol, Montreal, 1986;91. (Abstr.)

104. Reves JG, Kissin I, Fournier SE, et al. Additive negative inotropic effect of a combination of diazepam and fentanyl. Anesth Analg 1984;63:97–100.

105. Hamm D, Freedman B, Pellom G, et al. The maintenance of myocardial contractility by fentanyl during enflurane administration. Anesthesiology 1983;59:186.

106. Rendig SV, Amsterdam EA, Henderson GI, et al. Comparative cardiac contractile actions of six narcotic analgesics; morphine, meperidine, pentazocine, fentanyl, methadone, and L-α-acetylmethadol (LAAM). J Pharmacol Exp Ther 1980;215:259–265.

107. Mekhail NA, Estafanous FG, Khairallah PA, et al. Catecholamine-mediated positive inotropic response of narcotic anesthetics. Anesthesiology 1989;71:A522.

108. Stanley TH, Bennett GM, Loeser EA, et al. Cardiovascular effects of diazepam and droperidol during morphine anesthesia. Anesthesiology 1976;44:255–258.

109. Reves JG, Samuelson PN, Lewis S. Midazolam maleate induction in patients with ischaemic heart disease: haemodynamic observations. Can Anaesth Soc J 1979;26:402–409.

110. Jones DJ, Stehling LC, Zauder HL. Cardiovascular responses to diazepam and midazolam maleate in the dog. Anesthesiology 1979;51:430–434.

111. Samuelson PN, Reves JG, Smith LR, et al. Midazolam versus diazepam: different effects on systemic vascular resistance. Arzneim Forsch 1981;31:2268–2269.

112. Tomichek RC, Rosow CE, Schneider RC, et al. Cardiovascular effects of diazepam-fentanyl anesthesia in patients with coronary artery disease. Anesth Analg 1982;61:217–218.

113. Heikkila H, Jalonen J, Arola M, et al. Midazolam as adjunct to high-dose fentanyl anaesthesia for coronary artery bypass grafting operation. Acta Anaesthesiol Scand 1984; 28:683–689.

114. Sherlock S, Beann AG, Belling BH, et al. Splanchnic blood flow in man by the bromsulfalein method: the relation of peripheral plasma bromsulfalein level to calculated flow. J Lab Clin Med 1950;35:923–932.

115. Bower S, Hull CJ. Comparative pharmacokinetics of fentanyl and alfentanil. Br J Anaesth 1982;54:871–877.

116. Liddell D, Williams F, Briant R. Phenazone (antipyrine) metabolism and distribution in young and elderly adults. Clin Exp Pharmacol Physiol 1975;2:481–487.

117. Bentley JB, Borel JD, Nenad RE, et al. Age and fentanyl pharmacokinetics. Anesth Analg 1982;61:968–971.

118. Bovill JG, Sebel PS, Blackburn CL, et al. The pharmacokinetics of sufentanil in surgical patients. Anesthesiology 1984;61:502–506.

ritus. In this new approach, the hourly dose of bupivacaine was reduced to 5.7 mg. There was no postspinal headache.

Cesarean Section

According to many authors, women in labor need per segment one-third less of the local anesthetic than their nonpregnant counterparts. But no one can assess the precise dose needed. To adjust the dosage to the patient's needs, an epidural catheter is an absolute requisite. The cardiotoxicity of bupivacaine is related to the total dose, which is substantially reduced by the addition of sufentanil.

In more than 350 cases involving cesarean sections, we injected a mixture of bupivacaine 0.5%, epinephrine 1/200,000 (16 ml), and sufentanil 5 μg/ml (4 ml). From this mixture (warmed to about 35°C, and the operating table in a 10° Fowler position), 5 ml was given via the catheter. If inadvertently this dose (bupivacaine 20 mg/adreneline 20 μg/sufentanil 5 μg) is injected into the spinal fluid or into a vein, warning symptoms will appear, but no disaster will occur. This 5-ml test dose is nearly a full proof safety dose. If, within 5 minutes, no untoward effects have been observed, a further 10 to 15 ml of the mixture will be given. The table is placed in the horizontal position, the legs elevated 20°, the uterus being lifted and tipped to the left with the Kennedy device. The total dose of each—bupivacaine, epinephrine, and sufentanil—ranges respectively between 60 and 80 mg, 60 and 80 μg, and 15 and 20 μg. Injection by divided dose enhances safety. Motor blockade will be sufficient, provided anesthesia is adequate, because the gravid uterus has stretched the abdominal wall during the last weeks of pregnancy.

Surgery can start within 20 minutes. The duration of analgesia is between 3 and 6 hours. Blood pressure will be kept normal with a 500-ml warmed macromolecular starch solution given over a 15-minute period. There is no need for a larger volume of electrolytes. Oxygen 6 to 8 l/minute is given from the start through a transparent mask. Maternal and neonatal blood plasma levels of sufentanil after epidural administration of doses between 30 μg and 250 μg show clearly the low plasma content in mother and neonate at the time of delivery. Actually, the total sufentanil dose never exceeds 20 μg. No unwanted side effects (respiratory depression) have been observed. By warming up all drugs injected into the epidural space and the fast-transfused venous fluids, we reduced the shivering from 34 to 6%. Successful anesthesia was achieved in 96% of the patients.

Post-Cesarean Section Pain Relief

Since opioids have been injected into the spinal canal for pain relief, various complications have been observed, the most severe being respiratory depression and apnea. The classic opiate, morphine, injected epidurally provides effective and prolonged postoperative pain relief without sympathetic- or neuromuscular blockade. Unfortunately, morphine, a hydrophilic molecule, has a delayed onset time and a slow clearance from the CSF. This leaves more free drug available for supraspinal redistribution, with the potential risk of producing the common side effect, delayed respiratory depression. Less known is the association of epidural morphine injection for post-cesarean section pain relief, with an increased incidence of herpes simplex, type labialis. Herpes lesions appear between the second and the fifth day after morphine epidural injections. The lesions are located in the perioral and perinasal regions, sometimes over the whole face. The herpes simplex virus can spread to the infant and cause encephalitis.[10]

Post-cesarean section pain relief is provided by the epidural injection of 6 to 10 ml of bupivacaine (2.5 mg/ml), epinephrine (1.6 μg/ml), and sufentanil (1 μg/ml). This dose is tested and, if necessary, adjusted during the recovery room period. It will give comfort for 2 to 4 hours, and further injections are given on demand in the ward.

CONCLUSION

One may conclude that the addition of a minute dose of sufentanil to bupivacaine with epinephrine results in a decreased onset time, an improved incidence of satisfactory analgesia and anesthesia (cesarean section), a longer duration of analgesia, and an important reduction of bupivacaine. All these improvements contribute to greater safety and comfort for the mother and child, which are the ultimate goals.

REFERENCES

1. Nordberg G. (1984) Pharmacokinetic aspects of spinal morphine. Acta Anaesth Scand 1984;28(Suppl 79):1–38.
2. Handsdottir V, Hedner T, Nordberg G. CSF and plasma pharmacokinetics of sufentanil after epidural administration. Submitted for publication.
3. Handsdottir V, Hedner T, Nordberg G. CSF and plasma pharmacokinetics of sufentanil after intrathecal administration. Submitted for publication.
4. Reynolds F, O'Sullivan G. Epidural fentanyl and pain relief in labour. Anaesthesia 1989; 44:341–344.
5. Heytens L, Cammu H, Camu F. Extradural analgesia during labour using alfentanil. Br J Anaesth 1987;59:331–337.
6. Van Steenberge A, Debroux HC, Noorduin H. Extradural bupivacaine with sufentanil for vaginal delivery: a double-blind trial. Br J Anaesth 1987;59:1518–1522.
7. Little MS, McNitt JD, Choi HJ, et al. A pilot study of low-dose epidural sufentanil and bupivacaine for labor anesthesia. Anesthesiology 1987;67:A444.
8. Phillips GH. Epidural sufentanil-bupivacaine combinations for analgesia during labor: effect of varying sufentanil doses. Anesthesiology 1987;67:835–838.
9. McGrady EM, Brownhill DK, Davis AG. Epidural diamorphine and bupivacaine in labour. Anaesthesia 1989;44:400–403.
10. Naulty JS, Hertwig L, Hunt CO, et al. Duration of analgesia of epidural fentanyl following cesarian delivery: effects of local anesthetic drug selection. Anesthesiology 1986;65:A180.

Chapter 9 Discussion

GERARD W. OSTHEIMER: Opiate substances have been used to provide pain relief during childbirth for thousands of years. However, it was not until very recently that the site and mechanism of action of these compounds have begun to be understood. In the early 1970s, investigators began to identify and describe receptor sites for opioids in the mammalian central nervous system.

Following the identification of opioid receptors, the potent analgesic action of opioids when applied to these receptor sites was demonstrated in human studies as well as animal preparations. Naturally occurring peptides called enkephalins (from the Greek "in the head"), which exhibited opiatelike characteristics upon binding to these receptors, were discovered. Whereas local anesthetics interrupt the transmission of noxious stimuli via peripheral afferent nerves to the spinal cord, intraspinal opioids work by modification of these transmissions, most notably at the level of the dorsal horn of the spinal cord within the substantial gelatinosa. Both exogenous opioids and endogenous enkephalins alter the central release of neurotransmitters, thereby interfering with the first level of sensory integration and modifying the subjective interpretation of pain.

Intraspinal, i.e., subarachnoid and epidural, administration of opioids provides good to excellent pain relief for uterine contractions and cervical dilatation ("visceral pain") but poor analgesia at the time of delivery ("somatic pain"). Because of the character of post-cesarean pain, intraspinal opioids are an excellent choice for its management. Furthermore, the addition of opioids to varying concentrations of local anesthetics either in the epidural or subarachnoid space greatly enhances pain relief during labor and vaginal or cesarean delivery.

Morphine, a water-soluble and therefore long-acting opiate, gives prolonged pain relief but potentially produces several side effects such as pruritus, nausea, vomiting, drowsiness, urinary retention, and respiratory depression. The last is our main concern, particularly since it may be late in onset. For this reason, the use of the shorter-acting lipid-soluble opioids has been suggested. While the pain relief provided by a single intraspinal injection of highly lipid-soluble opioid is rapid in onset, it is also short-lived—less than 10 hours at maximum. Intermittent injection (which is labor-intensive) has been suggested; others have proposed continuous infusion, which has inherent problems. Some patients have preferred the use of local anesthetics alone for postoperative pain relief, either by intermittent injection or continuous infusion, since the minor side effects of intraspinal opioids, pruritus, nausea, and vomiting, were so disconcerting. In other cases, anesthesiologists have tried to circumvent the problems of side effects by using an infusion of naloxone, which can create another set of problems, including reversal of analgesia. The use of opioid–local anesthetic combinations has been suggested in order to decrease the side effects of both drugs and utilize their beneficial effects. Alternatively, the use of agonists-antagonist drugs offers pain relief of shorter duration than morphine but longer than the fentanyl derivatives, with diminished side effects except for unwanted sedation.

In many instances, the anesthesiologist must choose a method of pain relief that best fits the postpartum recovery and nursing circumstances because of concern about effective monitoring of patients who have received intraspinal opioids with or without local anesthetics. Pulse oximeters and apnea monitors are only as efficient as their observers. To date, we do not have the perfect intraspinal opioid. However, with the addition of patient-controlled analgesia for postoperative pain relief to the armamentarium of the anesthesiologist, a combination of drugs and techniques may be the answer.

While maternal effects of intraspinal opioids are well documented, the fetal and neonatal effects are still being evaluated and appear to be related to the standard concept of maternal and fetal pharmacokinetics applicable to opioids in general. Insignificant amounts of opioid have been found in breast milk, and no adverse effects have been demonstrated in the neonate of the nursing mother.

At present, it is my belief we have only begun to scratch the surface of the vast potential for intraspinal opioids with and without local anesthetics.

JEAN M. MILLAR: This is an interesting presentation of the use of sufentanil in obstetric analgesia and anesthesia. From the British point of view, it is difficult to comment constructively, as sufentanil is not available in the United Kingdom, and the combination of low concentrations of bupivacaine with opioids—principally fentanyl—has only recently been used to control recalcitrant pain.

The combination described by Dr. Van Steenberge seems to improve the quality and duration of analgesia while reducing the dosage of bupivacaine and its attendant motor block.

The combination of bupivacaine and fentanyl has been reported to be particularly effective for perineal pain,[1] which is difficult to treat and may result in increased instrumental delivery from large doses of bupivacaine. Alfentanil epidural infusions[2] and sufentanil[3-5] in varying doses added to bupivacaine have not shown striking advantages over fentanyl. Disappointingly, none of these combinations has reduced the incidence of instrumental delivery. Diamorphine[6] has also been used to good effect.

No comparison is made of cesarian section with and without the added sufentanil. The dose of bupivacaine with epinephrine could be expected to be sufficient alone but be of shorter duration. There is evidence that the presence of local anesthetic potentiates fentanyl analgesia postoperatively,[7] and this would presumably also apply to sufentanil.

The continued use of bupivacaine for post-cesarian section pain is generally avoided in the United Kingdom because of motor block and urinary retention. Fentanyl has been the most commonly used opioid, but because of its short action and tachyphylaxis it is increasingly being replaced by morphine despite morphine's slow onset. This provides 24 hours of analgesia. Is tachyphylaxis a problem with sufentanil?

It is clear that the combination of bupivacaine and opioids is better than the individual drugs alone, particularly for perineal or intractable pain. But it is unclear which opioid is the best.

REFERENCES

1. Reynolds F, O'Sullivan G. Epidural fentanyl and pain relief in labour. Anaesthesia 1989; 44:341–344.

2. Heytens L, Cammu H, Camu F. Extradural analgesia during labour using alfentanil. Br J Anaesth 1987;59:331–337.

3. Van Steenberge A, Debroux HC, Noorduin H. Extradural bupivacaine with sufentanil for vaginal delivery. A double blind trial. Br J Anaesth 1987;59:1518–1522.

4. Little MS, McNitt JD, Choi HJ, et al. A pilot study of low dose epidural sufentanil and bupivacaine for labor anesthesia. Anesthesiology 1987;67:A444.

5. Phillips GH. Epidural sufentanil/bupivacaine combinations for analgesia during labor: effect of varying sufentanil doses. Anesthesiology 1987;67:835–838.

6. McGrady EM, Brownhill DK, Davis AG. Epidural diamorphine and bupivacaine in labour. Anaesthesia 1989;44:400–403.

7. Naulty JS, Hertwig L, Hunt CO, et al. Duration of analgesia of epidural fentanyl following cesarian delivery—effects of local anesthetic drug selection. Anesthesiology 1986;65:A180.

10 NARCOTICS IN NEUROANESTHESIA

Robert W. McPherson and Marc A. Feldman

Anesthetic management of patients with neurological diseases, or those who are at risk of neurological injury, requires understanding of the interactions of drug effects with the patient's disease process. Drug effects that produce no important changes in a non-neurosurgical patient may cause life-threatening changes in the neurosurgical patient.

Patients at risk for neurological injury may have exhausted cerebral compensatory mechanisms and may require modification of anesthetic management. Specific requirements for neuroanesthesia include minimizing hypertensive responses and cerebral vasodilation, controlling intracranial pressure (ICP), supporting the cerebral perfusion pressure (CPP), and controlling drug effects on the postoperative neurological examination.

Volatile anesthetic gases produce dose-dependent cerebral hyperemia and decreased CPP, which may compromise the intracranial contents. Synthetic narcotics are very effective in decreasing the amount of those agents required to produce adequate anesthesia.

In both animals and humans, synthetic narcotics produce anesthesia as a single drug only in extremely high doses (compared to the amount that produces profound analgesia). Although synthetic narcotics appear to have minimal direct effects on the cerebral circulation, pure narcotic anesthesia could cause prolonged awakening and postoperative management problems. Thus, the optimal anesthetic management seems to be narcotic supplementation by other anesthetic agents.

Narcotics produce respiratory depression and may initially appear contraindicated in patients in whom increases in arterial carbon dioxide tension ($PaCO_2$) may cause intracranial decompensation due to increased cerebral blood flow (CBF) and ICP. Careful distinction must be made between direct and indirect drug effects. For instance, even large doses of narcotics have no effect on $PaCO_2$ and thus no indirect effects on CBF if ventilation is controlled.

Considerable controversy continues to exist concerning direct effects of synthetic narcotics on the cerebral circulation. This controversy seems to arise from different basal studies in frequently quoted animal studies. Therefore, we provide information here to allow evaluation of the basal anesthetic state.

EFFECT OF NARCOTICS ON REQUIREMENTS OF VOLATILE AGENTS AND OTHER INTRAVENOUS AGENTS

The response of the cerebral circulation to maintain normal blood flow with increases or decreases in perfusion pressure is termed autoregulation. Halothane, enflurane, and isoflurane cause dose-dependent decreases in cerebral autoregulation[1,2] and a dose-dependent hyperemia.[2] Intravenous supplementation decreases the inspired volatile anesthetic concentration necessary for adequate anesthesia and therefore should decrease the magnitude of cerebral hyperemia.

The use of narcotics is a reasonable method for decreasing the minimal alveolar concentration (MAC) of volatile agents. Synthetic narcotics have a theoretical advantage over both barbiturates and benzodiazepines because of the ease with which effects on level of consciousness can be reversed with a narcotic antagonist. The amount by which volatile gas anesthetic requirement can be decreased by narcotic is dose-related. Although there may be species and drug variability, synthetic narcotics such as fentanyl, alfentanil, and sufentanil decrease MAC by > 65% in the dog.[3–5] In the dog, enflurane MAC reduction is similar (about 75%) with alfentanil (32 μg/kg/min),[5] sufentanil (122 μg/kg/min),[6] and fentanyl (270 μg/kg).[3] Thus, the choice between alfentanil, fentanyl, and sufentanil seems to be influenced by pharmacokinetic properties of the drugs more than by differential effects on the cerebral vasculature.

Sprigge et al.[7] have suggested that in humans an arterial concentration of fentanyl that blocks response to stimulation is analogous to MAC for volatile anesthetic agents (serum fentanyl level about 15 ng/ml) and can be achieved with a loading dose of 50 μg/kg followed by an infusion of 0.5 μg/kg/min.

The lack of adverse effects on the upper and lower limits of cerebral autoregulation by fentanyl and alfentanil[8,9] suggests that peripheral vasoconstrictors may be used safely to increase mean arterial blood pressure (MABP) and CPP when decreased by intravenous narcotics. In this regard, synthetic narcotics may be more desirable than volatile anesthetics because at inspired concentrations that produce anesthesia, volatile gases may obtund cerebral autoregulation, and vasoconstrictor administered to maintain MABP may increase CBF and ICP.

Bristow et al.[10] studied the impact of low-dose narcotic infusion (fentanyl or sufentanil) during craniotomy with volatile gas anesthesia. They found that the narcotic infusion (fentanyl 1 μg/kg/hr; sufentanil 0.1 μg/kg/hr) increased brain relaxation and decreased the amount of brain retraction necessary. This effect did not appear to be due to a lower concentration of volatile anesthesia or a decrease in perfusion pressure. Notably, the narcotic infusion did not prolong emergence from anesthesia. The mechanism for the increased brain relaxation is unclear.

DIRECT RESPIRATORY AND CARDIOVASCULAR EFFECTS

Narcotics may elevate $PaCO_2$ in the spontaneously ventilating patient, which can increase CBF and ICP. The timing of narcotic administration should be adjusted to minimize carbon dioxide retention. In patients with intracranial mass effect, preoperative elevation of $PaCO_2$ might cause life-threatening brain stem herniation, whereas in the same patient a similar degree of $PaCO_2$ elevation following surgical decompression causes no more problem than in the non-neurosurgical patient.

Fentanyl directly affects function of brain stem respiratory neurons.[11] Inspiratory neurons of the tractus solitarius are caused by fentanyl to stop rhythmic firing and to begin a continuous and irregular discharge, whereas in neurons of the vertical respiratory group the activity of the neurons were totally abolished by fentanyl. This study indicates that synthetic narcotics have effects on the respiratory system exclusive of effects on peripheral chemoreceptors and suggests that patients with brain stem lesions might be very sensitive to the postoperative depressant effects of intraoperative narcotics.

The efficiency of narcotic supplementation in blunting the pressor response to intubation is particularly important in the neurosurgical patient. In the lightly anesthetized patient, endotracheal intubation results in a marked increase in MABP and ICP.[12] This acute rise in

lation prevent respiratory depression and un-mask direct effects of narcotics on the cerebral circulation.

The direct effect of synthetic narcotics on CBF is controversial, since their apparent effect depends on the pre-existing anesthetic level. McPherson and Traystman[8] found that fentanyl (25 µg/kg, IV bolus) in animals anesthetized with pentobarbital did not alter CBF, whereas Michenfelder and Theye[26] found that a smaller dose of fentanyl (6 µg/kg, IV bolus) decreased CBF by 47% and decreased cerebral metabolic rate of oxygen consumption ($CMRO_2$) by 18%. Perhaps in the latter study, the level of basal anesthetic was lighter. In a rat model, the decrease in CBF and $CMRO_2$ by fentanyl is greater in young rats than in older rats.[27] In young rats, fentanyl decreased CBF 49% and $CMRO_2$ 39%, while in old rats the same dose of fentanyl depressed CBF by only 37% (p < 0.05) and $CMRO_2$ by 34% (p < 0.05).

Yaster et al.[28] studied fentanyl alone and in combination with pentobarbital in the chronically instrumented lamb, thus avoiding basal anesthesia. In that study, high-dose fentanyl (3,000 µg/kg, IV bolus) produced severe respiratory depression, but the animals remained responsive to their environment. However, combination with subanesthetic doses of pentobarbital produced unconsciousness. High-dose fentanyl alone did not decrease CBF from the awake value, but combination with subanesthetic doses of pentobarbital caused unconsciousness and decreased CBF by 27% and $CMRO_2$ by a similar amount (19%), thus preserving the CBF/$CMRO_2$ ratio (Figure 10.3). Intravenous naloxone returned both CBF and $CMRO_2$ to control levels. The decrease in regional CBF was similar in both brain stem and hemispheric areas. This study is extremely helpful in clarifying the effect of fentanyl on the cerebral circulation. Clearly, synergistic effects of even small doses of other anesthetic drugs may alter the apparent effects of narcotics on the brain.

An important consideration in assessing the effects of narcotics on the cerebral vasculature is seizures, which have been described in an-

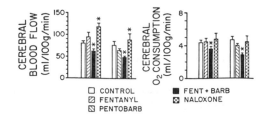

FIGURE 10.3 Hemispheric cerebral blood flow and cerebral oxygen consumption at control and after administration of 3 mg/kg fentanyl, 4 mg/kg pentobarbital, the combination of 3 mg/kg fentanyl and 4 mg/kg pentobarbital, and 0.1 mg/kg naloxone. (mean ± SEM) * denotes $p < 0.05$ compared to control. (Reprinted with permission of the authors and publisher from Yaster M, Koehler RC, Traystman RJ. Interaction of fentanyl and pentobarbital on peripheral and cerebral hemodynamics in newborn lambs. Anesthesiology 1989;70:461–469.)

imal studies. Synthetic narcotics may be similar to lidocaine in this effect on CBF, a dose-dependent decrease in CBF until seizures occur, which increases CBF. In the rat, fentanyl (100 µg/kg) decreases CBF by 30 to 50%,[29,30] whereas higher doses of fentanyl (400 µg/kg) cause seizures (Figure 10.4). With the lower doses of fentanyl,[30] $CMRO_2$ was depressed when CBF was depressed.

Maekawa et al.[31] studied regional CBF during fentanyl seizures in the rat using C^{14} iodoantipyrine autoradiography. During spike activity on EEG, CBF increased in all regions, with greater increases in superior colliculi, sensimotor cortex, and pineal body. With seizures, CBF increases significantly in all regions (58 to 231% of control). Thus, generalized increased flow occurs despite the fact that fentanyl seizures are usually subcortical.

Carlsson et al.[29] assessed the effects of fentanyl in rats and found that CBF was maximally decreased to 50% of control ($CMRO_2$ 65% of control) at 100 µg/kg (compared to nitrous oxide control). Higher doses of fentanyl did not further decrease either CBF or $CMRO_2$. However, they found seizure activity

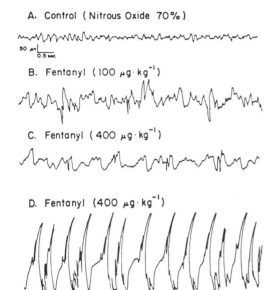

A. Control (Nitrous Oxide 70%)

B. Fentanyl (100 μg · kg⁻¹)

C. Fentanyl (400 μg · kg⁻¹)

D. Fentanyl (400 μg · kg⁻¹)

FIGURE 10.4 Representative frontoparietal electroencephalographic tracing for control (N₂O) rats and rats receiving either 100 or 400 μg/kg fentanyl, IV. Tracing B shows the slow-wave activity typically seen after 100 μg/kg fentanyl, while C shows waves with spikes, and D shows frank seizure activity. Both the spike and seizure occur after 400 μg/kg fentanyl. (Reprinted with permission of the authors and publisher from Safo Y, Young MI, Smith DS, et al. Effects of fentanyl on local cerebral blood flow in the rat. Acta Anaesthesiol Scand 1985;29:594–598.)

at 200 μg/kg and 400 μg/kg, which resolved with naloxone treatment. The seizures seem to increase $CMRO_2$ without increasing CBF. Young et al.[32] used the 2-deoxyglucose method to assess the effect of sufentanil on cortical and subcortical structures. They found that high-dose sufentanil (40 to 160 μg/kg) decreases cortical glucose utilization in cortex and caudate nucleus compared to halothane. However, increases in glucose utilization were found in amygdala and hippocampus.

With increasing doses of sufentanil in the rat, 80 μg/kg decreased CBF to 53% of control and $CMRO_2$ to 40% of control.[33] Larger doses of sufentanil did not further decrease CBF or

$CMRO_2$. Seizurelike activity was seen with increased dose, but no correlation between seizure activity and CBF or $CMRO_2$ was seen.

Despite evidence in animals that high-dose fentanyl causes seizures, Murkin et al.[34] showed that fentanyl (150 μg/kg, IV bolus) does not cause EEG evidence of seizures in humans despite characteristic truncal rigidity.

In summary, while narcotics produce parallel decreases in CBF and $CMRO_2$, with the induction of unconsciousness, especially in combination with other anesthetic drugs, the direct effects of synthetic narcotics given in the pharmacologic range would appear to be small.

EFFECT OF NARCOTICS ON ELECTROPHYSIOLOGICAL MONITORING

Intraoperative electrophysiological monitoring is widely used to diminish the risk of neurological injury. These monitors play the role of the only available neurologic examination for the recognition and prevention of neurologic injury in the anesthetized patient.

Brain electric activity is represented by the EEG. The averaged EEG response to repetitive peripheral nerve stimulation is termed the evoked potential or evoked response. Somatosensory evoked potentials (SSEP) or brain stem auditory evoked responses (BAER) may be measured dependent on the modality of the sensory stimulation. The changes in EEG and evoked potential that reflect oxygen deprivation and impending neural injury are slowing of the EEG and decreases in amplitude (size) and increases in latency (delay from stimulation) of the evoked potential.

Volatile anesthetic gases also cause EEG slowing and, at high concentration, flattening at the EEG signal. Inhalation anesthetics cause a dose-dependent decrease in amplitude and increase in latency of evoked potentials such that monitoring may be difficult, even in patients with a neurologically normal baseline. Narcotic anesthetics do not have the same depressant effect on electrophysiologic function. Smith et al.[35] compared the effects of fentanyl and sufentanil on the EEG. Generally, the effects were the same, with an increase in power in the low-frequency bands. Alfentanil also was found to increase slow-wave (δ) activity, decrease synchronization of the EEG, and produce spindle activity in 70% of patients.[36]

The effects of narcotics on evoked potentials are small and variable depending on the presence of other drugs. Koht et al.[37] found that fentanyl (10 μg/kg, IV bolus) added to etomidate increases SSEP latency and diminishes the augmentation effect of etomidate. When added to thiopental, fentanyl did not affect latency of SSEP but depressed amplitude. While fentanyl at a dose of 5 μg/kg was seen to decrease the amplitude of the long latency auditory P300 waveform,[38] Samra et al.[39] found that even a dose of 50 μg/kg does not alter the BAER wave latencies.

Unlike the effects of volatile anesthetics, the effects of narcotics on the EEG and evoked potentials are small and consistent and allow for reliable intraoperative neurologic monitoring.

PREMEDICATION

Narcotics may be used as premedication to reduce anxiety and relieve pain during transport to the operating room and insertion of vascular catheters. Because neurosurgical patients may have a depressed level of consciousness or may have decreased intracranial compliance, the amount of narcotic should be titrated to minimize carbon dioxide retention.

Invasive hemodynamic monitoring in this group of patients is frequent, and satisfactory methods of calming the patient and relieving discomfort during catheter insertion are necessary. Ideally, all catheters are placed prior to induction of anesthesia. Anesthesia induction may cause precipitous decreases in CPP, requiring immediate treatment. An attractive alternative to premedication on the ward is to administer intravenous medications while the patient is under the observation of the anesthesiologist. Small doses of short-acting barbiturates and synthetic narcotics meet these requirements.

The risk of carbon dioxide retention with small doses of narcotics is balanced against the possible adverse effects of hypertension associated with pain.

SPECIFIC OPERATIONS

Intracranial Mass Lesions

Intracranial mass lesions offer significant anesthetic management problems. These patients have frequently exhausted cerebral compensatory mechanisms, and relatively small cerebrovascular changes due to anesthetic drugs may adversely affect the cerebral circulation. Frequently the mass has grown sufficiently slowly so that there is impending brain stem herniation or midline shift. In those circumstances, decreases in cerebral perfusion may be detrimental to neural function. Preoperative preparation frequently includes osmotherapy (mannitol) so that the patient is mildly hypovolemic and hence sensitive to drugs that produce vasodilation. In this category of patients, surgical decompression during the middle of this operation greatly decreases the sensitivity of the patients to the adverse effects of volatile anesthetic gases. Thus, narcotics are best deleted from the latter parts of this anesthesia.

Bolus narcotic administration for anesthesia induction plus an infusion for maintenance until approximately 90 minutes prior to end of surgery will allow prompt awakening of the patient.

Ventriculoperitoneal Shunt

Cerebrospinal fluid diversion procedures are frequent procedures, either as primary procedures or following other intracranial procedures. These patients have elevated ICP, and decreases in arterial pressure will diminish CPP. These operations are relatively short (1 to 2 hours), so that narcotics with long-lasting effects are best avoided. Neurological complications, such as acute subdural hematoma, occur with some frequency; awakening must be prompt but without severe hypertension.

Neurovascular Procedures (Aneurysm, Arteriovenous Malformation)

Both intracranial aneurysm and cerebral arteriovenous malformations require careful control of CPP. These patients frequently present with subarachnoid hemorrhage, which causes both brain injury and vasomotor paralysis in the area of injury. These patients are at risk of neural injury because of decreased CPP produced by arterial hypotension (prior to skull opening), increased pressure due to brain retractors, and hypoperfusion due to cerebral vasospasm. Continuous monitoring of neural function by EEG and evoked potentials has been shown to decrease intraoperative injury. Fentanyl produces only small effects on evoked potentials, and successful monitoring is possible even in the presence of high doses.

Posterior Fossa Surgery

Surgery of the posterior fossa may produce dysfunction of both lower cranial nerves and brain stem respiratory dysfunction, which may contribute to postoperative respiratory dysfunction. If high-dose narcotic anesthesia is used, the patient may be awake and responsive while stimulated, including adequate airway maintenance. However, if the patient is unstimulated, unconsciousness may return and upper airway obstruction may occur because of lack of response to hypercapnia or hypoxia. Shupak et al.[40] assessed fentanyl (100 μg/kg) by rapid infusion in patients undergoing suboccipital craniectomy in the sitting position. The operation lasted approximately 4 hours. Naloxone (1.5 μg/kg, IV bolus) plus an infusion was required in the immediate postoperative period. A 20% decrease in cardiac output was found in the seated position. Naloxone was required for 18 hrs (6,775 μg total dose/

patient). Thus, high-dose fentanyl alone is best avoided.

Spinal Cord Procedures

The impact of narcotics on neurological monitoring is particularly important in these procedures.

Spinal cord operations are indicated for tumor, stenosis, vascular abnormalities, and developmental abnormalities like Arnold-Chiari malformation and scoliosis. These operations put the spinal cord at risk. Blood flow to the spinal cord seems to be controlled in a similar manner to blood flow to the brain. The spinal cord possesses the ability to autoregulate flow and to respond to changes in PaO_2 and $PaCO_2$.

Although few comparison studies are available, probably drugs affect the spinal cord in a similar fashion to the brain.

NARCOTIC ANTAGONISTS

Optimal management of intraoperative narcotic administration would be such that narcotic antagonists are seldom required. However, the availability of a relatively safe and specific antagonist is an important asset to these drugs. Narcotic reversal may be indicated for treatment of postoperative respiratory depression or sedation. Prolonged postoperative narcosis is seen in patients with unanticipated brief surgical procedures or in patients unusually sensitive to usual narcotic doses. Certain neurosurgical procedures, such as those requiring frontal lobe retraction, are associated with altered levels of consciousness postoperatively. These patients may be sensitive to the sedative effects of narcotics even at levels not depressing ventilation, as evidenced by a normal $PaCO_2$. Administration of a narcotic antagonist may be used to rapidly reverse the effects of narcotics.

The direct effects of the narcotic antagonist naloxone are negligible in the absence of opioid drugs. At doses of greater than 300 μg/kg, normal subjects show only some increase in systolic blood pressure and decreased perform-ance on memory tests.[41] Administration of na-loxone to reverse narcotic analgesia, however, has been associated with undesirable effects such as acute hypertension and cardiac ar-rhythmia. Small doses of naloxone given to narcotic-dependent patients may precipitate acute withdrawal. Naloxone reversal of nar-cotics should always be titrated to effect with starting doses of 0.5 to 1.0 μg/kg. A mainte-nance infusion may be necessary to prevent the return of narcosis in cases of large overdose.

Naloxone in large doses has been postulated in some animal models to have a protective effect against neural ischemia and injury. Har-iri et al.[42] assessed the effect of naloxone (1 mg/kg) given at the time of total global is-chemia in the rat. They found that naloxone prevented a decrease in cardiac output asso-ciated with ischemia as well as blocking the hyperemia followed by oligemia, which pro-gressed to stroke in untreated animals. They hypothesized that opiate receptor blockade prevents stimulation of vagally mediated brain stem centers secondary to ischemia and pre-vents a vagal decrease in cardiac output. No-tably, in that study, MABP was not increased by naloxone. Hosobuchi et al.[43] found in ger-bils subjected to carotid occlusion that nalox-one caused reversal of neurological deficit, hemiparesis, although it did not improve outcome.

The possible role of naloxone as a neuro-protective agent is controversial. No role for narcotic antagonists has been established in neurological injury. Certainly, there is no evi-dence that exogenous narcotics are detrimen-tal for patients at risk of neurological injury.

PHARMACOLOGIC HORIZONS

The synthetic narcotics have proved to be use-ful components to neuroanesthetic manage-ment. Their rapid popularity is evidence of their efficacy. New developments in receptor pharmacology promise the availability of agents of even greater safety and effectiveness.

Opioid drugs act as brain receptors impor-tant for the modulation of pain stimuli. These narcotic receptors have been grouped into var-ious types. Drugs such as morphine, fentanyl, and their derivatives all act at the μ opioid receptor. This receptor subtype is responsible for analgesia and respiratory depression (Ta-ble 10.1).

TABLE 10.1   Subtypes of prototypic drugs and their proposed actions

Subtype	Prototypic Drugs	Proposed Actions
μ_1	Opiates and most opioid peptides	Supraspinal analgesia, including periaqueductal gray, nucleus raphe magnus, and locus ceruleus Prolactin release Catalepsy
μ_2	Morphine sulfate	Respiratory depression Gastrointestinal tract transit Most cardiovascular effects
κ	Ketocyclazocine and dynorphin	Spinal analgesia Inhibition of antidiuretic hormone release Sedation
δ	Enkephalins	Spinal analgesia Dopamine turnover in the brain
ϵ	β-endorphin	Rat vas deferens bioassay
σ	N-allylnormetazocine (SKF-10,047)	Psychotomimetic effects Linked to N-methyl-D-aspartate

Source: Adapted from Pasternak GW. Multiple morphine and enkephalin receptors and the relief of pain. JAMA 1988;259:1362–1367.

The κ receptor also mediates analgesia but without respiratory depression. This receptor is the primary mediator of spinal analgesia. κ agonist drugs may also be weak μ agonists or may be μ antagonists. The agonist-antagonist drugs cause some respiratory depression, but the effect is not dose-related and a ceiling effect occurs.[44] The benzomorphan analogue bremozocrine causes potent analgesia without respiratory depression. In doses up to 40 μg/kg it has no significant cardiovascular or respiratory effects. A dose-dependent decrease in high-frequency EEG activity was reversed by a κ antagonist. This study suggests that κ receptor sites distinct from those interacting with other opioids (μ receptors) are responsible for the effects of bremozocrine.

Althaus et al.[45] studied U-50,488H, a selective κ receptor agonist, and found that it reduced halothane MAC by 70%. The decrease in MAC was not reversed by naloxone. Because naloxone has a much higher affinity for μ receptors than for κ receptors, this suggests that the decrease in MAC was not due to μ receptor stimulation.

Castillo et al.[46] found that U-50,488H when administered by intracerebroventricular injection caused a dose-dependent increase in threshold to noxious stimulation without respiratory depression. Thus, a κ agonist may be used to provide spinal (epidural) analgesia without respiratory depression.

In rat studies, the specific κ agonist U-50,488H decreased the postischemia neuronal loss from 80 to 20%.[47] Those authors hypothesize that κ receptor stimulation actually improves postischemia neuronal preservation. Heath et al.[48] assessed the effect of the κ agonist in rhesus monkeys prepared with chronic electrodes. They found that κ agonists cause behavioral changes and slow-wave EEG changes.

κ agonists are not ideal drugs, however. Gautret and Schmitt[49] found that the κ agonist ethylketocyclazocine causes bradycardia and hypotension, which is not altered by atropine but is inhibited by naloxone.

Pasternak[50] has suggested that there may be subtypes of μ receptors: the μ_1 receptor, responsible for analgesia; and μ_2, responsible for

respiratory depression.[51] When naloxonazine, a relatively specific μ_1 blocker, was used, the analgesic effects of morphine could be blocked in rats, with no change in respiratory depression. The possibility of a safe and effective μ_1 agonist would offer a drug with all the analgesic effects of morphine but without cardiovascular or respiratory side effects.

Ideal neuroanesthetic management requires the maintenance of cerebral perfusion pressure, control of cerebral vasodilation and intracranial pressure, reliable electrophysiologic monitoring, and a rapid return to consciousness for neurologic examination. The availability of the synthetic narcotics makes these goals realistic, and newer drugs may bring us even closer to the ideal.

REFERENCES

1. Miletich DH, Ivankovich AD, Albrecht RF, et al. Absence of the autoregulation of cerebral blood flow during halothane and enflurane anesthesia. Anesth Analg (Cleve) 1976; 55:100–109.

2. McPherson RW, Traystman RJ. Effects of isoflurane on cerebral autoregulation in dogs. Anesthesiology 1988;69:493–499.

3. Murphy MR, Hug CC, Jr. The anesthetic potency of fentanyl in terms of its reduction of enflurane MAC. Anesthesiology 1982;57:485–488.

4. Hecker BR, Lake CL, DiFazio CA, et al. The decrease of the minimum alveolar anesthetic concentration produced by sufentanil in rats. Anesth Analg 1983;62:987–990.

5. Hall RI, Szlam F, Hug CC Jr. The enflurane-sparing effect of alfentanil in dogs. Anesth Analg 1987;66:1287–1291.

6. Hall RI, Murphy MR, Hug CC Jr. The enflurane-sparing effect of sufentanil in dogs. Anesthesiology 1987;67:518–525.

7. Sprigge JS, Wynands JE, Whalley DG, et al. Fentanyl infusion anesthesia for aortocoronary bypass surgery: plasma levels and hemodynamic response. Anesth Analg 1982;61:972–978.

8. McPherson RW, Traystman RJ. Fentanyl and cerebral vascular responsivity in dogs. Anesthesiology 1984;60:180–186.

9. McPherson RW, Krempasanka E, Eimerl D, et al. Effects of alfentanil on cerebral vascular reactivity in dogs. Br J Anaesth 1985;57:1232–1238.

10. Bristow A, Shalev D, Rice B, et al. Low-dose synthetic narcotic infusions for cerebral relaxation during craniotomies. Anesth Analg 1987;66:413–416.

11. Tabatabai M, Kitahata LM, Collins JG. Disruption of the rhythmic activity of the medullary inspiratory neurons and phrenic nerve by fentanyl and reversal with nalbuphine. Anesthesiology 1989;70:489–495.

12. Bedfor RF, Persina JA, Pobereskin L, et al. Lidocaine or thiopental for rapid control of intracranial hypertension? Anesth Analg (Cleve)1980;59:435–437.

13. Bennett GM, Stanley TH. Human cardiovascular responses to endotracheal intubation during morphine-N_2O and fentanyl-N_2O anesthesia. Anesthesiology 1980;52:520–522.

14. Cork RC, Weiss JL, Hameroff SR, et al. Fentanyl preloading for rapid-sequence induction of anesthesia. Anesth Analg (Cleve) 1984;63:60–64.

15. Chung F, Evans D. Low-dose fentanyl: haemodynamic response during induction and intubation in geriatic patients. Can Anaesth Soc J 1985;32:622–628.

16. Payne KA, Murray WB, Oosthuizen JH. Obtunding the sympathetic response to intubation. S Afr Med J 1988;73:584–586.

17. Wynands JE, Townsend GE, Wong P, et al. Blood pressure response and plasma fentanyl concentrations during high- and very-high-dose fentanyl anesthesia for coronary artery surgery. Anesth Analg 1983;62:661–665.

18. Freye E, Arndt JO. Perfusion of the fourth cerebral ventricle with fentanyl induces naloxone-reversible bradycardia, hypotension, and EEG synchronization in conscious dogs. Naunyn Schmiedebergs Arch Pharmacol 1979;307:123–128.

19. Spiess BD, Sathoff RH, El-Ganzouri AR, et al. High-dose sufentanil: four cases of sudden hypotension on induction. Anesth Analg 1986;65:703–705.

20. McPherson RW, Koehler RC, Traystman RJ. Cerebral autoregulation with increased venous pressure or intracranial pressure or decreased arterial pressure. AJP 1988;255:H516–524.

21. Artru AA. Reduction of cerebrospinal fluid pressure by hypocapnia: changes in cerebral blood volume, cerebrospinal fluid volume, and brain tissue water and electrolytes. II Effects of anesthetics. J Cereb Blood Flow Metab 1988;8:750–756.

22. Artru AA. Effects of halothane and fentanyl on the rate of CSF production in dogs. Anesth Analg 1983;62:581–585.

23. Benthuysen JL, Kien ND, Quam DD. Intracranial pressure increases during alfentanil-induced rigidity. Anesthesiology 1988;68:438–440.

24. Tiznado E, James HE, Moore S. The effects of acute high-dose fentanyl administration on experimental brain edema: analysis of intracranial pressure, systemic arterial pressure, central venous pressure, and brain water content. Pharmacol Biochem Behav 1986;24:785–789.

25. Moss E, Powell D, Gibson RM, et al. Effects of fentanyl on intracranial pressure and cerebral perfusion pressure during hypocapnia. Br J Anaesth 1978;50:779–784.

26. Michenfelder JD, Theye RA. Effects of fentanyl, droperidol, and innovar on canine cerebral metabolism and blood flood. Br J Anaesth 1971;43:630–635.

27. Baughman VL, Hoffman WE, Albrecht RF, et al. Cerebral vascular and metabolic effects of fentanyl and midazolam in young and aged rats. Anesthesiology 1987;67:314–319.

28. Yaster M, Koehler RC, Traystman RJ. Interaction of fentanyl and pentobarbital on peripheral and cerebral hemodynamics in newborn lambs. Anesthesiology 1989;70:461–469.

29. Carlsson C, Smith DS. Keykhah M, et al. The effects of high-dose fentanyl on cerebral circulation and metabolism in rats. Anesthesiology 1982;57:375–380.

30. Safo Y, Young M, Smith DS, et al. Effects of fentanyl on local cerebral blood flow in the rat. Acta Anaesthesiol Scand 1985;29:594–598.

31. Maekawa T, Tommasino C, Shapiro HM. Local cerebral blood flow with fentanyl-induced seizures. J Cereb Blood Flow Metab 1984;4:88–95.

32. Young M, Smith DS, Greenberg J, et al. Effects of sufentanil on regional cerebral glucose utilization in rats. Anesthesiology 1984;61:564–568.

33. Keykhah M, Smith DS, Carlsson C, et al. Influence of sufentanil on cerebral metabolism and circulation in the rat. Anesthesiology 1985;63:274–277.

34. Murkin JM, Moldenhauer CC, Hug CC Jr, et al. Absence of seizures during induction of anesthesia with high-dose fentanyl. Anesth Analg 1984;63:489–494.

35. Smith NT, Dec-Silver H, Sanford TJ, et al. EEG's during high-dose fentanyl-, sufentanil-, or morphine-oxygen anesthesia. Anesth Analg 1984;63:386–393.

36. Bovill JG, Sebel PS. Wauquier A, et al. Influence of high-dose alfentanil anaesthesia on the electroencephalogram: correlation with plasma concentrations. Br J Anaesth 1983; 55:199S–209S.

37. Koht A, Schutz W, Schmidt G, et al. Effects of etomidate, midazolam, and thiopental on median nerve somatosensory evoked potentials and the additive effects of fentanyl and nitrous oxide. Anesth Analg 1988;67:435–441.

38. Velasco M, Velasco F, Castaneda R, et al. Effect of fentanyl and naloxone on the P300 auditory potential. Neuropharmacology 1984; 23:931–938.

39. Samra SK, Lilly DJ, Rush NL, et al. Fentanyl anesthesia and human brain stem auditory evoked potentials. Anesthesiology 1984;61: 261–265.

40. Shupak RC, Harp JR, Stevenson-Smith W, et al. High-dose fentanyl for neuroanesthesia. Anesthesiology 1983;58:579–582.

41. Cohen MR, Cohen RM, Pickar D, et al. High-dose naloxone infusions in normals. Arch Gen Psychiatry 1983;40:613–619.

42. Hariri RJ, Supra EL, Roberts JP, et al. Effect of naloxone on cerebral perfusion and cardiac performance during experimental cerebral ischemia. J Neurosurg 1986;64:780–786.

43. Hosobuchi Y, Baskin DS. Woo SK. Reversal of neurological deficits by opiate antagonist naloxone after cerebral ischemia in animals and humans. J Cereb Blood Flow Metab 1982; 2(suppl 1):S98–S100.

44. Bovill JG. Which potent opioid? Important criteria and selection. Drugs 1987;33:520–530.

45. Althaus JS, Von Voigtlander PF, DiFazio CA, et al. Effects of U-50,488H, a selective κ analgesic, on the minimum anesthetic concentration (MAC) of halothane in the rat. Anesth Analg 1987;66:391–394.

46. Castillo R, Kissin I, Bradley EL. Selective κ opioid agonist for spinal analgesia without the risk of respiratory depression. Anesth Analg 1986;65:350–354.

47. Hall ED. Pazara KE. Quantitative analysis of effects of κ opioid agonists on postischemic hippocampal CAI neuronal necrosis in gerbils. Stroke 1988;19:1008–1012.

48. Heath RG, Fitzjarrell AT, Walker CF. κ opiate receptor agonists: effects on behavior and on brain function and structure in rhesus monkeys. Biol Psychiatry 1984;19:1045–1074.

49. Gautret B, Schmitt H. Cardiac slowing induced by peripheral κ opiate receptor stimulation in rats. Eur J Pharmacol 1984;102:159–163.

50. Pasternak GW. Multiple μ opiate receptors: biochemical and pharmacological evidence for multiplicity. Biochem Pharmacol 1986;35:361–364.

51. Ling GSF, Spiegel K, Lockhart SH, et al. Separation of opioid analgesia from respiratory depression: evidence for different receptor mechanisms. J Pharmacol Exp Ther 1985;232:149–155.

Chapter 10 Discussion

JEAN M. MILLAR: This presentation reinforces the reasons for the key position that opioids currently occupy in neuroanesthesia. It rightly emphasizes the importance of cerebral perfusion pressure (CPP) rather than intracranial pressure (ICP).

Particularly important are the reduction in minimal alveolar concentration of volatile agents while maintaining cardiovascular stability, and the reduction in the pressor response to intubation. The combination of fentanyl and thiopentone is particularly beneficial to cerebral blood flow and cerebral metabolic rate of oxygen consumption.

What is the ideal short-acting narcotic is debatable. Alfentanil has the advantage of rapid onset and is effective at obtunding the pressor response to intubation. It may be given by infusion, producing better control preoperatively, with more rapid return of consciousness. However, Marx and colleagues[1] compared the effects of fentanyl (5 µg/kg), sufentanil (1 µg/kg), and alfentanil (50 µg/kg followed by infusion of 1 µg/kg/min) on CSF cerebrospinal fluid pressure (CSFP). The effect of fentanyl on CSFP was negligible, and its effect on CPP least of the three agents. Sufentanil resulted in the greatest increases in CSFP, and alfentanil produced the greatest reduction in CPP because of a significant fall in mean arterial blood pressure. They suggest that sufentanil acts as a cerebral vasodilator and concluded that fentanyl is the preferred opioid in patients with compromised intracranial compliance.

REFERENCE

1. Marx V, Shah N, Long C, et al. Sufentanil, alfentanil, and fentanyl: impact on CSF pressure in patients with brain tumors. Anesthesiology 1988;98:A627.

11 OPIOIDS AND OUTCOME IN PERIPHERAL VASCULAR SURGERY

David J. Benefiel and Michael F. Roizen

The occurrence of morbidity associated with cardiovascular surgery may be influenced by many factors, including pre-existing organic disease, the procedure performed, skill of the surgeon and anesthesiologist, postoperative management, and anesthetic agent. Most studies in this area have focused on coronary artery surgery, since usually only one endpoint, myocardial ischemia and infarction, is of interest, and many more coronary than vascular procedures are performed at any given institution.

Prior studies in coronary artery surgery patients have failed to show that anesthetic agents alter outcome,[1-6] although control of heart rate[3] and the incidence of perioperative ischemia[7,8] have been shown to be of importance. Surgical factors such as aortic cross-clamp time and number of grafts also play a role in coronary artery surgery and, of course, have no parallels in vascular surgery.

In aortic vascular surgery, the organs distal to the clamp are subjected to ischemia during the cross-clamp and those above, including the heart, are subjected to wide swings in perfusion pressure. The heart experiences dramatic changes in preload and afterload associated with clamping and release. Therefore, in aortic vascular surgery, not only is the heart subject to stress but other organs experience wide swings in perfusion associated with clamping and release. Any study of patients undergoing aortic vascular surgery should then examine morbidity associated not only with myocardial ischemia but also morbidity involving the kidneys, liver, brain, and lungs.

Two studies have been reported that examined outcome in patients undergoing major peripheral vascular surgery. Both report a decrease in morbidity associated with a reduction in stress attributable to the anesthetic agents used. These studies are reviewed here.

EPIDURAL ANESTHESIA AND ANALGESIA IN HIGH-RISK SURGICAL PATIENTS

Yeager et al.[9] studied patients scheduled for intrathoracic, intra-abdominal, or major peripheral vascular surgery. The patients were randomly assigned to epidural anesthesia and analgesia (EAA, group I), or general anesthesia and parenteral narcotic administration for postoperative pain relief (group II). In group I, patients were maintained with light levels of general anesthesia and received in-

TABLE 11.4   Serum and urine cortisol

	Group I (n)	Group II (n)	p Value
Serum cortisol (μg/dl)[a]			
1 hour after incision	12.6 $\pm$ 11.3 (20)	17.7 $\pm$ 19.2 (21)	NS
ICU arrival	14.6 $\pm$ 8.3 (19)	16.2 $\pm$ 14.5 (16)	NS
Urine cortisol excretion rate (μg/hr)[a]			
Total first 24 hours	37.2 $\pm$ 27.0 (16)	73.8 $\pm$ 61.9 (13)	0.025
Total second 24 hours	34.9 $\pm$ 58.0 (7)	30.3 $\pm$ 45.4 (8)	NS

NS, not significant. Data are mean $\pm$ standard deviation.
[a]Expressed as excess above baseline.

tient's anesthetic group. Plasma samples for catecholamine levels were drawn from an arterial line at 15 intervals beginning 20 minutes after the arterial line was inserted and before anesthetic induction, and ending with samples drawn on arrival in the recovery room. These intervals included periods of anticipated maximum stress, such as 3 minutes following incision, 3 and 7 minutes after aortic occlusion, and after removal of the aortic cross-clamp.

Results

Although the incidence or severity of preoperative disease and the volume of intraoperative fluid did not differ between groups, we found that fewer patients in the sufentanil group developed postoperative congestive heart failure on renal insufficiency (Table 11.5). When comparing the number of patients experiencing at least one complication, we found fewer in the sufentanil group than in the isoflurane group.

Of patients who developed renal insufficiency or congestive heart failure in the postoperative period, the mean of the highest norepinephrine levels of each patient was 730 $\pm$ 569 and 669 $\pm$ 560 (mean $\pm$ 1 SD), respectively, both greater than that of patients who did not have a complication (429 $\pm$ 320), $p \leq 0.001$ and $p \leq 0.05$, respectively. Of patients who developed renal insufficiency or

congestive heart failure in the postoperative period, the mean of the highest epinephrine levels was 1131 $\pm$ 550 and 754 $\pm$ 684 (mean $\pm$ 1 SD), respectively, both greater than that of patients who did not develop a complication, 264 $\pm$ 224, $p \leq 0.0005$ and $p \leq 0.001$, respectively.

The association of postoperative complications with greater intraoperative catecholamine levels occurred independently of the choice of anesthetic.

TABLE 11.5   Number of patients with postoperative complications

	Isoflurane (n = 50)	Sufentanil (n = 46)
Renal insufficiency	16	4[a]
Congestive heart failure	13	4[a]
Ventilation	9	4
Pneumonia	2	1
Renal failure (dialysis)	3	1
Stroke	2	0
Death	2	1
Jaundice	1	0
Myocardial infarction	0	1
Important or severe complication	20	9[a]
Severe complication	5	2
Important or severe complication and suprarenal clamp	17	7[a]

[a]$p \leq 0.05$ by Fisher's exact test (two sided).

Discussion

There are several similarities between the study by Yeager et al. and ours. In both studies, the anesthetic that led to a lower level of stress, as indicated by urinary cortisol in Yeager's study and by plasma catechols in our study, resulted in a lower incidence of morbidity. In both studies, congestive heart failure and the need for postoperative mechanical ventilation was higher in the group of patients experiencing the higher degree of stress. It is interesting to note that more patients in our isoflurane group required mechanical ventilation, even though one might expect patients receiving a moderately high dose of narcotic to be more likely to require postoperative mechanical ventilation than those receiving a volatile anesthetic.

Another factor in the outcome difference in our study may be the way our anesthetic techniques were planned and administered. Unlike the usual clinical practice of today, only morphine premedication added narcotic to the regimen in the isoflurane group. Usually, larger doses of narcotics are administered in conjunction with isoflurane. The addition of a narcotic to isoflurane blunts the stress response, whereas isoflurane alone is often ineffective, a fact not known at the time of this study. Perhaps if this study were repeated with additional narcotic administered to the patients in the isoflurane group, outcome might have been different. As a result of the study by Yeager et al. as well as ours, we must believe that even when anesthetic techniques or common anesthetic drugs are administered to the same hemodynamic endpoints, outcomes may be different.

REFERENCES

1. Tuman KJ, McCarthy RJ, Spiess BD, et al. Does choice of anesthetic agent significantly affect outcome after coronary artery surgery? Anesthesiology 1989;70:189–198.

2. Conahan TJ III, Ominsky AJ, Wollman H, et al. A prospective random comparison of halothane and morphine for open-heart anesthesia: one year's experience. Anesthesiology 1973;38:528–535.

3. Slogoff S, Keats AS. Randomized trial of primary anesthetic agents on outcome of coronary artery bypass operations. Anesthesiology 1989;70:179–188.

4. Kistner JR, Miller ED, Lake CL, et al. Indices of myocardial oxygenation during coronary-artery revascularization in man with morphine versus halothane anesthesia. Anesthesiology 1979;50:324–330.

5. Wilkinson PL, Hamilton WK, Moyers JR, et al. Halothane and morphine–nitrous oxide anesthesia in patients undergoing coronary artery bypass operation. Patterns of intraoperative ischemia. J Thorac Cardiovasc Surg 1981;82:372–382.

6. Moffitt EA, Sethna DH, Bussell JA, et al. Myocardial metabolism and hemodynamic responses to halothane or morphine anesthesia for coronary artery surgery. Anesth Analg 1982;61:979–985.

7. Slogoff S, Keats AS. Does perioperative myocardial ischemia lead to postoperative myocardial infarction? Anesthesiology 1985;62:107–114.

8. Knight AA, Hollenberg M, London MJ, et al. Perioperative myocardial ischemia: importance of the preoperative ischemic pattern. Anesthesiology 1988;68:681–688.

9. Yeager MP, Glass DD, Neff RK, et al. Epidural anesthesia and analgesia in high-risk surgical patients. Anesthesiology 1987;66:729–736.

10. Benefiel DJ, Roizen MF, Lampe GH, et al. Morbidity after aortic surgery with sufentanil vs. isoflurane anesthesia. Anesthesiology 1986;65:A516.

11. Roizen MF, Lampe GH, Benefiel DJ, et al. Is increased operative stress associated with worse outcome? Anesthesiology 1987;67:A1. (Abstr.)

As the sole anesthetic agent in combination with pancuronium, high doses of these narcotics are well tolerated in children of all ages with few hemodynamic effects. A recent study of ejection fraction and shortening fraction of fentanyl and sufentanil, compared with inhalation agents, in children with congenital heart disease showed minimal effects of myocardial depression with sufentanil and fentanyl compared to halothane.[18]

In addition to preserving hemodynamic stability when properly used, large doses of potent narcotics are also effective in blunting the marked stress responses that occur in neonates and in older children undergoing major surgery.[8-10] Suppression of these stress responses may be important in decreasing the morbidity of anesthesia and surgery.[8]

Both the amount of opioids needed for maximal suppression of stress in young children and the timing of opioid doses are somewhat controversial.[19] However, recent pharmacokinetic data suggest a more rational approach to the pediatric administration of potent narcotics. Pharmacokinetic data from several sources suggest that sufentanil and fentanyl can have a markedly prolonged and variable duration of action in neonates because of decreased clearance.[20-22] This is particularly true in premature infants. Clearance of potent narcotics then rapidly changes during the first month of life. It appears that by 1 month of age, the ability to clear sufentanil and fentanyl has markedly increased. By this age the duration of action of sufentanil and fentanyl is actually shorter in infants than in older children and adults.[23-25] Infants and young children thus may need more frequent doses and higher infusion rates of sufentanil and other narcotics than older children and adults.

Data on opioid-induced ventilatory depression, at least that with fentanyl, support these pharmacokinetic data. Ventilatory depression, measured by the incidence of apnea and episodes of apnea, increased with age in a recent study of infants, children, and adults.[26] An exception to this was the very young infant, under 2 months, who seems somewhat more susceptible to apnea. This suggests that fentanyl and probably the other potent synthetic narcotics can be used in older infants and children without undue fear of exaggerated respiratory depression. This may be particularly true in the case of alfentanil. Recent pharmacokinetic studies of alfentanil in children suggest that this narcotic may be particularly useful for pediatric ambulatory surgical cases. Its elimination half-life in young children is similar to, and may even be shorten than, that reported in adults.[27,28]

In the postoperative period, critical hemodynamic crises may be triggered by inadequate pain control. Following cardiac surgery, high-risk infants who have had complex intracardiac repairs and high pulmonary vascular resistance frequently have pulmonary hypertensive crises early postoperatively. These pulmonary hypertensive crises result in severe systemic hypotension and sometimes sudden death. They occur most frequently in agitated children and often respond to sedative and analgesic agents that block the stress of tracheal suctioning.[29] One potent narcotic, fentanyl, has been shown to block the stress responses to endotracheal suctioning in the pulmonary circulation of infants.[30] Thus, control of pain and stress with opioids in the postoperative period can potentially prevent deleterious hemodynamic crises leading to death postoperatively. This is in addition to the role of opioids in attenuating intraoperative metabolic and hormonal stress responses.

ROLE OF OPIOIDS IN MINOR PROCEDURES

The importance of stress responses in small children with minor surgical procedures is less certain, and few data are available. Certainly studies of circumcision in neonates have shown that substantial stress responses to this "minor" procedure occur, but their significance is unknown, other than documented short-term behavioral changes.[11] Deleterious decreases in arterial oxygen saturation and increases in serum cortisol levels result even from the stress of this procedure in the unanesthetized infant.[31,32]

Because the mechanisms by which stress may affect perioperative morbidity and recovery are poorly understood, it is difficult to detect subtle effects of inadequate stress protection during minor procedures on the perioperative clinical course and outcome. Whether perioperative control of pain and stress are equally valuable and important factors for the reduction of morbidity in minor surgical procedures in infants is less certain; this will require considerable investigation. However, smaller doses of opioids, particularly those with short half-lives like alfentanil, can help produce a smoother intraoperative course and still allow prompt awakening without clinically important respiratory depression.

PRELIMINARY EVIDENCE FOR EFFECTS ON OUTCOME

Some preliminary evidence from our institution suggests that in cases of extreme stress in very young neonates, even hospital mortality may be affected by the perioperative control of pain and stress. Effects of extremes of stress and pain on the immune system, protein synthesis and wound healing, coagulation, and tissue energy stores all have been shown in isolated systems, and some of these mechanisms might mediate effects on mortality and morbidity. Present evidence clearly shows that hormonal and metabolic stress responses to operation in children can be markedly attenuated using potent opioids. However, opioids by themselves, even at the highest doses that have been used clinically, do not totally block stress responses, even in neonates.[9,10] Other anesthetic agents probably will have to be added to opioids if the goal of complete, temporary suppression of stress responses is to be achieved.

Further research is required to investigate if effects of stress other than hormonal and metabolic responses can also be attenuated by opioids. The role of other agents added to opioids in further suppression of stress responses also needs to be investigated in children. However, there is mounting evidence that outcome of anesthesia and operation in pediatric patients undergoing extreme stress may be favorably influenced by even partial control of such stress using opioids alone.

REFERENCES

1. Beecher HK, Todd DP. A study of the deaths associated with anesthesia and surgery. Ann Surg 1954;140:2–34.
2. Graff TD, et al. Baltimore anesthesia study committee: factors in pediatric anesthesia mortality. Anesth Analg (Cleve) 1964;43:407–410.
3. West JP. Cardiac arrest during anaesthesia and surgery. Ann Surg 1954;140:623–629.
4. Harrison GG. Death attributable to anaesthesia: a ten-year survey. Br J Anaesth 1978;50:1041–1046.
5. Yeager MP, Glass DD, Neff RK, et al. Epidural anesthesia and analgesia in high-risk surgical patients. Anesthesiology 1987;66:729–736.
6. Roizen MF, Lampe GH, Benefiel DJ, et al. Is increased operative stress associated with worse outcome? Anesthesiology 1987;67:A1. (Abstr.)
7. Moyer E, Cerra F, Chenier R, et al. Multiple systems organ failure. IV death predictors in the trauma septic state—the most critical determinants. J Trauma 1981;21:862–869.
8. Anand KJS, Sippell WG, Aynsley-Green A. Randomized trial of fentanyl anaesthesia in preterm babies undergoing surgery: effects on the stress response. Lancet 1987;1:243–248.
9. Anand KJS, Hickey PR. Randomized trial of high-dose sufentanil anesthesia in neonates undergoing cardiac surgery: effects on the metabolic stress response. Anesthesiology 1987;67:A502. (Abstr.)
10. Anand KJS, Carr DB, Hickey PR. Randomized trial of high-dose sufentanil anesthesia in neonates undergoing cardiac surgery: hormonal and hemodynamic stress responses. Anesthesiology 1987;67:A501. (Abstr.)
11. Anand KJS, Hickey PR. Pain and its effects in the human fetus and neonate. N Engl J Med 1987;317:1321–1329.
12. Berry FA, Gregory GA. Do premature infants require anesthesia for surgery? Anesthesiology 1987;67:291–293.

13. Hickey PR, Hansen DH. Fentanyl- and sufentanyl-oxygen-pancuronium anesthesia for cardiac surgery in infants. Anesth Analg 1984;63:117–124.

14. Moore RA, Yang SS, McNicholas KW, et al. Hemodynamic and anesthetic effects of sufentanil as the sole anesthetic for pediatric cardiovascular surgery. Anesthesiology 1985;62:725–731.

15. Hickey PR, Hansen DD, Wessel DW, et al. Pulmonary and systemic hemodynamic responses to fentanyl in infants. Anesth Analg 1985;64:483–486.

16. Yaster M, Koehler RC, Traystman RJ. Effects of fentanyl on peripheral and cerebral hemodynamics in neonatal lambs. Anesthesiology 1987;66:524–530.

17. Hansen DD, Hickey PR. Anesthesia for hypoplastic left-heart syndrome: use of high-dose fentanyl in 30 neonates. Anesth Analg 1986;65:127–132.

18. Glenski JA, Feisen RH, Bergund NL, et al. Comparison of the hemodynamic and echocardiographic effects of sufentanil, fentanyl, isoflurane, and halothane for pediatric cardiovascular surgery. J Cardiothorac Anesth 1988;2:147–155.

19. Yaster M. The dose response of fentanyl in neonatal anesthesia. Anesthesiology 1987;66:433–435.

20. Greeley WJ, De Bruijn NP. Changes in sufentanil pharmacokinetics within the neonatal period. Anesth Analg 1988;67:86–90.

21. Koehntop DE, Rodman JH, Brundage DM, et al. Pharmacokinetics of fentanyl in neonates. Anesth Analg 1986;65:227–232.

22. Collins C, Koren G, Crean P, et al. Fentanyl pharmacokinetics and hemodynamics effects in preterm infants during ligation of patent ductus arteriosus. Anesth Analg 1985;64:1078–1080.

23. Singleton MA, Rosen JI, Fisher DM. Plasma concentration of fentanyl in infants, children, and adults. Can Anaesth Soc J 1987;34:152–155.

24. Greeley WJ, De Bruijn NP, Davis DP. Sufentanil pharmacokinetics in pediatric cardiovascular patients. Anesth Analg 1987;66:1067–1072.

25. Davis PJ, Cook DR, Stiller RL, et al. Pharmacodynamics and pharmacokinetics of high-dose sufentanil in infants and children undergoing cardiac surgery. Anesth Analg 1987;66:203–208.

26. Hertzka RE, Gauntlett IS, Fisher DM, et al. Fentanyl-induced ventilatory depression: effects of age. Anesthesiology 1989;70:213–218.

27. Meistelman C, Saint-Maurice C, Lepaul M, et al. A comparison of alfentanil pharmacokinetics in children and adults. Anesthesiology 1987;66:13–16.

28. Goresky GV, Koren G, Sabourin MA, et al. The pharmacokinetics of alfentanil in children. Anesthesiology 1987;67:654–659.

29. Del Nido PJ, Williams WG, Villamater J, et al. Changes in pericardial surface pressure during pulmonary hypertensive crises after cardiac surgery. Circulation 1987;76 (suppl 3):93–96.

30. Hickey PR, Hansen DD, Wessel DL, et al. Blunting of stress responses in the pulmonary circulation of infants by fentanyl. Anesth Analg 1985;64:1137–1142.

31. Maxwell LG, Yaster M, Witzel RC, et al. Penile nerve block for circumcision. Obstet Gynecol 1987;70:415–419.

32. Stang HJ, Gummar AR, Snellman L, et al. Local anesthesia for circumcision: stress and cortisol responses. JAMA 1988;259:1507–1511.

13 OPIOIDS AND SAME-DAY SURGERY

Surinder K. Kallar and Gareth W. Jones

The ideal anesthetic agent for outpatient surgery should be able to produce a rapid and smooth onset of action, intraoperative analgesia and amnesia, good surgical conditions, and a short recovery period with minimal or no side effects. In addition, the ideal technique should be flexible enough for use in surgical procedures ranging in duration and degree of surgical stimulation from a 10-minute dilatation and curettage to a lengthier surgical procedure like a 6-hour plastic surgery operation. The technique would also be required to blunt cardiovascular responses to tracheal intubation, skin incision, and noxious intraoperative stimuli without compromising the recovery period, and to provide deep anesthesia for short procedures when necessary but still allow patients to recover quickly and be home-ready within 2 hours or less.

It is clear that at this time no single anesthetic agent is available to meet these demands. Inhaled anesthetic agents remain extremely popular in outpatient anesthesia, as they are considered to be controllable and easy to use during surgery, but the introduction of intravenous anesthetic agents with rapid onset of action and short elimination half-lives has

The authors thank Annette H. Jackson for her expertise in typing this manuscript.

provided an alternative technique for induction and maintenance of anesthesia in the outpatient facility. The intravenous agents can be used alone (total intravenous anesthesia) or in combination with volatile agents to achieve rapid recovery from anesthesia. Whether used alone or in conjunction with volatile agents, either an intermittent intravenous (IV) bolus or infusion technique can be selected. Epstein et al.[1] have shown that pretreatment with a rapid and short-acting opioid analgesic (fentanyl 1 to 2 µg/kg) significantly reduces anesthetic requirements during brief outpatient procedures and therefore decreases recovery time. In addition, the use of intravenous agents satisfies increasing concern over environmental pollution caused by the volatile anesthetic agents.

Intermittent bolus administration of intravenous agents results in rapid increases and decreases in blood concentrations of these drugs. As a result, the depth of anesthesia and analgesia oscillates above and below the effective level. These peaks and valleys of blood concentration can be minimized by using intravenous infusions of short-acting agents, which also decreases the total amount of drug administered.

The opioids fentanyl and alfentanil are the two most widely used narcotic analgesics in outpatient anesthesia. Compared with the older narcotic analgesics, both have rapid onset of action and relatively short elimination half-lives. Alfentanil, however, has the more appropriate pharmacokinetic profile for use as a continuous infusion. In this chapter, we discuss pharmacokinetics of the opioids as they effect the choice of agent in outpatient surgery, different regimens utilizing opioids, and their side effects.

PHARMACOKINETICS

Fentanyl and alfentanil are the two most frequently used opioids in outpatient anesthesia because in addition to being short-acting narcotic analgesics they also exert minimal cardiovascular depression, are metabolized without generating toxic compounds, and blunt the cardiovascular and hormonal responses to noxious stimuli. Alfentanil has a shorter duration of action than fentanyl because of its elimination half-life of 94 minutes as compared to fentanyl's 180 minutes.[2] Fentanyl is in fact cleared from the serum five times as fast as alfentanil, but the prolonged half-life results from the much larger volume of distribution (V_d fentanyl 4 l/kg, V_d alfentanil 0.6 l/kg). This is a result of fentanyl's much greater lipid solubility compared to alfentanil.

The ionization constant (pka) for alfentanil is 6.5, compared to 8.4 for fentanyl;[3,4] therefore at physiologic pH, 89% of alfentanil will be unionized compared to 9% for fentanyl. The unionized form of a drug is more freely diffusible, and therefore alfentanil is able to cross membranes rapidly and produce a more rapid onset of action than fentanyl.

These pharmacokinetic characteristics make these agents well suited for use in ambulatory surgery units, where quick emergence and rapid recovery from anesthesia are desirable. The agents can be used in an intermittent bolus technique or by continuous infusion. The shorter elimination half-life of alfentanil makes it the more suitable of the two agents for continuous infusion techniques.

Ausems et al.[5] have shown that different infusion rates are required to adequately inhibit the responses to the varying perioperative stimuli. The highest plasma levels were required to obtund the intubation response, with lower levels to cover the effects of wound incision and closure: in the presence of nitrous oxide a lower plasma level, and hence a lower infusion rate, was required for wound closure than was required for spontaneous ventilation. It is therefore necessary for the anesthesiologist to vary the infusion rates or administer intermittent boluses depending on the degree of stimulus and the response of the patient.

Several investigators have noted that the pharmacokinetics of alfentanil are not totally predictable. Maitre et al.[6] studied 45 patients who received 50 µg/kg bolus alfentanil and reported that the interindividual variability for the initial distribution was approximately 30% and the variability for total body clearance was approximately 50%. Some of this variability can be attributed to age. Sitar et al.[7] have shown that older patients metabolize alfentanil more slowly but with less interindividual variability. Clearance is also decreased in obese patients and patients with liver disease. It is important, therefore, when utilizing these techniques, that the anesthesiologist remain vigilant and adjust the regimen to suit the patient.

COMPARISON OF RECOVERY TIMES AND DOSAGES

A rapid and complete recovery of the patient is essential for the effective running of an outpatient surgery facility. In order to maintain an efficient flow of patients without overburdening the postanesthesia care unit, the patients need to become alert and clear-headed as quickly as possible. For this reason, short-acting anesthetic agents have become popular in the outpatient facility. Fentanyl has been widely used and is still popular in outpatient surgery but is being replaced more frequently by alfentanil because of the latter's more favorable pharmacokinetics, which result in rapid recovery.

Several investigators have reported the results of their studies of alfentanil and fentanyl for induction or maintenance of anesthesia during short surgical procedures.[8–16] Depending on the amount of drug administered, recovery times following the use of alfentanil were either similar[8,13,14] or shorter[9,12,15,16] than those reported following the use of fentanyl[8,14,16] or halothane.[15]

Kallar and Keenan[16] studied 43 outpatients presenting for dilatation and evacuation who were treated with intravenous bolus doses of either fentanyl or alfentanil as the supplement to methohexital, nitrous oxide in oxygen anesthesia. They evaluated both the speed and quality of patients' recovery. The patients were given either 2 μg/kg fentanyl or 6 to 8 μg/kg alfentanil as a loading dose and supplemented with either 0.5 to 1.5 μg/kg fentanyl or 2 to 5 μg/kg alfentanil as required. Recovery time was evaluated on the basis of the time elapsed from the end of the maintenance phase to the time to respond to command, to establish alertness, and to complete the finger-to-nose test. Quality of the recovery was assessed using a recovery score of 0 to 2 for two parameters: respiration and consciousness. The results showed a significant reduction in time to establish alertness with alfentanil (16 minutes) as compared with fentanyl (25 minutes) (Figure 13.1). Figure 13.2 demonstrates the evaluation of patients' recovery during the first postoperative hour. A significantly greater number of patients in the alfentanil group had complete recovery at 20 minutes ($p = 0.03$) and 30 minutes ($p = 0.05$). The median time for complete recovery of respiration and consciousness was significantly shorter with alfentanil (13 minutes) than with fentanyl (35 minutes) ($p = 0.007$).

White and coworkers[17] compared alfentanil and fentanyl infusions in addition to bolus administration in a study of 100 outpatients presenting for dilatation and extraction. The patients were subdivided into four groups: group 1 received a bolus dose of 100 μg fen-

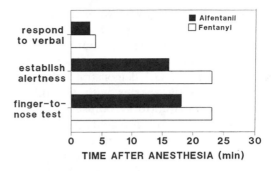

FIGURE 13.1 Median times for recovery parameters for anesthesia. (Reprinted with permission of the publisher from Kallar SK, Keenan RL. Evaluation and comparison of recovery time from alfentanil and fentanyl for short surgical procedures. Anesthesiology 1984;61:A379.)

tanyl at induction with supplements of 50 μg IV; group 2 received 100 μg fentanyl at induction and an infusion of 10 μg/min fentanyl; group 3 received a bolus dose of 500 μg alfentanil at induction with supplements of 250 μg; group 4 received 500 μg alfentanil at induction with an infusion of 50 μg/min. All patients received thiopental sodium (4 mg/kg) and nitrous oxide (70%) in oxygen. The following

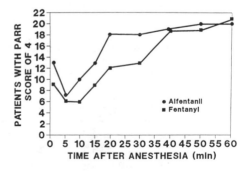

FIGURE 13.2 Proportion of patients receiving the best possible combined score for quality of consciousness and respiration. (Reprinted with permission of the publisher from Kallar SK, Keenan RL. Evaluation and comparison of recovery time from alfentanil and fentanyl for short surgical procedures. Anesthesiology 1984;61:A379.)

measurements of recovery were made: awakening time (time to respond to simple commands), orientation time (orientated in time and place), and ambulation time (time to walk unassisted). Table 13.1 demonstrates that times were significantly shorter with the infusion technique compared to IV boluses in three of the comparisons and also that the use of alfentanil resulted in significantly shorter recovery times than fentanyl in all the comparisons. In addition, the patients in the alfentanil infusion group had significantly lower Trieger scores (measurement of psychomotor function) and lower sedation analog scores than those in the fentanyl infusion groups in the early postoperative period. The authors concluded that alfentanil has some clinically significant advantages over fentanyl as a supplement to outpatient anesthesia and that dose requirements can be reduced by the use of infusions, thereby reducing recovery times.

The dosage of alfentanil should be adjusted to different anesthetic techniques (e.g., mask versus intubation) and to the length and type of surgery (e.g., a superficial procedure versus intra-abdominal procedure). Therefore, in establishing the initial drug dosage, both the technique used by the anesthesiologist and the experience of the surgeon should be taken into consideration. Although the time to complete

TABLE 13.1 Postoperative recovery times of fentanyl and alfentanil

Drug Group	Recovery Times (min)[a]		
	Awake	Oriented	Ambulatory
FB	5.2 ± 0.9	7.7 ± 1.1	67 ± 5
FI	3.7 ± 0.8[b]	6.1 ± 1.2	55 ± 5
AB	2.5 ± 0.8[c]	3.5 ± 0.4[c]	48 ± 4[c]
AI	1.2 ± 0.1[b,c]	2.6 ± 0.3[b,c]	41 ± 3[c]

Source: Reprinted with permission of the publisher from White PF, Coe V, Shafer A, et al. Comparison of alfentanil with fentanyl for outpatient anesthesia. Anesthesiology 1986;64:99–106.

[a]Mean values ± SEM.

[b]AI or FI group significantly different from AB or FB group ($p < 0.05$), respectively.

[c]AB or AI group significantly different from FB or FI group ($p < 0.05$), respectively.

recovery is slightly shorter with infusion techniques, intermittent boluses remain popular in the outpatient facility because of familiarity with the technique and simplicity of use. An initial dose of 10 to 20 µg/kg alfentanil can be used for procedures lasting less than 30 minutes. For longer procedures and those requiring intubation, 20 to 50 µg/kg alfentanil given slowly in divided doses is recommended. Incremental doses should range from 3 to 7 µg/kg.[18] Administering alfentanil slowly minimizes the incidence of chest wall rigidity and hypotension while ensuring loss of consciousness and hemodynamic stability during laryngoscopy and intubation. The use of a small dose of nondepolarizing muscle relaxant as a pretreatment would be expected to further decrease the incidence of chest wall rigidity. Droperidol (0.625 to 1.25 mg, IV) should be administered before induction of anesthesia to prevent postoperative nausea and vomiting. The dose of alfentanil should be reduced in elderly and debilitated patients.

For continuous infusion, alfentanil should be started at a rate of 0.5 to 1.5 µg/kg/min immediately following a loading dose of 25 to 50 µg/kg in the average patient.[19] During the operation, the alfentanil maintenance infusion rate should be varied depending on the clinical responses to the surgical stimuli. In patients with signs of inadequate hypnosis, small bolus doses of 25 to 50 mg thiopental or 10 to 20 mg methohexital can be administered. If clinical signs of inadequate analgesia are noted, e.g., acute hypertensive episodes, pupillary dilatation, lacrimation, or diaphoresis, a small bolus dose of 5 to 10 µg/kg alfentanil, followed by an increase in the maintenance infusion rate, would be recommended.

Conscious sedation is another technique gaining increasing popularity for outpatients; short-acting opioids are an integral part of any drug combination used for this technique to supplement local or regional anesthesia. Boldy et al.[20] have shown that when a benzodiazepine is supplemented with a narcotic analgesic, there is a significant improvement in patient cooperation during the procedure and more profound sedation than with benzodiazepine alone.

At the Medical College of Virginia,[21] the conscious sedation technique includes administration of 2 to 3 mg midazolam followed by a bolus dose of 250 to 500 μg alfentanil or 50 to 100 μg fentanyl along with 20 to 30 mg methohexital. With these doses, the patient should be able to obey commands but not otherwise respond to the surroundings. Incremental doses of alfentanil (250 μg), or methohexital (10 to 20 mg) are given to maintain this subanesthetic level. It is essential that the patient be monitored with a pulse oximeter during conscious sedation technique.

SIDE EFFECTS

The side effects of opioids are primarily dose-dependent and include nausea, vomiting, bradycardia, and respiratory and cardiovascular depression. The incidence of side effects associated with alfentanil is reported to be similar to that associated with fentanyl (Table 13.2).[8,10,12,17]

The inclusion of narcotics in the anesthetic technique has been shown to increase postoperative nausea and vomiting.[22] Pollard,[23] however, has demonstrated that the addition of droperidol to a narcotic-based anesthetic technique can reduce the incidence of postoperative nausea and vomiting so that it is comparable to that seen with isoflurane anesthesia. In some circumstances, analgesics may reduce postoperative nausea and vomiting,[24] e.g., if related to pain. Prophylactic use of droperidol (0.625 to 1.25 mg, IV) administered before induction of anesthesia markedly reduces the incidence of postoperative nausea and vomiting.[25]

Fentanyl and alfentanil cause vagally mediated bradycardia, especially after larger bolus doses.[26] Large doses of alfentanil (250 μg/kg) have been administered to healthy patients without untoward cardiovascular effects, but in the presence of antihypertensive medication, 40 μg/kg alfentanil has produced hypotension and bradycardia.[27] Furthermore, there have been case reports of severe bradycardia and asystole occurring after small doses of alfentanil (20 μg/kg) used in combination with succinylcholine.[28,29]

Andrews et al.[30] have demonstrated that both fentanyl and alfentanil produce similar depression of ventilation when administered in equipotent continuous infusions. Because of the shorter β elimination half-life of alfentanil, the effect diminishes much more quickly than with fentanyl, but even in the case of fentanyl the effect was negligible 1 hour after cessation of the infusion. Scamman et al.[31] measured respiratory depression following intravenous bolus injections of fentanyl and alfentanil. The doses used were similar to those employed in outpatient anesthesia (1.5 or 3 μg/kg fentanyl and 7.5 or 15 μg/kg alfentanil). The results also demonstrated more prolonged respiratory depression with fentanyl. Depression of respiratory function was detectable up to 80 minutes after the larger dose of fentanyl and for 30 minutes with the lower dose. For alfentanil, depression of respiration was present for up to 4 minutes with the larger dose and not at all with the lower dose. Scamman et al.[31] also concluded that fentanyl was 13 times as potent as alfentanil as a respiratory depressant on a milligram-for-milligram basis, whereas an analgesic potency ratio of 10 has been reported.

The risk of significant respiratory depression, therefore, disappears much more quickly with alfentanil, but several investigators have noted the greater interindividual variability of

TABLE 13.2 Side effects of fentanyl and alfentanil

Drug Group	Side Effects (%)			
	Nausea	Vomit	Dizzy	Drowsy
FB	60	48	52	36
FI	68	60	24	28
AB	52	36	24	16
AI	68	60	28	8[a]

Source: Reprinted with permission of the publisher from White PF, Coe V, Shafer A, et al. Comparison of alfentanil with fentanyl for outpatient anesthesia. Anesthesiology 1986;64:99–106.

[a]AI group significantly different from FI group ($p < 0.05$).

effect with alfentanil,[6,30] and there has been a recent case report of respiratory depression occurring 15 minutes after the return of adequate ventilation in a patient who received an alfentanil infusion.[32] The authors were unable to explain the event but postulate that patients who exhibit abnormal pharmacokinetics may be at risk of late respiratory depression.

Increasing age does effect metabolism of alfentanil. Sitar et al.[7] have demonstrated that older patients have a prolonged β elimination half-life and are therefore at risk of respiratory depression for a longer period of time. The effect in infants and young children is unclear, but Hertzka et al.[33] have demonstrated that there is no difference between the degree of respiratory depression from fentanyl seen in infants greater than 3 months or young children and that seen in adults.

If respiratory depression requires treatment, the opioid antagonist naloxone in increments of 0.4 mg is effective; in addition, Bailey et al.[34] have shown that the partial antagonist nalbuphine (2.5 mg) is equally effective in reversing respiratory depression but has less effect on reversing analgesia. Because respiratory depression may last longer than the action of the opioid antagonist, it is important to emphasize that appropriate postoperative monitoring (e.g., pulse oximetry) should be employed with the use of alfentanil, particularly after infusion and large doses, to ensure that adequate spontaneous breathing is established and maintained in the absence of stimulation prior to discharging the patient from the recovery area. It has been observed that increasing familiarity with the characteristics of alfentanil may reduce the need for reversal.

Chest wall rigidity has been demonstrated with fentanyl[31] and alfentanil[32] but requires large doses. Scamman[35] found that chest rigidity occurred with a mean fentanyl dose of 17 μg/kg. Benthuysen et al.[36] used a dose of 175 μg/kg alfentanil in their study of rigidity. It was also demonstrated that all muscle groups are affected and reflect a neurohumeral mechanism. Scamman et al.[31] postulate that glottic rigidity may be responsible for the difficulty in ventilation. In all cases, rigidity was abol-ished by neuromuscular blockade. These large doses of opioids are inappropriate for outpatient use, and it is unlikely that muscle rigidity will cause problems in the outpatient facility. The mental effects of alfentanil and fentanyl have been studied by Scamman and coworkers,[31] who demonstrated that in small doses (fentanyl 1.5 to 3.0 μg/kg; alfentanil 7.5 to 15 μg/kg) opioids do not specifically impair memory, and any decrease in learning ability is due to decreased alertness and attention. However, larger doses of fentanyl do decrease motor coordination and control. As is not the case with diazepam, the inability to perform motor tests was perceived by the subject.

DRUG INTERACTIONS

Opioids may potentiate the action of other anesthetic agents, particularly sedatives. This interaction, however, can be beneficial in that total doses of the agents can be reduced to produce a faster recovery period. Dundee et al.[37] have shown that pretreatment with either 100 μg fentanyl or 300 μg alfentanil reduced the induction dose of thiopental sodium from a mean of 4.6 mg/kg in the control group to 3.3 mg/kg for the fentanyl pretreatment group and 3.76 μg/kg for the alfentanil group. In addition, pretreatment with opioids reduces the time taken to induce anesthesia with an induction dose of midazolam.[38]

Patients receiving erythromycin may demonstrate prolonged β elimination half-lives with alfentanil. Bartkowski et al.[39] have postulated that this is due to an inhibition of alfentanil's metabolism by the erythromycin.

CONCLUSION

In the past, it is probable that all the opioids have been used in the anesthetic management of outpatients; however, the pharmacokinetics of fentanyl and particularly alfentanil make these the most rational choice in the ambulatory patient. Opioids are required in outpatient anesthesia to provide analgesia, obtund stress response during surgical stimulation, and reduce the amount of other anesthetics required in order to provide a rapid return to home-readiness. Furthermore, as has been outlined in this chapter, although they may cause nausea and vomiting as side effects, opioids can also reduce the incidence of nausea and vomiting where these are due to postoperative pain.

With the pressure from hospital administration, medical insurance companies, and surgeons to undertake more complex surgery and to operate on patients in the ASA physical status III, the need for and use of potent short-acting opioids in the outpatient facility will expand. We have outlined possible therapeutic regimens incorporating opioids that have been used successfully for outpatient surgery but would emphasize the need for vigilant monitoring and continuous assessment of the patient, so that the prescribed regimens can be tailored to the individual and therefore limit the total dose of opioids (and other agents) to achieve the primary aim of ambulatory surgery, that is, to produce a rapid return to home-readiness.

REFERENCES

1. Epstein BS, Levy M, Thein MH, et al. Evaluation of fentanyl as an adjunct to thiopental-N_2O-O_2 anesthesia for short surgical procedures. Anesthesiol Rev 1975;2:24.

2. Bovill JG, Sebel PS, Blackburn CL, et al. The pharmacokinetics of alfentanil (R39209): a new opioid analgesic. Anesthesiology 1982;57:439–443.

3. Hull CJ. The pharmacokinetics of alfentanil. Br J Anaesth 1983;55:157S.

4. Meuldermans WEG, Hurkmans RMA, et al. Plasma protein binding and distribution of fentanyl, sufentanil, alfentanil, and lofentanil in blood. Arch Int Pharmacodyn Ther 1982;257:4–19.

5. Ausems ME, Hug CC Jr, de Lange S. Variable rate infusion of alfentanil as a supplement to nitrous oxide anesthesia for general surgery. Anesth Analg 1983;62:982–986.

6. Maitre PO, Vezeh S, Heykants J, et al. Population pharmacokinetics of alfentanil: the average dose–plasma concentration relationship and interindividual variability in patients. Anesthesiology 1987;66:3–12.

7. Sitar DS, Duke PC, Benthuysen JL, et al. Aging and alfentanil disposition in healthy volunteers and surgical patients. Can Anaesth Soc J 1989;36:149–154.

8. Rosow CE, Latta WB, Keegan CR, et al. Alfentanil and fentanyl in short surgical procedures. Anesthesiology 1983;59:A345. (Abstr.)

9. Patrick M, Eagar B, Toft DF, et al. Alfentanil-supplemented anesthesia for short procedures: a double-blind comparison with fentanyl. Anesthesiology 1983;59:A346. (Abstr.)

10. Coe V, Shafer A, White PF. Techniques for administering alfentanil during outpatient anesthesia: a comparison with fentanyl. Anesthesiology 1983;59:A347. (Abstr.)

11. Kay B, Cohen AT. Intravenous anaesthesia for minor surgery: a comparison of etomidate or althesin with fentanyl and alfentanil. Br J Anaesth 1983;55:165S–167S.

12. Kay B, Venkataraman P. Recovery after fentanyl and alfentanil in anaesthesia for minor surgery. Br J Anaesth 1983;55:169S–171S.

13. Hull CJ, Jacobson L. A clinical trial of alfentanil as an adjuvant for short anaesthetic procedures. Br J Anaesth 1983;55:173S–178S.

14. Cooper GM, O'Connor M, Mark J, et al. Effect of alfentanil and fentanyl on recovery from brief anaesthesia. Br J Anaesth 1983;55:179S–182S.

15. Youngberg JA, Subaiya C, Graybar GB, et al. Alfentanil for day-stay surgery in children: an evaluation. Anesth Analg 1984;63:A284. (Abstr.)

16. Kallar SK, Keenan RL. Evaluation and comparison of recovery time from alfentanil and fentanyl for short surgical procedures. Anesthesiology 1984;61:A379. (Abstr.)

17. White PF, Coe V, Shafer A, et al. Comparison of alfentanil with fentanyl for outpatient anesthesia. Anesthesiology 1986;64:99–106.

18. Kallar SK. Opioid anesthesia for ambulatory surgery utilizing an intermittent bolus technique. Piscataway, N.J.: Janssen Pharmaceutica, 1987.

19. White PF. Opioid anesthesia for ambulatory surgery utilizing continuous infusion techniques. Piscataway, N.J.: Janssen Pharmaceutica, 1987.

20. Boldy DAR, English JSC, Lang GS, et al.

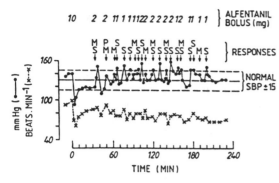

FIGURE 13.4 Course of anesthesia during administration of multiple alfentanil boluses, showing alfentanil doses and patient responses. Reprinted with permission of the authors and publisher from Ausems ME, Vuyk J, Hug CC Jr, Stanski DR. Comparison of a computer-assisted infusion versus intermittent bolus administration of alfentanil as a supplement to nitrous oxide for lower abdominal surgery. Anesthesiology 1988;68:851–861.)

continuous variable infusion technique. Especially for shorter cases, use of a continuous variable infusion has additional convenience. The administration of alfentanil by infusion is much simpler than by repeated, multiple boluses. To enable rapid adjustment of opioid blood levels during variable continuous infusion, the drug administration technique consists of a loading dose, given by bolus(es) or rapid infusion, followed by a maintenance infusion.

Both of the opioids commonly used for same-day surgery have been investigated and used by variable continuous infusion: fentanyl[3] and alfentanil.[2] Alfentanil in particular is appropriate for administration by continuous infusion because of the drug's pharmacokinetic properties, which include rapid opioid equilibration between plasma and site of action, rapid redistribution from brain to nonresponsive tissues, and rapid elimination from the body without the formation of active metabolites.[2]

The theoretical advantages of alfentanil administration by variable rate infusion have been borne out in patient studies. Some of these data have been presented by Dr. Kallar in her discussion of White et al.[4] Those authors compared the administration of fentanyl and alfentanil by infusion or intermittent bolus in brief outpatient gynecologic

procedures. The patients who received opioid by infusion required lower total doses and had fewer intraoperative side effects such as chest wall rigidity (requiring succinylcholine), apnea, or slowed respiration (< 5 breaths/minute). The infusion patients also had significantly shorter recovery times for awakening, orientation, and ambulation. These results are complemented by the data from general surgical patients studied by Ausems et al.[1] Patients who received opioid by infusion rather than by intermittent bolus had a smoother intraoperative course. They demonstrated a significantly lower incidence of hemodynamic, autonomic, and somatic responses to stimuli and a lower incidence of rigidity. In addition, the plasma concentrations of alfentanil at skin closure and awakening were significantly lower in the infusion group, and the number of patients who required naloxone to sustain adequate postoperative ventilation after discontinuation of N_2O was significantly smaller.

On the basis of these data, we prefer to give alfentanil to day-surgery patients at Brigham and Women's Hospital by continuous variable infusion.[5] A variety of equipment can be used for infusion, from an in-line burette to a computer-controlled volumetric infusion pump. We primarily use a syringe pump, the Bard Alfentanil Infuser. The syringe pump has the advantages of using undiluted drug, being calibrated for commonly used alfentanil dosage increments, and avoiding the need for intraoperative calculations. Adjustment of the pump controls for opioid infusion rate and intermittent bolus is directly analogous to adjusting a volatile anesthetic agent vaporizer.

The anesthetic technique we employ for day-surgery patients may begin with mild premedication. If a benzodiazepine is used, the dose should be reduced so as not to compound postoperative sedation. Alfentanil administration is started during the application of monitoring devices in the operating room (Table 13.4). A 10 μg/kg alfentanil bolus is given and the infusion is begun at a rate of 0.5 μg/kg/min. An additional 5 to 10 μg/kg initial bolus

TABLE 13.4 Dosage of alfentanil by infusion for day surgery

Initial bolus	10 μg/kg
Initial infusion	0.5 μg/kg/min
Incremental bolus	5–10 μg/kg
Incremental infusion	+0.5 μg/kg/min
	−0.25 μg/kg/min

is given after assessing the patient's respiratory rate and sedation. Anesthetic induction is performed with barbiturate or equivalent agent in reduced, titrated doses and 75% N_2O is administered. Neuromuscular blocking drugs are used if endotracheal intubation is planned. During the operation, additional alfentanil is given for signs of light anesthesia or in anticipation of significant surgical stimulation. At that time, an additional 5 to 10 μg/kg bolus is given alone or with an increase in the infusion rate to 1.0 μg/kg/min. The latter infusion rate is often needed for more intrusive surgery. If the patient exhibits no response to intraoperative stimuli, the infusion rate is titrated downward until the minimal effective dose is reached. Alfentanil infusion is terminated within 5 to 10 minutes of the end of the procedure, depending on its duration. A total intravenous anesthesia technique for day-surgery patients has been reported by others,[6] using a combination of alfentanil and a hypnotic such as midazolam; however, we recommend its use only for long cases.

Alfentanil given as a component of general anesthesia for day surgery may produce a drop in heart rate. This bradycardia is due to increased vagal activity, possibly secondary to stimulation of the central vagal nucleus, and has been observed with all opioids except meperidine. When alfentanil-induced increased vagal tone is enhanced by other vagal stimuli, sinus arrest has been reported. Maryniak and Bishop[7] gave 30 μg/kg alfentanil followed by the stimulus of lidocaine spray to the laryngeal mucosa. Two patients experienced sinus arrests of 10 and 12 seconds, which spontaneously reverted to nodal and then sinus rhythm. A third patient developed a sinus bradycardia of 37 beats per minute. Rivard and Lebowitz[8] reported similar occurrences with alfentanil (22 μg/kg) given in conjunction with succinylcholine for intubation. Sinus arrest has also occurred with sufentanil-succinylcholine. During alfentanil-containing anesthetics, a definite bradycardia is common in the absence of significant surgical stimulus; it responds well to atropine if needed.

An additional comment should be made concerning the use of naloxone to reverse opioid-induced respiratory depression. In order to avoid the problem of excessive reversal of analgesia, naloxone should preferably be titrated in small increments of 0.04 mg, and the effect of each dose assessed. Also, a syndrome of hypertension, pulmonary edema, ventricular extrasystoles, and cardiac arrest has been reported in young healthy adults who have received low-dose naloxone, as little as 0.08 mg.[9] As the authors point out, the duration of acton of naloxone is relatively short. The serum half-life of naloxone is approximately 1 hour, and if the original opioid dose was large, reappearance of narcotic effect may occur. The importance of continued postoperative observation and monitoring cannot be overemphasized.

REFERENCES

1. Ausems ME, Vuyk J, Hug CC Jr, et al. Comparison of a computer-assisted infusion versus intermittent bolus administration of alfentanil as a supplement to nitrous oxide for lower abdominal surgery. Anesthesiology 1988;68:851–861.
2. Ausems ME, Hug CC Jr, Stanski DR, et al. Plasma concentrations of alfentanil required to supplement nitrous oxide anesthesia for general surgery. Anesthesiology 1986;65:362–373.
3. White PF. Clinical uses of intravenous anesthetic and analgesic infusions. Anesth Analg 1989;68:161–171.
4. White PF, Coe V, Shafer A, et al. Comparison of alfentanil with fentanyl for outpatient anesthesia. Anesthesiology 1986;64:99–106.
5. Philip BK. Dilatation and curettage. In: Anesthesia and outpatient surgery. Piscataway, N.J.: Janssen Pharmaceutica, 1988.
6. Holmes CM, Galletly DG. Midazolam/fentanyl: a total intravenous technique for short procedures. Anaesthesia 1982;37:761–765.
7. Maryniak JK, Bishop VA. Sinus arrest after alfentanil. Br J Anaesth 1987;59:390–391.
8. Rivard JC, Lebowitz PW. Bradycardia after alfentanil-succinylcholine. Anesth Analg 1988; 67:907.
9. Partridge BL, Ward CF. Pulmonary edema following low-dose naloxone administration. Anesthesiology 1986;65:709–710.

JEAN M. MILLAR: This chapter displays an excellent understanding of the logistics of same-day surgery and the place of opioids in improving perioperative conditions and postoperative recovery.

From the British point of view, some of the practices mentioned need qualifying:

- It is generally considered that 30 to 45 minutes is the upper limit for day-surgery procedures, although the use of propofol undoubtedly extends this. Anesthetic and surgical turnover is probably faster, so this is not as restrictive as

equal the rates of distribution and elimination.[1] Thus, complex and continuous alterations in drug receptor–membrane interaction are partly responsible for our inability either to define or to measure the depth of anesthesia.

To minimize the effect of this uncertainty, anesthesia can be alternatively viewed as a three-state phenomenon: light-moderate-deep,[2] or inadequate-adequate-excessive.[3] This tristate approach avoids the unnecessary complexities associated with attempted measurement of small incremental changes in anesthetic effect and allows the formulation of a set of specific, objective, measurable criteria for adequate anesthesia. The addition of a classification scheme for intravenous anesthetics (Table 14.1) implies that the objectives of anesthesia cannot be equally or effectively met by sole reliance on a single anesthetic agent from any one class. The anesthetic classification scheme, based on available monitoring modalities, defines the minimal configuration of measurements necessary to reliably document anesthetic adequacy. The classification also helps focus attention on the aspects of

anesthetic polypharmacy that may complicate determination of adequate anesthesia. For example, class I and II agents tend to decrease mean electroencephalographic (EEG) frequency, while class III and IV agents may have the opposite effect. Thus, the resultant EEG effects of coadministration of class I and II agents with class III and IV agents are complex and require sophisticated techniques to separate them out. Fortunately, these techniques are available.

ASSESSMENT OF NEUROMUSCULAR SYSTEMS

The concept of anesthetic depth was originally developed for use with inhalation agents. A primary goal of depth assessment was to avoid the potentially fatal overdosage that accompanied hydrocarbon anesthetics with low therapeutic indices (ratio of median anesthetic to median lethal dose). However, many modern intravenous anesthetic agents have a much larger margin of safety. Concomitantly, the

TABLE 14.1 Clinical classification of intravenous anesthetics based on some commercially available monitoring modalities

	Class I	Class II	Class III	Class IV
Central nervous system (cerebrocortical)				
EEG mean frequency	−	−	±	+
EEG mean amplitude	−	+	±	±
EEG seizures	−	+	−	+
Conscious awareness	−	−	0	±
Consciousness recall	−	0	−	−
Central nervous system (subcortical)				
Upper facial EMG	−	−	−	+
CO_2 responsiveness	−	−	0	0
Autonomic responsiveness	−	0	+	+
Neuromuscular function	−	±	−	±
Examples	Thiopental Propanidid Alphadione	Fentanyl Morphine Alfentanil	Diazepam Lorazepam Midazolam	Ketamine Etomidate Propofol

Source: Couture LJ, Edmonds JL Jr. Monitoring responsiveness during anesthesia. In: Jones G, ed. Bailliere's clinical anaesthesiology: depth of anaesthesia. London: W.B. Saunders, 1989, p. 552.
−, depression; +, stimulation; ±, mixed; 0, little or no effect.

discrimination between adequate and excessive has become less emphasized than that between adequate and inadequate. This emphasis is best illustrated by the recent flurry of interest in awareness during anesthesia and surgery. The importance of this topic is made clear by the recent publication of a book, *Consciousness, Awareness, and Pain in General Anesthesia*, devoted entirely to the subject of awareness.[4] (The reader is referred to this important book to supplement the material in this chapter.)

These concerns are greatest with opioid/relaxant anesthesia, which has been most often associated with the conscious postoperative recall of stressful intraoperative events.[5] However, episodes of unintended awareness occurring during opioid anesthesia do not necessarily represent a limitation of the technique. Rather, these events dramatically illustrate the importance of appropriate monitoring. Inadequate opioid anesthesia can be successfully avoided by continuous, objective functional assessment of physiologic systems.

Muscular Contraction

Opioids, when used alone, are often unable to achieve all the objectives of general anesthesia. Perhaps most important, they lack the ability to induce marked relaxation of skeletal muscles. In fact, they may even increase muscular tone, leading to potentially hazardous chest wall rigidity. Thus, opioid anesthetic techniques frequently include a neuromuscular blocking agent. Although partial chemical paralysis may be necessary, injudicious overuse of the relaxants can make more difficult the detection of inadequate anesthesia.[1] Maintenance of some residual neuromuscular transmission (NMT) after effective, but incomplete, relaxation helps in the accurate monitoring of opioid anesthetic adequacy.[1]

Skeletal Muscles

NMT is easily assessed in accessible skeletal muscles either by visual estimation of mechanical twitches or by electromyographic (EMG) recording of responses evoked by electrical stimulation of peripheral motor nerves. The most widely used technique employs a train-of-four (TOF), 2-Hz stimulation by a hand-held, battery-powered device. Visual detection of the number of twitches provides a crude index of neuromuscular blockade. This minimal documentation of relaxant effect is necessary if one wishes to characterize opioid effects on the striated nonskeletal mimic muscles of the upper face (see next section).

Despite its ubiquity, the technique of NMT measurement by estimation of visual twitches is error-prone and thus potentially misleading. There are numerous sources of error. First, there is marked interobserver variability in twitch counting.[6] This large variation means that clinically significant NMT depression can be overlooked. Second, valid interpretation of TOF responses assumes a supramaximal stimulus intensity to activate completely all subserving motor fibers.[7] Lower intensities lead to unacceptably large response variation. However, currents of 50 to 60 mA are often required to achieve supramaximal stimulation. Many of the hand-held stimulators cannot achieve this high intensity, even with fresh batteries. Third, twitch counting is a relatively insensitive NMT measure. The amplitude of evoked EMG responses may still be 20 to 25% of prerelaxant reference at the disappearance of the last visible TOF twitch.[8] Because of these technical limitations, Ali[7] and others[9] advocate the routine use of evoked EMG responses to objectively quantify NMT. The current generation of commercial EMG monitors designed for this purpose seems to have overcome the limitations of visual twitch counting.

Regardless of the device chosen for NMT monitoring, other technical factors may interfere with accurate measurement. For example, the NMT monitoring site is often chosen without careful consideration. TOF responses obtained from sites that are either distal to a blood pressure cuff or cold may overestimate the degree of chemical paralysis. Furthermore, it should be recognized that striated muscles differentially respond to relaxants.[10] Muscular responses evoked from different sites during neuromuscular blockade are not interchangeable. TOF responses may be evoked in frontalis muscles with doses of nondepolarizing blockers that completely obliterate hypothenar responsiveness.[11] The relative insensitivity of the upper facial muscles to NMT blockade seems due in part to their unusually low innervation ratios.[12] This observation is important because it means that upper facial muscle responsiveness persists during the near-complete relaxation of skeletal and abdominal muscles. Thus, opioid anesthetic adequacy can be objectively assessed by monitoring the reactivity of the relaxant-resistant facial muscles.[12]

Reflex skeletal or facial muscle contractions may occur in the absence of visual or EMG-detectable TOF responses. Clear demonstration of this phenomenon is provided through the use of transcranial magnetic motor-evoked potentials (tcMMEP). A powerful magnet induces depolarizing electrical currents in the motor cortex, which results in limb movements. During opioid anesthesia, low-limb tcMMEP may be recorded even though relaxants have virtually eliminated hypothenar responses to electrical stimulation of the ulnar nerve.[13] Single stimuli applied to motor cortex result in repetitive discharges within the anterior horn cell region.[14] Through spatial and temporal recruitment, this centrally mediated facilitation can overcome an apparently complete drug-induced NMT block. Thus, unexpected movement may signify inadequate anesthesia rather than insufficient relaxation.[1]

Upper Facial Muscles

The upper facial muscles provide a simple means for assessing the adequacy of opioid anesthesia. Phasic reactivity of these unique muscles is controlled largely by visceral efferents of the VII cranial nerve. Thus, in most cases they provide easy access for the measurement of autonomic response to noxious stimuli. Involuntary reflex facial muscular contraction occurs during moderate (frown with procerus or corrugator supercilii) and extreme (wince or grimace with orbicularis oculi) negative affect (stress, pain). With careful inspection, these facial changes may be visible during opioid anesthesia. However, objective documentation of facial hyperactivity signifying inadequate anesthesia requires some form of EMG monitoring.

Facial muscles are also unique because they lack a γ negative feedback control system, and their strength of contraction is modulated primarily by the firing rate of motor neurons rather than by the motor unit recruitment typical of skeletal muscles.[15] The normal high resting tone in the fatigue-resistant, slow-twitch facial muscle fibers is maintained by vigilance control centers within the reticular activating system. This process is readily apparent in the universally characteristic upper facial expression of drowsiness. Therefore, phasic (abrupt) increases in facial EMG (FEMG) amplitude signal involuntary autonomic discharge,[16,17] while the tonic (baseline) amplitude provides an objective index of vigilance.[18]

The utility of FEMG monitoring for the assessment of opioid effects and anesthetic adequacy has been demonstrated in both laboratory[19] and clinical[7] settings. Edmonds et al.[12] measured FEMG amplitude during opioid administration for postoperative pain. Near-complete suppression of tonic FEMG activity accompanied the analgesic and depressant effects of subanesthetic doses of morphine, fentanyl, and butorphanol. The FEMG amplitude appeared exquisitely sensitive to the low doses of opioids used in these somnolent, but arousable, patients. Responsiveness was consistently characterized by abrupt phasic increases in FEMG amplitude (Figure 14.1).

Since subanesthetic opioid levels may virtually eliminate tonic FEMG activity, this measure alone is insufficient to document inadequate anesthesia. However, in the absence of artifact, a large phasic FEMG increase emerging from a baseline of low tonic activity reliably signifies some patient responsiveness and awareness. Such events may or may not be consciously recalled later by the patient. For example, in scoliosis surgery with opioid anesthesia, the FEMG predicts patient re-

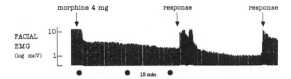

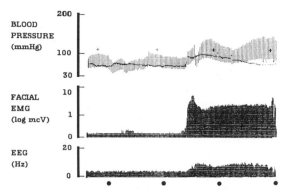

FIGURE 14.1 A subanesthetic dose of morphine depresses tonic (baseline) upper facial electromyograph (EMG) in this somnolent patient postoperatively. Abrupt phasic increases demonstrate patient responsiveness to questioning. The tracing is composed of a compact series of thin vertical bars, each of which represents a 10-second average of the mean integrated EMG amplitude obtained from upper facial muscles. Amplitude is displayed on a logarithmic scale.

FIGURE 14.2 This graph, made during a wake-up test, characterizes the changes in systolic-diastolic arterial pressure (vertical bars, top trace), heart rate (dots, top trace), EMG (middle trace), and frontomastoid electroencephalogram (EEG) (mean zero-cross frequency of successive 10-second epochs on linear scale). Although all these measures eventually indicated patient responsiveness, the earliest and most prominent increases were observed in the EMG.

sponsiveness to voice command occurring during a standardized wake-up test[20] (Figure 14.2). Results such as these illustrate the clinical utility of objective measurement of facial muscle activity. The high sensitivity of this monitor makes it well suited for the discrimination between adequate and inadequate anesthesia. However, it is generally not a useful measure of excessive anesthesia, since both spontaneous (tonic) and evoked (phasic) FEMG amplitudes may be suppressed to the amplifier noise level during adequate anesthesia.

Nonstriated Smooth Muscles

Like the atypical striated muscles of the upper face, the nonstriated smooth muscle of the lower esophagus is relatively unaffected by neuromuscular blocking drugs.[21] In another similarity, activity of this muscle increases during stress.[22] Evans et al.[23] reported that the frequency of spontaneous lower esophageal contractions (SLEC) in patients anesthetized with nitrous oxide appeared to be inversely related to the infusion rate of fentanyl. More recently, Silvay et al.[24] recorded hemodynamic, electrocortical, and SLEC changes during open-heart surgery in 23 patients, half of whom were anesthetized with high-dose fen-

tanyl. Based on hemodynamic criteria, 23 episodes of inadequate anesthesia were detected. Nearly 80% of these were accompanied by electrocortical or SLEC increases. However, only one-third of the 55 episodes based on SLEC had either hemodynamic or electrocortical concomitants. These findings suggest that increased SLEC may provide a useful monitor for opioid anesthetic adequacy. However, until more information is available, prudence dictates additional hemodynamic and electrocortical measurement to minimize the incidence of false positives. Many factors affect lower esophageal contractility. For example, Maccioli et al.[25] concluded that lower esophageal contractility might be an indicator of depth of anesthesia with inhaled agents, as reflected by MAC, but that further studies are needed to quantify the effects of surgical stimulus, intravenous anesthetics, vasodilators, anticholinergics, calcium channel blockers, β-adrenergic agonists, and the presence of a nasogastric tube. Schweiger et al.[26] studied this monitor versus somatic signs. They observed that the rate of spontaneous contractions was significantly greater at times of somatic response than when there was no somatic response, although there was no significant difference in the amplitude of provoked contractions. The most favorable cutoff point was determined to be a rate of six contractions per 3-minute period. This produced a false positive rate of 11.9% and a sensitivity (true positive rate) of 52.2%. They concluded that lower esophageal contractility was less reliable for detection of inadequate anesthesia when an opioid was used as the primary anesthetic agent than when an inhaled agent was the primary agent.

MONITORING ANESTHETIC ACTION ON THE BRAIN

Central Nervous System

During general anesthesia, the objectives of analgesia, anxiolysis, and amnesia are accomplished by lowering the patient's vigilance level to the point of unresponsiveness. Since vigilance is a cerebral function, all general anesthetics may reasonably be expected to alter measures of brain activity. Anesthetic-induced changes in cerebral metabolic activity have been both quantified and visualized through the use of 2-deoxyglucose autoradiography in animals and 15-oxygen or 18-fluorine positron emission tomography in humans. When coupled with electrophysiologic monitoring, these techniques depict the generalized metabolic and functional depression accompanying administration of the volatile halogenated[27] and class I (Table 14.1) intravenous anesthetics.[28] In contrast, anesthetics from classes II to IV have complex regional actions on neuronal oxygen utilization, glucose uptake, and electrophysiologic responsiveness. For example, although μ agonist opioids depress cortical metabolic and functional activity, reactivity of the auditory pathway is relatively uninfluenced.[29] Metabolic and electrographic maps, our psychophysiologic anesthetic classification scheme (Table

14.1), and common clinical impression all demonstrate that the altered states of consciousness produced by general central nervous system (CNS) depressants (class I) and opioids (class II) are distinctly different. Therefore, it seems inappropriate to use a uniform set of criteria to assess anesthetic adequacy. Rather, configuration of the monitoring system for anesthetic adequacy should be guided by the choice of anesthetic.

Spontaneous Cerebrocortical Electrical Activity (EEG)

Of the available techniques for the objective monitoring of anesthetic action on the brain, practical considerations limit intraoperative measurement to recordings of spontaneous (EEG) or evoked (EP) electrical potentials obtained from scalp electrodes. The conventional, unprocessed EEG may be viewed as a graph of signal amplitude (voltage) as a function of time. Scalp electrodes provide a distance-weighted average of the electrical currents produced over large areas of cortex. During high levels of vigilance, this averaging is depicted as a series of low-amplitude waves of short period (high frequency) due to the differential activation of individual cortical columns.[30] Conversely, with diminished vigilance the highly regionalized columnar activity is absent. The synchronized discharge of large populations of cortical neurons is reflected in the EEG as high-amplitude waves of long period (low frequency). The diffuse decrease in neuronal metabolism and synaptic activity associated with hypothermia, hypoxia/ischemia, or excessive doses of CNS depressants leads to decreases in both EEG amplitude and frequency, ultimately progressing to electrocortical silence (flat EEG).

Amplitude analysis in the time domain (period) is appropriate if the EEG is viewed as a series of discrete events like fast or slow waves, K-complexes, etc.[31] However, conventional EEG recording is not often used intraoperatively because its interpretation is complex and costly. With the advent of inexpensive microprocessors, several commercial devices now utilize period-amplitude analysis to display EEG information in compressed, simplified formats.[3,32-37] Alternatively, the EEG over one brief interval can be thought of as the algebraic summation of outputs from a group of oscillators, each with a fixed frequency characteristic, but variable amplitude.[31] In this case, the appropriate frequency domain analysis expresses amplitude as a function of frequency. To enhance the dynamic range of the display, most commercial monitors of this type measure amplitude in volts,[2] or power, the so-called power spectrum analysis. The essential third dimension, time, is typically plotted on the z axis. Aperiodic analysis works differently from the averaging techniques that are used in most EEG monitors. The latter are typified by the Fourier transform. Aperiodic analysis[38,39] detects every waveform in the EEG and compresses the information on the waveform as three values: frequency, amplitude (µv), and time. To gather this information, the computer detects wave peaks, valleys, zero-crossings, and length of time between valleys. A wave is defined by detecting a valley, then a peak, then another valley. The period of the wave is the time between valleys. Frequency is the reciprocal of the period. Slow and fast waves are detected differently. Detection of slow waves requires the presence of zero-crossings between the highest peaks and lowest valleys; detection of fast waves requires only consecutive peaks and valleys. On the screen, this information is displayed as a large number of telephone poles, one for each EEG wave (Figure 14.3).

Dutton et al.[40] felt that the patient movement endpoint is important from the standpoint of awareness, since unparalyzed patients who do not move during surgery rarely have any memory of awareness during surgery. This means that an EEG system that predicts patient movement might be used to titrate administration of anesthetic agents. This EEG system might be useful while general anesthesia is maintained in paralyzed patients. In a manner analogous to studies of MAC, in which the concentration of anesthetic agent is used to describe the probability that patients

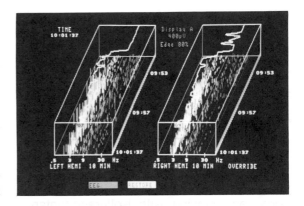

FIGURE 14.3 The electroencephalogram (EEG) during induction with alfentanil (175 µg/kg, IV) as interpreted by aperiodic analysis. The color displays were produced by a Lifescan EEG monitor. Frequency is displayed on the x axis; the scale is nonlinear and compressed at the higher frequencies. The amplitude of each mapped EEG wave (y axis) is the height of a vertical "pole" and is referred to the top of the transparent box, which is 400 µv. Time is displayed on the z axis; as time advances, the display moves up from the bottom of the box, where the current time and results appear. "Edge 80%" refers to the activity edge, the line below which 80% of the EEG activity occurs. This is displayed as the white line floating over the "poles." Notice the sharp shift to the left of both the pattern and the line, around 0954, reflecting the sudden onset of anesthesia with this rapidly acting opioid.

will move, the EEG was used to plot curves to predict patient movement. The first step was the development of a method to express the EEG in the form of a single-number score. The EEG was analyzed by parametric analysis[41] to obtain 13 variables for describing the EEG power frequency spectrum. A computer analysis technique, called discriminant analysis, was then used to determine the best method to use these 13 variables to predict patient movement. These scores were then employed to generate probability-of-movement curves (Figures 14.4 and 14.5), similar to quantal re-

Autonomic Nervous System

Respiration
The common use of chemical paralysis and attendant mechanical ventilation makes respiratory patterns unsuitable for the assessment of opioid anesthetic adequacy.

Heart Rate
Because of the nonspecificity of cardiovascular changes, heart rate and blood pressure changes alone are insufficient to reliably judge the level of anesthesia.[57] In addition, the frequent use of autonomic drugs and β-adrenergic blocking agents make it difficult to trust the heart rate as a monitor.

Blood Pressure
Mean arterial pressure can serve as a crude indicator of global perfusion but is an inappropriate descriptor of opioid anesthetic adequacy.[58] Matilla[59] reported on the usefulness of finger pulse amplitude, obtained from uncorrected oximetric waveforms, for the detection of insufficient anesthesia. Rantala et al.[60] both confirmed this observation and compared pulse changes with those seen in facial muscle, EEG, and hemodynamic variables. In the absence of drugs affecting vascular tone, pulse amplitude changes closely paralleled those seen in the facial EMG. Either of these measures appeared to be more reliable than blood pressure, heart rate, or mean EEG amplitude/frequency changes. However, pulse amplitude alone is unlikely to provide a reliable measure of anesthetic adequacy, since it is markedly influenced by vascular pathology, temperature, blood volume, and a wide variety of drugs used during surgery.

Pupil Diameter, Sweating, and Lacrimation
These commonly employed clinical signs are inconsistent and unreliable indices of anesthetic adequacy because of their lack of specificity.[61] Nevertheless, if present, sweating or lacrimation should be considered a sign of inadequate depth until proved otherwise.

OPIOID EXCESS

The opioid dose required to achieve and maintain adequate anesthesia varies enormously among patients. Thus, despite the high therapeutic indices of these compounds, excessive administration has led to serious consequences. The profound respiratory depression that accompanies high doses of μ agonist opioids may complicate postoperative recovery by requiring ventilatory assistance. Undetected renarcotization of patients in the recovery room has resulted in catastrophic brain damage. Thoughtful use of the reliable monitors of anesthetic adequacy previously discussed to guide individualized opioid titration can help avoid unnecessary excessive dosing with its attendant hazards. It appears that of all the methods discussed, the EEG shows the greatest promise to succeed in this area.

REFERENCES

1. Hug CC Jr. Monitoring. In: Miller RD, ed. Anesthesia. New York: Churchill Livingstone, 1986;1:411–464.
2. Cullen SC, Larson CP Jr. Evaluation of anesthetic depth. Anesthesiol Rev 1975;2:18–25.
3. Edmonds HL Jr, Wauquier A. Computerized EEG monitoring in anesthesia and critical care. Helsinki: Instrumentarium Science Foundation, 1986;82–89.
4. Rosen M, Lunn JN, eds. Consciousness, awareness, and pain in general anesthesia. London: Butterworths, 1987.
5. Jones JG. Awareness under anaesthesia. In: Anaesthesia rounds. London: ICI Pharmaceuticals, 1988;21:1–28.
6. Viby-Mogensen J, Jensen NH, Engbaek J, et al. Tactile and visual evaluation of the response to train-of-four nerve stimulation. Anesthesiology 1985;63:440–447.
7. Ali HH, Savarese JJ. Monitoring of neuromuscular function. Anesthesiology 1976; 45:216–249.
8. Edmonds HL Jr, Couture LJ, Stolzy SL, et al. Quantitative surface electromyography in anesthesia and critical care. Int J Clin Monit Comput 1986;3:135–145.
9. Lee C, Katz RL, Lee ASJ, et al. A new

instrument for continuous recording of the evoked compound electromyogram in the clinical setting. Anesth Analg (Cleve) 1977;56:260–270.

10. Stiffel P, Hameroff SR, Blitt CD, et al. Variability in assessment of neuromuscular blockade. Anesthesiology 1980;52:436–437.

11. Paloheimo M, Wilson RC, Edmonds HL Jr, et al. Comparison of neuromuscular blockade in upper facial and hypothenar muscles. J Clin Monit 1988;4:256–260.

12. Edmonds HL Jr, Couture LJ, Paloheimo M, et al. Objective assessment of opioid action by facial muscle surface electromyography (SEMG). Prog Neuropsychopharmacol Biol Psychiatry 1988;12:727–738.

13. Edmonds HL Jr, Paloheimo M, Backman MH, et al. Transcranial magnetic motor-evoked potentials (tcMMEP) for functional monitoring of motor pathways during scoliosis surgery. Spine 1989;14(7):683–686.

14. Day BL, Rothwell JC, Thompson PD, et al. Motor cortex stimulation in intact man. II Multiple descending volleys. Brain 1987; 110:1119–1120.

15. Van Boxtel A, Schomaker LRB. Motor unit firing rate during static contraction indicated by the surface EMG power. IEEE Trans Biomed Eng 1983;BME30:601–608.

16. Cobb CR, De Vries HA, Urban RT, et al. Electrical activity in muscle pain. Am J Phys Med 1975;54:80–87.

17. Harmel MH, Klein FF, Davis DA. The EEMG: a practical index of cortical activity and muscular relaxation. Acta Anaesthesiol Scand 1978;70:97–102.

18. Edmonds HL Jr, Stolzy SL, Couture LJ. Surface electromyography during low-vigilance states. In: Rosen M, Lunn JN, eds. Consciousness, awareness, and pain in general anesthesia. London: Butterworths, 1987;89–98.

19. Menon MK, Tseng L-F, Loh HH, et al. An electromyographic method for the quantitative evaluation of narcotic analgesic in rats. Neuropharmacology, 1980;19:231–236.

20. Couture LJ, Edmonds HL Jr. Monitoring responsiveness during anesthesia. In: Jones G, ed. Bailliere's clinical anaesthesiology: depth of anaesthesia. London: W.B. Saunders, 1989; 547–558.

21. Evans JM, Davies WL, Wise CC. Lower oesophageal contractility: a new monitor of anaesthesia. Lancet 1984;2:1151–1154.

22. Rubin J, Nagler R, Spiro HM, et al. Measur-

ing the effect of emotions on esophageal motility. Psychosom Med 1962;24:170–176.

23. Evans JM, Fraser A, Wise CC, et al. Computer-controlled anaesthesia. In: Prakash O, ed. Computing in anaesthesia and intensive care. The Hague: Martinus Nijhoff, 1983;279–291.

24. Silvay G, Grossbarth D, Kuni D, et al. Lower esophageal contractility and assessment of depth of anesthesia during open-heart surgery. Anesth Analg 1988;67:S209.

25. Maccioli GA, Kuni DR, Silvay G, et al. Response of lower esophageal contractility to changing concentrations of halothane or isoflurane: a multicenter study. J Clin Monit 1988;4:247–255.

26. Schweiger IM, Hug CC Jr, Hall RI, et al. Is lower esophageal contractility a reliable indicator of the adequacy of opioid anesthesia? J Clin Monit 1989;5:164–169.

27. Hawkins RA, Maziotta JC, Phelps ME. Applications of PET in the brain. Prog Neuropsychopharmacol Biol Psychiat 1987;11:165–172.

28. Sokoloff L. Localization of functional activity in the central nervous system by measurement of glucose utilization with radioactive deoxyglucose. J Cereb Blood Flow Metabol 1981;1:7–21.

29. Samra SK, Lilly DJ, Rush NL, et al. Fentanyl anesthesia and human brain stem auditory evoked potentials. Anesthesiology 1984; 61:261–265.

30. Mountcastle VB. Sleep, wakefulness, and the conscious state. In: Mountcastle VB, ed. Medical physiology. 14th ed. St. Louis: C.V. Mosby, 1980:1:299–323.

31. Bergmann BM, Mistlberger RE, Rechtschaffen A. Period-amplitude analysis of rat electroencephalogram: stage and diurnal variations and effects of suprachiasmatic nuclei lesions. Sleep 1987;10:523–536.

32. Fleming RA, Smith NT. Density modulation: a technique for the display of three-variable data in patient monitoring. Anesthesiology 1979;50:543–546.

33. Smith NT. Monitoring. The medical turn key. In: Benumof LJ, ed. Clinical frontiers in anesthesiology. New York: Grune & Stratton, 1983;245–252.

34. Smith NT, Rampil IJ. The use of computer-generated numbers in interpreting the EEG. In: Prakash O. Computing in anaesthesia and intensive care. The Hague: Martinus Nijhoff, 1983;214–226.

35. Levy WJ, Grundy B, Smith NT. The electro-encephalogram. In: Saidman LJ, Smith NT, eds. Monitoring in anesthesia. 2d ed. London: Butterworths, 1984;441–496.
36. Smith NT. Principles of computerized EEG monitoring. J Clin Monit 1987;3:318.
37. Smith NT. New developments in monitoring animals for evidence of pain control. J Am Vet Med Assoc 1987;191(10):1269–1272.
38. Demetrescu M, Kavan E, Smith NT. Monitoring the brain condition by advanced EEG. Anesthesiology 1981;55:A130. (Abstr.)
39. Gregory TK, Pettus DC. An electroencephalographic processing algorithm specifically intended for analysis of cerebral electrical activity. J Clin Monit 1986;2:190–197.
40. Dutton RC, Smith WD, Smith NT. The use of EEG to predict patient movement during anaesthesia. In: Rosen M, Lunn JN, eds. Consciousness, awareness, and pain in general anesthesia. London: Butterworths, 1987;72–82.
41. Smith WD, Lager DL. Evaluation of simple algorithms for spectral parameter analysis of the electroencephalogram. IEEE Trans Biomed Eng 1986;33:352–358.
42. Waud DR. On biological assays involving quantal responses. J Pharmacol Exp Ther 1972;183:577–607.
43. Lopez da Silva FH, Smith NT, Zwart A, et al. Spectral analysis of the EEG during halothane anesthesia: input-output relations. Electroencephalogr Clin Neurophysiol 1972;33:311–319.
44. Smith NT, Calverley RK, Coles JR, et al. The EEG as an indicator of changing anesthetic depth in man. Proc Annu Meet Am Soc Anesthesiologists, 1976;192–193. (Abstr.)
45. Smith NT, Rampil IJ, Sasse FJ, et al. EEG during rapidly changing halothane or enflurane. Anesthesiology 1979;51:S4.
46. Smith NT, Demetrescu M. The EEG during high-dose fentanyl anesthesia. Anesthesiology 1980;53(suppl 3):S7. (Abstr.)
47. Smith NT, Silver H, Sanford TJ, et al. The EEG during high-dose fentanyl, sufentanil, or morphine-oxygen anesthesia. Anesth Analg 1984;63:386–393.
48. Smith NT, Dec-Silver H, Sanford TJ Jr, et al. Changes in the electroencephalogram during high-dose narcotic anesthesia. In: Estafanous FG, ed. Opioids in anesthesia. Boston: Butterworths, 1984;61–66.

49. Smith NT, Westover CJ Jr, Quinn ML, et al. The EEG of alfentanil: a comparison with other narcotics and with thiopental. J Clin Monit 1985;1:236–243.
50. Rampil IJ, Smith NT. Comparison of EEG indices during halothane anesthesia. J Clin Monit 1985;1:89.
51. Hudson RJ, Stanski DR, Saidman LJ, et al. A model for studying the depth of anesthesia and acute tolerance to thiopental. Anesthesiology 1983;59:301–308.
52. Scott JC, Ponganis KV, Stanski DR. EEG quantitation of narcotic effect: the comparative pharmacodynamics of fentanyl and alfentanil. Anesthesiology 1985;62:234–241.
53. Wauquier A. Monitoring depth of anesthesia with the EEG. In: Stanley TH, Petty WC, eds. Anesthesiology. Boston: Martinus Nijhoff, 1986;242–254.
54. Arndt JO, Bednarski B, Parasher C. Alfentanil's analgesic, respiratory, and cardiovascular actions in relation to dose and plasma concentration in unanesthetized dogs. Anesthesiology 1986;64:345–352.
55. Wauquier A, De Ryck M, Van den Broeck W, et al. Relationships between quantitative EEG measures and pharmacodynamics of alfentanil in dogs. Electroencephalogr Clin Neurophysiol 1988;69:550–560.
56. Velasco M, Velasco F, Castaneda R, et al. Effect of fentanyl and naloxone on human somatic and auditory evoked potential components. Neuropharmacology 1984;23:359–366.
57. Gravenstein JS, Paulus DA. Clinical monitoring practice. 2d ed. Philadelphia: Lippincott, 1987;242–281.
58. Cullen DJ. Interpretation of blood-pressure measurements in anesthesias. Anesthesiology 1974;40:6–12.
59. Matilla M. Pulsewave oximetry and capnography in monitoring depth of anaesthesia. Proc 1st Int Symp on Memory and Awareness in Anaesthesia. Amsterdam: Swets Zeitlinger, 1989.
60. Rantala B, Makelainen A, Paloheimo M. Assessing the depth of anesthesia: a comparison of clinical parameters. J Clin Monit 1989;5(4):300 (Abstr).
61. Thornton C, Konieczko K, Jones JG, et al. Effect of surgical stimulation on the auditory evoked response. Br J Anaesth 1988;60:372–378.

Chapter 14 Discussion

HELMUT F. CASCORBI: Edmonds and Smith review various monitors to assess the adequacy of opioid anesthesia, a notoriously difficult task in patients with paralyzed myoneural junctions. Facial EMG is a monitoring technique that should be assessed more widely for its usefulness.

However, in the final analysis, the end organ for the production of anesthesia is the brain. It is my opinion that more easily applied, less expensive, and more easily understandable monitors of EEG and evoked potentials should be used for the rational assessment of the effect of all anesthetics, including opioids. Here the work of Edmonds and Smith and others is notable, and I am looking forward to the day when brain functions can be assessed almost as easily as oxygen saturation of the blood is assessed today.

15 POSTOPERATIVE MYOCARDIAL ISCHEMIA: MECHANISMS AND THERAPIES

Deanna Siliciano and Dennis T. Mangano

Perioperative cardiac morbidity (PCM) continues to complicate both cardiac and noncardiac surgical procedures. In noncardiac surgical patients with a history of, or risk factors for, coronary artery disease (CAD), postoperative myocardial infarction (PMI) occurs in 1 to 40% and death in up to 2%.[1-6] In cardiac surgical patients, PMI occurs in 2 to 40% and death in 0.5 to 15%.[1] These figures will most likely increase in the coming years as the patient population presenting for surgery becomes older, with more advanced CAD. In order to prevent that occurrence, reversible predictors of PCM must be identified and their physiologic mechanisms understood. Therapeutic trials can then be undertaken to test our understanding of these predictors.

Until 1985, only current congestive heart failure, intraoperative tachycardia, and hypotension[1,7-9] had been clearly identified as predictors of adverse cardiac outcome that could be modified by clinical management. Other proven predictors in noncardiac surgical patients (e.g., age, hypertension, type and duration of anesthesia, valvular heart disease,

history of recent myocardial infarction) and cardiac surgical patients (e.g., age, sex, preoperative ejection fraction, aortic cross-clamp and bypass time) were irreversible, unaffected by clinical care, or were controversial.[1]

In 1985, a dynamic intraoperative predictor, which can be reversible, was identified. Slogoff and Keats[10] examined 1,023 patients undergoing coronary artery surgery (CAS) for evidence of myocardial ischemia prior to bypass and for myocardial infarction on the first postoperative day. Of 377 patients with ST-segment changes consistent with myocardial ischemia in the prebypass period, 6.9% had PMIs compared with 2.5% for the 646 patients without prebypass myocardial ischemia. But Slogoff and Keats did not include the postbypass or postoperative period in their study; therefore, the relative importance of the prebypass period was not assessed.

The emphasis on the intraoperative prebypass period was questioned in recent studies in cardiac[11] and noncardiac[12] surgical patients, suggesting that, when corrected for duration of monitoring, the intraoperative incidence of myocardial ischemia is no different than the preoperative incidence. Knight et al.[11] found that the mean number of ischemic episodes

Supported in part by a grant from the National Institutes of Health (ROI-HL36744).

per hour monitored was 0.09 in the preoperative and 0.11 in the intraoperative period. What then is the role of the postoperative period? We examine this crucial time period in this chapter.

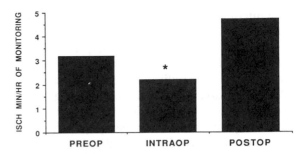

FIGURE 15.1 The incidence of preoperative (PREOP), intraoperative (INTRAOP), and postoperative (POSTOP) ischemia occurring during the measurement periods. (Adapted with permission of the publisher from Knight AA, Hollenberg M, London MJ, et al. Perioperative myocardial ischemia: importance of the preoperative ischemic pattern. Anesthesiology 1988;68:681–688.)

NONCARDIAC SURGICAL PATIENTS

In studies of patients with CAD, or with risk factors for CAD, undergoing noncardiac surgery, myocardial ischemia was found to occur more commonly in the postoperative period (38%) than in the preoperative (24%) or intraoperative (21%) periods.[13] The myocardial ischemia detected in the postoperative period was silent (97%), occurred at higher heart rates (90 versus 74 beats/min), and lasted longer than in the preoperative period (51 versus 30 minutes). Myocardial ischemia occurred throughout the first week after surgery, with peak incidence at 2 to 3 days and again at 6 to 7 days.[14] Recent evidence in noncardiac surgical patients also suggests that myocardial ischemia may be related to outcome.[12]

CARDIAC SURGICAL PATIENTS

In patients undergoing CAS, Knight et al.,[11] using continuous ECG (Holter monitoring), showed that, as in noncardiac surgical patients, myocardial ischemia occurs more commonly during the postoperative period [40% postoperative versus 18% prebypass (Figure 15.1)] and has longer duration than in the prebypass period (41 versus 19 minutes, median episode duration). The majority of the episodes appear to be silent. In another study of 40 patients, the maximum ST-segment deviations also were shown to be larger in the postoperative than the intraoperative period (0.23 versus 0.15 mV).[15] This apparent increased severity of postoperative ischemia occurs despite the intervening, apparently successful, coronary revascularization.

Unlike noncardiac surgical patients, though, the incidence of myocardial ischemia following cardiopulmonary bypass (CPB) was highest (42%) in the first hour postbypass, then decreased gradually such that by 18 hours postbypass (the morning of the first postoperative day) fewer than 5% of patients were ischemic (Figure 15.2).[11,15] No data exist on patterns of ischemia following CAS after 48 hours.

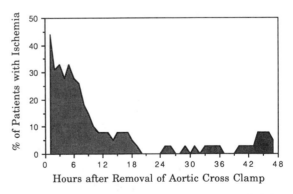

FIGURE 15.2 Incidence of myocardial ischemia as a function of time after aortic cross-clamp release. (Reprinted with permission of the authors from Siliciano D, Hollenberg M, Mangano DT. Myocardial ischemia following coronary revascularization. Proc 27th Annual West Anesthesia Residents Conf, April 1989.)

the greatest perioperative stress occurs in the postoperative period, not with intubation or surgical stimulation.

Halter et al.[19] found similar activation of the sympathetic nervous system in eight patients undergoing abdominal surgery with halothane–nitrous oxide anesthesia. Anesthesia alone suppressed plasma epinephrine (70 to 20 pg/ml), while norepinephrine remained constant, but levels of both catecholamines rose in all patients with surgical stimulation. The peak elevation, though, occurred from extubation to the early recovery period (epinephrine 70 to 300 pg/ml; norepinephrine 180 to 490 pg/ml).

These two studies demonstrate a generalized activation of the sympathetic nervous system with stimulation of both the adrenal medulla and the peripheral sympathetic neurons, which are marked following the end of surgical stimulation and anesthesia. The factors known to activate the sympathetic nervous system are hypothermia, hypotension, hypoxia, and hypercarbia. In the study by Halter et al.,[19] there was a strong positive correlation between changes in catecholamines and changes in mean arterial pressure ($r = 0.73$ for epinephrine; $r = 0.68$ for norepinephrine), and changes in catecholamines were unrelated to changes in temperature or arterial blood gases. These negative findings are compatible with the hypothesis that this adrenergic activation is a response to afferent signals from the site of trauma, a hypothesis supported by reports of intraoperative suppression of growth hormone and cortisol by morphine anesthesia (1 mg/kg) compared with halothane.[20] That intraoperative stress adversely affects outcome was shown by Roizen et al.[21] who measured intraoperative plasma catecholamine levels and postoperative outcomes in 100 patients undergoing vascular surgery. They found that elevated levels of plasma epinephrine and norepinephrine in the intraoperative period were associated with postoperative renal insufficiency and congestive heart failure.[21] Much of current intraoperative management is focused on suppressing this stress response.[22]

For patients with CAD undergoing cardiac surgical procedures, there has been interest in suppressing the stress response to anesthesia and surgery. But unlike the success demonstrated by Udelsman et al.[18] with "modern anesthetics" in noncardiac surgery, suppression of stress responses has been difficult, if not impossible, in cardiac surgical patients. This difference is accounted for by the influence of CPB. Whereas many different anesthetic techniques have been shown to block the stress response prior to CPB (halothane,[23] isoflurane,[24] morphine 4 mg/kg,[20] fentanyl 75 μg/kg,[25] sufentanil 50 μg/kg[26]), this benefit is confined to the prebypass period.

Many anesthetic techniques have been tested for their ability to block the adrenergic response to CPB with its resultant hormonal, metabolic, and hemodynamic changes. Although several studies have shown the ability of higher concentrations of sufentanil (25 versus 15 μg/kg)[27] to blunt the increases in epinephrine, and of higher concentrations of isoflurane (2 versus 1%)[28] to blunt the increases in cortisol on CPB, no anesthetic regimen tested has been able to block the marked adrenergic response to CPB, characterized by a five- to tenfold increase in plasma epinephrine.[29]

Is this response due to inadequate analgesia, as a result of changes in drug-protein binding during hemodilution? Okatuni et al.[26] tested this hypothesis by anesthetizing ten patients with 40 μg/kg sufentanil followed by an infusion of 12 μg/kg/hr until CPB. In these patients, plasma sufentanil concentrations remained greater than 4 ng/ml throughout CPB, when plasma epinephrine concentrations had increased by 250%. The authors concluded that the catecholamine responses during CPB were not related to adequacy of analgesia but to other factors, such as hypothermia or hemodilution.

Few studies have examined the time course of these effects following CPB. Flacke et al.[30] showed that in ten patients anesthetized with 12 μg/kg sufentanil and isoflurane, epinephrine levels remained markedly elevated (>

300%), compared with preinduction values, for 3 hours after arrival in the intensive care unit (ICU). Walsh et al.[31] showed that in 16 patients undergoing aortic valve replacement with 75 μg/kg fentanyl or papaveretum, the increases in plasma cortisol and growth hormone that occurred with CPB did not resolve until at least 48 hours following surgery. Thus, it appears that the stimulation of the sympathetic nervous system that occurs with CPB continues well into the postoperative period.

Parasympathetic Nervous System

Activation of the sympathetic nervous system, and its effects, predominate in the postoperative period in noncardiac surgical patients, and following CPB in cardiac surgical patients; however, there are also changes in the parasympathetic nervous system.

Noninvasive tests of cardiac parasympathetic activity have shown that impairment of parasympathetic nervous function is common in patients with CAD.[32] Airaksinen et al.[33] reported that a further impairment of parasympathetic heart-rate control is common when patients are tested 6 weeks after CAS. The heart-rate response to both standing (14.5 versus 10 beats/min) and deep breathing (1.22 versus 1.12; 30:15 ratio) was significantly lower after CAS than preoperatively.[33] This may result from inadequate myocardial preservation, direct injury to nerve fibers or the sinus node, or central nervous system complications during surgery. The importance of this reduction in parasympathetic nervous system activity is in the unopposed activity of the sympathetic nervous system, both in vasoregulatory mechanisms and in modulating the ventricular fibrillatory threshold.[34] Therefore, in patients with CAD undergoing noncardiac surgery or, to a more marked extent, cardiac surgery, the early postoperative period is characterized by significant stimulation of the sympathetic nervous system, which is modulated to a lesser degree by an impaired parasympathetic nervous system.

Left Ventricular Function

Stimulation of the sympathetic nervous system typically results in an increase in myocardial contractility with an increase in ejection fraction. In the postoperative period, this is not the case for patients with CAD. Coriat et al.[35] showed that immediately after extubation left ventricular ejection fraction decreased significantly (20%) in patients with mild angina. These changes occurred in the absence of ST changes and resolved by 3 hours after extubation.

In cardiac surgical patients, numerous studies have shown that, despite apparently successful revascularization, left ventricular function, as determined by scintigraphic ejection fractions[36-38] and ventricular function curves,[39] decreased with respect to preoperative values immediately after CPB (Figure 15.5). This decrease from control values was seen in patients with normal ventricular func-

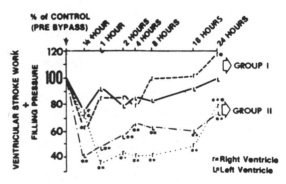

FIGURE 15.5 Mean values for LVSWI/ PCWP and RVSWI/CVP for group 1 patients (normal preoperative ejection fraction) and group 2 patients (depressed preoperative ejection fraction) for each measurement period are compared with control values (100%). (Reprinted with permission of the publisher from Mangano DT. Biventricular function after myocardial revascularization in humans: deterioration and recovery patterns during the first 24 hours. Anesthesiology 1985;62:571–577.)

tion (25%) and with depressed ventricular function (60%)[39] with pulsatile (35%) or non-pulsatile flow (27%).[38] These changes resolved within 4 to 24 hours.

Hemostasis

It is known that a hypercoagulable state follows surgery, which can predispose patients to venous and arterial thrombosis. In 89 general surgical patients, Mansfield[40] demonstrated a biphasic fibrinolytic response. There was a significant increase in fibrinolysis during the surgical procedure as measured by the euglobulin lysis time (decreased by 29%). In contrast, fibrinolysis decreased in the postoperative period for up to 5 days (increase in euglobulin lysis time of 168 to 200%).[40] Britton et al.[41] also showed an increase in Factor VIII levels (182%) during, and for up to 7 days, after surgery, as well as a decrease in the thromboelastogram (28%) and an increase in euglobulin lysis time (196%) at the end of surgery compared with preoperative levels. This hypercoaguability has been associated with the trauma of surgery, in particular with the activation of the sympathetic nervous system. In 1916, Grabfield[42] demonstrated a reduction in coagulation time of blood in patients given epinephrine as well as in patients likely to have high levels of endogenous epinephrine, such as those with fear, pain, and anxiety. Epinephrine has been shown to cause activation of platelets via their α_2-adrenergic receptors.[43] Britton et al.[41] examined this association in healthy patients undergoing graded exercise. They found that Factor VIII (fivefold) and epinephrine (11-fold) both rose with maximal exercise in ten volunteers with a correlation of $r = 0.77$. Thus, sympathoadrenal stimulation may play a significant role in the hypercoagulable state that follows surgery.

In patients undergoing cardiac surgery, hemostasis is more complex, because of the influence of heparin, protamine, and the effects of CPB on hemodilution, contact activation of platelets,[44] and sympathetic nervous system stimulation. As in noncardiac surgery, there is evidence for increased coagulability. As previously mentioned, there is an exaggerated activation of the sympathetic nervous system, with increases in plasma epinephrine due to CPB. Other factors are particular to cardiac surgery. Sternotomy can cause embolization of bone marrow that has thromboplastin activity.[45] Contact of blood with the bypass circuit can cause Factor XII activation, leading to thrombin formation.[46] And hemodilution of the heparin-Antithrombin III complex may make inhibition of any thrombin formed inadequate. These factors can result in the generation of microthrombi in the microcirculation, as well as on the arterial filter of the bypass machine.[44]

However, a number of factors act to decrease coagulability during and after cardiac surgery. These include residual heparin, excess protamine, and dilution of clotting factors and platelets.[47] On bypass, there is increased fibrinolytic activity, as measured by decreased kaolin-activated euglobulin activity (to 40% of baseline levels) and by increased levels (threefold) of tissue plasminogen activator (tPA).[48] tPA is thought to be released from vascular walls during bypass, with activation of plasminogen at the site of thrombin formation in the microcirculation, preserving flow.

Coagulation is also impaired because of a transient reduction in platelet function as well as concentration. Platelet aggregability to adenosine diphosphate (ADP) or collagen decreases with the onset of bypass, reaching minimal responsiveness (28 and 23% of initial values) immediately after protamine administration. Platelet aggregability slowly improves to 68% (in response to ADP) and 40% (in response to collagen) of baseline levels at 24 hours after surgery.[44]

It appears that opposing factors serve to maintain the integrity of the microcirculation during bypass. After CPB, platelet dysfunction persists, as does sympathetic nervous system activation. The precise interaction of these factors in the postoperative period following cardiac surgery is still unclear.

Oxygen Delivery

Oxygen content of the blood is often reduced in the postoperative period. Depressed postoperative cardiac output with increased oxygen extraction peripherally results in decreased mixed venous oxygen saturation. Postoperative changes in pulmonary function due to atelectasis, with decreased functional residual capacity and ventilation perfusion mismatching; decreased hypoxic pulmonary vasoconstriction; and hypoventilation due to pain or residual anesthetics can result in reduced PaO_2 and decreased hemoglobin saturation. Content can be further decreased by reductions in hemoglobin due to blood lost during the surgical procedure. This decrease in hemoglobin is less likely to be treated with heterologous blood transfusion because of the risk of bloodborne infections.

Pain Perception

There are many factors during the postoperative period that alter the normal perception of pain. That pain perception is in fact altered in the postoperative period is suggested by the high incidence of silent myocardial infarctions (> 60%) in postoperative patients compared with the incidence of silent infarctions (10 to 15%) in nonsurgical patients.[49] Postoperative factors that might influence pain perception include the effects of residual anesthetics, which can be either analgesic or antianalgesic, depending on the residual concentration[50,51] as well as supplemental analgesics received after surgery. Competing somatic stimuli (such as incisional pain) also modulate pain perception via spinal and supraspinal pathways. These interactions are complex, and a more thorough understanding of pain perception in the postoperative period awaits further study.

Hemodynamics

Hemodynamic changes in the postoperative period depend on many factors, including pain,

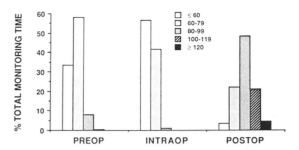

FIGURE 15.6 Heart rate distribution for the three periods. (Reprinted with permission of the publisher from Knight AA, Hollenberg M, London MJ, et al. Perioperative myocardial ischemia: importance of the preoperative ischemic pattern. Anesthesiology, 1988;68: 681–688.)

temperature, fluid balance, and catecholamines. In both cardiac and noncardiac surgical patients, postoperative heart rates increase 25 to 50% over preoperative levels, and up to 25% of patients have heart rates over 100 (Figure 15.6).[11]

MECHANISMS OF MYOCARDIAL ISCHEMIA IN THE POSTOPERATIVE PERIOD

Myocardial ischemia results from an imbalance of myocardial oxygen supply and demand. The physiologic changes seen in the postoperative period directly influence myocardial oxygen supply and demand, and thus can precipitate ischemia. The many potential causes of myocardial ischemia in the postoperative period divide into those related to decreased supply and those related to increased demand.

Reduced Supply

Decreases in myocardial oxygen supply can result from either acute narrowing of the coronary lumen, reduction in oxygen content, or reductions in coronary blood flow without luminal narrowing. Current theories[52,53] about the genesis of acute myocardial ischemia include rapid progression of atherosclerosis, platelet aggregation, plaque fissure or rupture, abnormal arachidonic acid metabolism, and coronary artery spasm.

Rapid progression of atherosclerosis as determined by coronary angiography was seen in 75% of patients with unstable angina compared with 30% of patients with stable angina,[54] but both the sensitivity and specificity of these angiographic results are questionable. That platelets have a role in the genesis of acute myocardial ischemia was shown by Folts et al.[55] Their studies in dogs with constricted coronary arteries demonstrated pathologically that cyclic reductions in coronary blood flow and distal coronary perfusion pressure was associated with platelet aggregation at the site of the coronary narrowing. The aggregation of platelets at the site of turbulent flow and stasis is thought to occur in severely stenosed coronary arteries ($> 75\%$).[52]

Platelets are also thought to play a role in less stenotic coronary arteries, where plaque fissure or rupture occurs because of wall-shear stresses, allowing blood to come in contact with collagen. This stimulates arachidonic acid release and conversion to leukotrienes. Leukotrienes C4 and D4 are potent coronary vasoconstrictors, especially in disrupted vessels. These leukotrienes also decrease the threshold for platelet aggregation to low concentrations of epinephrine, a phenomenon that has been described in patients with unstable angina.[56]

Aggregated platelets release thromboxane A_2 and serotonin,[57] which further promotes platelet aggregation and thrombus formation. Activated platelets also release platelet-derived growth factor, which causes progression in atherosclerosis, and β-thromboglobulin and platelet factor 4, which increase endothelial permeability and decrease levels of the vasodilator prostacyclin.[52] Impaired fibrinolytic ability also appears to be a factor in patients with CAD,[58] allowing the generation of thrombus to go unchecked. It appears that dynamic coronary vasoconstriction and thrombus formation at the site of an atherosclerotic plaque

occurs because of plaque rupture, with enhanced platelet aggregation, in the setting of an abnormal fibrinolytic system.[56]

Ischemia does occur in the absence of atherosclerotic coronary arteries and is thought to result from coronary artery spasm. Increases in plasma calcium and withdrawal of calcium channel blockers and nitrates have been implicated in the triggering of spasm, but studies of patients following CAS did not support the latter theory.[59]

Changes in oxygen content, particularly in the setting of fixed flow, can precipitate myocardial ischemia. Decreased oxygen content can be due to decreased hemoglobin or decreased oxygen saturation. Reductions in coronary blood flow without changes in luminal diameter are a result of either decreased diastolic filling time or decreased coronary perfusion pressure. Tachycardia, which is commonly seen in the postoperative period, produces decreases in diastolic filling time. Coronary perfusion pressure decreases either because of decreases in diastolic blood pressure or increases in left ventricular end-diastolic pressure, the latter seen with ventricular dysfunction or ischemia postoperatively in both cardiac and noncardiac surgical patients. Several mechanisms of reduction in myocardial oxygen supply are limited to patients after CAS. These include incomplete revascularization, acute vein graft thrombosis, and embolization of air or particulate matter into the coronary arteries.

Increased Demand

Increased myocardial oxygen consumption (MVO_2) is a hallmark of the postoperative period, and all three determinants of MVO_2 contribute to the increase. Elevated heart rates are well documented in the postoperative period and are commonly increased 25 to 50% over preoperative levels (Figure 15.6). Many factors contribute to postoperative tachycardia: increased sympathetic nervous system activity, pain, anxiety, hypovolemia, hyperthermia, β blocker and anesthetic withdrawal, and the use of adrenergic agonists. Elevated wall tension occurs because of the reduced left ventricular function seen in the postoperative period.[35–39] Elevated afterload also contributes to wall stress and can be due to hypothermia, increased sympathetic tone, anxiety, pain, or drugs. Finally, contractility could be increased as a result of the increased catecholamines postoperatively, but studies of postoperative left ventricular function do not support this. However, therapy with exogenous ionotropes will certainly increase MVO_2 on this basis.

DETECTION AND PREVENTION OF POSTOPERATIVE MYOCARDIAL ISCHEMIA

Myocardial ischemia is common in the postoperative period, which is not surprising given an understanding of the physiologic changes of the postoperative period and their interactions with myocardial oxygen supply and demand. Clearly, detection of myocardial ischemia is an important goal in prevention. How, then, can myocardial ischemia be detected in the postoperative period? Clinically, the most common detectors of ischemia are the patients themselves. But in the postoperative period, 90 to 100% of myocardial ischemic episodes are silent, either because of altered pain perception or competing somatic stimuli.

The 12-lead ECG is commonly used to detect ischemia,[60] but in the absence of discrete signs or symptoms, it is an impractical screening tool. Continuous 2-lead ECG monitoring is more practical, but electronic filters narrow the frequency range of clinical monitors, producing distortion of the ST segment.[61] Holter recorders have two channels and frequency ranges from 0.5 to 100 Hz, which is recommended by the American Heart Association for ST-segment analysis. However, Holter monitors require lengthy analysis and are not suitable for clinical monitoring. TEE is a sensitive detector of SWMAs, but it is impractical for lengthy monitoring and uncomfortable in awake patients; also, its usefulness as a real-

time monitor has been questioned. Myocardial ischemia has also been associated with changes in hemodynamics, such as tachycardia and increases in pulmonary capillary wedge pressures.[62] The correlation with hemodynamic changes, however, is poor, with only 30% of SWMAs occurring in the ICU preceded by elevations ($> 20\%$) in heart rate, systolic blood pressure, or pulmonary artery diastolic pressure, or by reductions ($> 20\%$) in diastolic blood pressure.[63] Real-time detection of myocardial ischemia in the postoperative period holds promise but awaits further development.

As such, prevention of ischemia is paramount. Myocardial oxygen demand can be decreased by decreasing heart rate, pain, catecholamines, and wall tension; or supply can be improved by decreasing heart rate, wall tension (to prevent plaque rupture), and epinephrine-induced platelet aggregation (as well as increasing PaO_2 and hemoglobin).

Several pharmacologic classes of drugs may play an important role. Vasodilators such as nitroprusside and nitroglycerin can decrease wall tension by decreasing systemic vascular resistance. However, the use of nitroprusside can result in a reflex tachycardia, as can nitroglycerin, but only with hypovolemia. They do not influence catecholamines, pain, or platelet aggregation. β blockers like esmolol[64] have been used to treat tachycardia and hypertension in the postoperative period, but their negative ionotropic effects can cause significant decreases in left ventricular function in a period already characterized by reduced function. Like vasodilators, β blockers have no effect on pain, catecholamines, or platelet aggregation. Opioids, however, can decrease heart rate, wall tension, and catecholamines without compromising left ventricular function. These characteristics of narcotics suggest that they might be useful in the prevention of myocardial ischemia in the postoperative period.

Currently, postoperative management includes small intermittent doses of a narcotic, usually morphine, given in response to complaints of pain or signs such as tachycardia or hypertension. These signs reflect significant sympathetic stimulation and, as such, small intermittent doses of narcotic can only blunt the peak effects. To prevent myocardial ischemia in the postoperative period, with the increased sensitivity of platelets to epinephrine, the decreased fibrinolysis, and the decreased left ventricular function, it is probably necessary to fully suppress activation of the sympathetic nervous system.

PRELIMINARY STUDIES

Anesthesia may suppress intraoperative ischemia[65] compared to the preoperative pattern,[13,66] and the suppression of this ischemia may be able to reduce postoperative morbidity and mortality.[10] Therefore, extending anesthesia into the stressful postoperative period may decrease the severity of postoperative ischemia. To assess the effects of prolonging anesthesia into the postoperative period, we compared a continuous high-dose sufentanil infusion to intermittent small doses of morphine.[67] We assessed the difference between these techniques by measurement of the incidence and severity of ECG-ST abnormalities consistent with ischemia following CAS. Sixty-three men undergoing elective CAS were studied. Patients with uninterpretable ECGs (e.g., left bundle branch block) were excluded. Anesthesia was 5 to 10 μg/kg sufentanil for induction followed by an infusion of 4.2 to 6.0 μg/kg/hr, and up to 0.5 mg/kg of valium. Following bypass, patients were randomized to receive either 1 μg/kg sufentanil as a bolus, given after protamine, followed by an infusion of 1 μg/kg/hr (group S, n = 32) or morphine up to 2 mg/kg in divided doses (group M, n = 31). In the ICU, group S continued to receive the infusion of 1 μg/kg/hr, while group M received intermittent doses of morphine (1 to 10 mg IV every 30 minutes prn). Both groups received midazolam 1 to 4 mg IV every 20 minutes prn. Sedation was discontinued at 04:00. No other aspects of clinical care were dictated by protocol. Patients were monitored continuously with two-channel (CM5, CC5) Holter monitors. Ischemic episodes (IE) were defined as a ≥ 1mm ST depression at J + 60

or a ≥ 2mm elevation at J, which was transient and lasted for at least 60 seconds. Hemodynamics were recorded every minute by a computer interfaced with the bedside monitor.

Preoperatively, patients in groups S and M were similar in weight, age, ejection fraction (< .40), left-main disease, unstable angina, hypertension and β blocker use. However, fewer diabetics were in group S than in group M (13 versus 37%; $p = 0.02$). The two groups received similar amounts of sufentanil (26.1 ± 5.4 versus 24.3 ± 4.1 μg/kg) and valium (0.43 ± 0.09 versus 0.42 ± 0.09 mg/kg) in the operating room, and fluids in the ICU (3,872 ± 1,031 versus 4,110 ± 1,422 cc). Time to extubation was also similar for both groups (615 ± 447 versus 512 ± 397 minutes after discontinuing sedation). In the ICU (mean study time = 14 hours), group S received a total of 14.1 ± 2.9 μg/kg sufentanil, compared with 0.44 ± 0.33 mg/kg of morphine (mean dose = 3 mg/hr) for group M. Group S received less midazolam than group M (0.11 ± 0.1 versus 0.23 ± 0.22 mg/kg; $p < 0.005$). In group S (versus group M), there was a trend toward lower mean heart rates (86 ± 7 versus 92 ± 13) and lower systolic pressures (116 ± 8 versus 124 ± 12) and a significantly lower double product (10,006 ± 1,114 versus 11,515 ± 2,203, $p < 0.05$).

In the operating room, the incidence (41 versus 42%) and severity of IEs postbypass was similar in the two groups, as was the incidence (28 versus 29%) of new IEs in the ICU. However, in group S, the IEs that occurred in the ICU tended to be shorter and had significantly smaller ST deviation and area under the ST-segment time curve (AUC) than in group M (Table 15.1).

These data demonstrate that continuous administration of high doses of sufentanil, versus prn administration of morphine, can blunt the severity of ischemic episodes that occur in the ICU following CAS.

CONCLUSION

New approaches to the prevention of PCM are needed in the coming years as the patient pop-

TABLE 15.1 Severity of ischemic episodes in the intensive care unit

	Group S	Group M	p Value
Incidence of ischemia	28%	29%	
Duration of ischemic episode (min)	71 ± 76	153 ± 122	$p = 0.07$
Maximum ST segment deviation (mm)	1.5 ± 0.5	2.1 ± 0.7	$p = 0.04$
Area under the ST segment time curve (mm²)	64 ± 87	405 ± 535	$p = 0.05$

Source: Reprinted with permission of the publisher from Siliciano D, Hollenberg M, Goehner P, et al. Use of continuous versus intermittent narcotic after CABG surgery: effects on myocardial ischemia. Anesth Analg 1990;70(Suppl):S371. (Abstr.)
Data are mean ± standard deviation.

ulation presenting for cardiac and noncardiac surgery ages, bringing more advanced CAD and its complications to the operating room. Postoperative myocardial ischemia appears to be a strong predictor of PCM and, as such, the new theories of mechanisms of postoperative ischemia are particularly timely. Preliminary data show that, by maintaining a continuous infusion of a high dose of narcotic, postoperative myocardial ischemia can be modified. The implication is that by blunting activation of the sympathetic nervous system in the postoperative period, and preventing the resultant endocrine, metabolic, and hemodynamic changes, the imbalance of myocardial oxygen supply and demand can be shifted away from ischemia. Further investigation is needed to confirm this, and to address the effects of modification of postoperative myocardial ischemia on eventual postoperative cardiac outcomes.

REFERENCES

1. Mangano DT. Perioperative cardiac morbidity. Anesthesiology 1990;72:153–184.
2. Luchi RJ, Scott SM, Deupree RH, et al. Comparison of medical and surgical treatment for unstable angina pectoris: results of a Veterans Administration Cooperative Study. N Engl J Med 1987;316:977–984.
3. Varnauskas E, European Coronary Surgery Study Group. Survival, myocardial infarction, and employment status in a prospective randomized study of coronary bypass surgery. Circulation 1985;72(suppl 5):V90–V101.
4. Teoh KH, Christakis GT, Weisel RD, et al. Increased risk of urgent revascularization. J Thorac Cardiovasc Surg 1987;93:291–299.
5. Junod FL, Harlan BJ, Payne J, et al. Preoperative risk assessment in cardiac surgery: comparison of predicted and observed results. Ann Thorac Surg 1987;43:59–64.
6. Kouchoukos NT, Ebert PA, Grover FL, et al. Report of the ad hoc committee on risk factors for coronary artery bypass surgery. Ann Thorac Surg 1988;45:348–349.
7. Rao TK, Jacobs KH, El-Etr AA. Reinfarction following anesthesia in patients with myocardial infarction. Anesthesiology 1983;59:499–505.
8. Goldman L, Caldera DL, Nussbaum SR, et al. Multifactorial index of cardiac risk in noncardiac surgical procedures. N Engl J Med 1977;297:845–850.
9. Steen PA, Tinker JH, Tanhan S. Myocardial reinfarction after anesthesia and surgery. JAMA 1987;239:2566–2575.
10. Slogoff S, Keats AS. Does perioperative myocardial ischemia lead to postoperative myocardial infarction? Anesthesiology 1985;62:107–114.
11. Knight AA, Hollenberg M, London MJ, et al. Perioperative myocardial ischemia: importance of the preoperative ischemic pattern. Anesthesiology 1988;68:681–688.
12. Fegert G, Hollenberg M, Browner W, et al. Perioperative myocardial ischemia in the noncardiac surgical patient. Anesthesiology 1988; 69:A49. (Abstr.)
13. Mangano DT, SPI Research Group. Characteristics of electrocardiographic ischemia in high-risk patients undergoing surgery. J Electrocardiol 1990; in press.
14. Wong MG, Wellington YC, London MJ, et al. Prolonged postoperative myocardial ischemia in high-risk patients undergoing non-

cardiac surgery. Anesthesiology 1988;69:A56. (Abstr.)

15. Siliciano D, Hollenberg M, Mangano DT. Myocardial ischemia following coronary revascularization. Proc 27th Annual West Anesthesia Residents Conf, 1989. (Abstr.)

16. Smith JS, Cahalan MK, Benefiel DJ, et al. Intraoperative detection of myocardial ischemia in high-risk patients: electrocardiography versus two-dimensional transesophageal echocardiography. Circulation 1985;72:1015–1021.

17. Leung J, O'Kelly B, Browner W, et al. Prognostic importance of postbypass regional wall-motion abnormalities in patients undergoing coronary artery bypass graft surgery. Anesthesiology 1989;71:16–25.

18. Udelsman R, Norton JA, Jelenich SE, et al. Responses of the hypothalamic-pituitary-adrenal and renin-angiotensin axes and the sympathetic system during controlled surgical and anesthetic stress. J Clin Endocrinol Metab 1987;64:986–994.

19. Halter J, Pflug A, Porte D. Mechanism of plasma catecholamine increase during surgical stress in man. J Clin Endocrinol Metab 1977;45:936–944.

20. George JM, Reier CE, Lanese RR, et al. Morphine anesthesia blocks cortisol and growth hormone response to surgical stress in humans. J Clin Endocrinol Metab 1974;38:736–741.

21. Roizen M, Lampe G, Benefiel D, et al. Is increased operative stress associated with worse outcome? Anesthesiology 1987;67:A1. (Abstr.)

22. Roizen M. Should we all have a sympathectomy at birth? Or at least preoperatively? Anesthesiology 1988;68:482–484.

23. Stanley T, Isern-Anmaral J, Lathrop G. Urine norepinephrine excretion in patients undergoing mitral or aortic valve replacement with morphine anesthesia. Anesth Analg 1975;54:509–517.

24. Flezzani P, Croughwell N, McIntyre RW, et al. Isoflurane blunts the norepinephrine response to cardiopulmonary bypass. Anesth Analg 1987;66 (Suppl):S59.

25. Stanley TH, Berman L, Green O, et al. Plasma catecholamine and cortisol responses to fentanyl-oxygen anesthesia for coronary-artery operations. Anesthesiology 1980;53:250–253.

26. Okutani R, Philbin DM, Rosow CE, et al. Effect of hypothermic hemodilutional cardiopulmonary bypass on plasma sufentanil and catecholamine concentrations in humans. Anesth Analg 1988;67:667–670.

27. Samuelson PN, Reves JG, Kirklin JK, et al. Comparison of sufentanil and enflurane–nitrous oxide anesthesia for myocardial revascularization. Anesth Analg 1986;65:217–226.

28. Flezzani P, Croughwell ND, McIntyre RW, et al. Isoflurane decreases the cortisol response to cardiopulmonary bypass. Anesth Analg 1986;65:1117–1122.

29. Reves JG, Karp RB, Buttner EE, et al. Neuronal and adrenomedullary catecholamine release in response to cardiopulmonary bypass in man. Circulation 1982;66:49–55.

30. Flacke JW, Bloor BC, Flacke WE, et al. Reduced narcotic requirement by clonidine with improved hemodynamic and adrenergic stability in patients undergoing coronary bypass surgery. Anesthesiology 1987;67:11–19.

31. Walsh E, Paterson J, O'Riordan J, et al. Effect of high-dose fentanyl anaesthesia on the metabolic and endocrine response to cardiac surgery. Br J Anaesth 1981;53:1155–1164.

32. Airaksinen K, Ikaheimo M, Linnaluoto M, et al. Impaired vagal heart rate control in coronary artery disease. Br Heart J 1987;58:592–597.

33. Airaksinen K, Ikaheimo M, Takkunen J. Heart rate after coronary artery bypass grafting. Am J Cardiol 1987;60:1395–1397.

34. Hohnloser S, Verrier R, Lown B. Effects of adrenergic and muscarinic receptor stimulation on serum potassium concentrations and myocardial electrical stability. Cardiovasc Res 1986;20:891–896.

35. Coriat P, Mundler O, Bousseau D, et al. Response of left ventricular ejection to recovery from general anesthesia. Anesth Analg 1986;65:593–600.

36. Gray R, Maddahi J, Berman D, et al. Scintigraphic and hemodynamic demonstration of transient left ventricular dysfunction immediately after uncomplicated coronary artery bypass grafting. J Thorac Cardiovasc Surg 1979;77:504–510.

37. Roberts AJ, Spies SM, Sanders JH, et al. Serial assessment of left ventricular performance following coronary artery bypass grafting. J Thorac Cardiovasc Surg 1981;81:69–84.

38. Levine F, Phillips H, Carter J, et al. The effect of pulsatile perfusion on preservation of left ventricular function after aortocoronary by-

pass grafting. Circulation 1981;64(Suppl 2):40–44.

39. Mangano DT. Biventricular function after myocardial revascularization in humans: deterioration and recovery patterns during the first 24 hours. Anesthesiology 1985;62:571–577.

40. Mansfield A. Alteration in fibrinolysis associated with surgery and venous thrombosis. Br J Surg 1972;59:754–757.

41. Britton B, Hawkey C, Wood W, et al. Stress: a significant factor in venous thrombosis? Br J Surg 1974;61:814–820.

42. Grabfield G. Factors affecting the coagulation time of blood. IX. The effect of adrenalin on the factors of coagulation. Am J Physiol 1916;42:46–55.

43. Hoffman BB, Michel T, Brenneman TB, et al. Interactions of agonists with platelet α-adrenergic receptors. Endocrinology 1982;110:926–932.

44. Zilla P, Fasol R, Groscurth P, et al. Blood platelets in cardiopulmonary bypass operations. J Thorac Cardiovasc Surg 1989;97:379–388.

45. Milam J, Austin S, Martin R, et al. Alteration of coagulation and selected clinical chemistry parameters in patients undergoing open-heart surgery without transfusions. Am J Clin Pathol 1981;76:155–162.

46. Griffin JH. Role of surface in surface-dependent activation of Hageman factor (blood coagulation factor XII). Proc Nat Acad Sci 1978;75:1998–2002.

47. Kalter R, Saul C, Wetstein L, et al. Cardiopulmonary bypass: associated hemostatic abnormalities. J Thorac Cardiovasc Surg 1979;77:427–435.

48. Tanaka K, Takao M, Yada I, et al. Alterations in coagulation and fibrinolysis associated with cardiopulmonary bypass during open-heart surgery. J Cardiothorac Anesth 1989;3:181–188.

49. Kannel WB, McGee D, Gordon T. A general cardiovascular risk profile: the Framingham study. Am J Cardiol 1976;38:46–51.

50. Clutton-Brock J. Pain and the barbiturates. Anaesthesia 1961;16:80–88.

51. Dundee W. Alterations in response to somatic pain associated with anaesthesia. II: The effect of thiopentone and pentobarbitone. Br J Anaesth 1960;32:407–414.

52. Conti CR, Mehta JL. Acute myocardial ischemia: role of atherosclerosis, thrombosis, platelet activation, coronary vasospasm, and altered arachidonic acid metabolism. Circulation 1987;75 (suppl 5):V84–V95.

53. Willerson JT, Hillis LD, Winniford M, et al. Speculation regarding mechanisms responsible for acute ischemia heart disease syndromes [editorial]. J Am Coll Cardiol 1986;8:245–250.

54. Moise A, Therous P, Taeymans Y, et al. Unstable angina and progression of coronary atherosclerosis. N Engl J Med 1983;309:685–692.

55. Folts J, Crowell E, Rowe L. Platelet aggregation in partially obstructed vessels and its elimination with aspirin. Circulation 1976;54:365–371.

56. Mehta J, Mehta P, Ostrowski N. Increase in human platelet α 2-adrenergic receptor affinity for agonist in unstable angina. J Lab Clin Med 1985;106:661–662.

57. Bush LR, Campbell WB, Buja LM, et al. Effects of the selective thromboxane synthetase inhibitor dazoxiben on variations in cyclic blood flow in stenosed canine coronary arteries. Circulation 1984;69:1161–1170.

58. Payamo J, Colucci M, Collen D, et al. Plasminogen activator inhibitor in the blood of patients with coronary artery disease. Br Med J 1985;291:573–578.

59. Lockerman Z, Rose D, Cunningham J, et al. Postoperative ST-segment elevation in coronary artery bypass surgery. Chest 1986;89:647–651.

60. London MJ, Hollenberg M, Wong MG, et al. Intraoperative myocardial ischemia: localization by continuous 12-lead electrocardiography. Anesthesiology 1988;69:232–241.

61. Arbeit S, Rubin I, Gross H. Dangers in interpreting the electrocardiogram from the oscilloscope monitor. JAMA 1970;211:453–456.

62. Kaplan JA, Wells PH. Early diagnosis of myocardial ischemia using the pulmonary arterial catheter. Anesth Analg 1981;60:789–793.

63. Leung J, O'Kelly B, Browner W, et al. Are regional wall motion abnormalities detected by transesophageal echocardiography triggered by acute changes in supply and demand? Anesthesiology 1988;69:A801. (Abstr.)

64. Gray R, Bateman T, Czer L, et al. Use of esmolol in hypertension after cardiac surgery. Am J Cardiol 1985;56:49F–56F.

65. Tarnow J, Markschies-Hornung A, Schulte-Sasse U. Isoflurane improves the tolerance to

TABLE 16.1 Complications in relation to anesthetic technique

Technique	No. of Patients	Complications	Incidence (Patients)
Local only	10,169	38	1/268
Local and sedation	10,229	96	1/106
General	61,299	513	1/120
Regional block	1,936	7	1/277
Other	462	1	1/462

Source: FASA Special Study. I. 1985. Reprinted with permission of the Federated Ambulatory Surgery Association, Alexandria, Va.

opioid.[2] Many of these patients were having diagnostic endoscopic procedures performed by endoscopists outside an operating room setting without anesthesia personnel in attendance. Yet in a recent study of 100,000 anesthetics,[3] monitored anesthesia care was associated with the highest rate of mortality (208.85 per 10,000 anesthetics) even though an anesthesiologist was in attendance. Unfortunately, as is the problem with many studies, specific data on agents, doses, and events were lacking. Specific doses were provided, however, in a closed claims analysis of 14 cases of cardiac arrest in healthy patients under spinal anesthesia.[4] One of the recurring patterns of management believed to be contributory was the intraoperative use of sedation. In 9 of these cases, fentanyl was administered. In all 14 cases, an anesthesiologist was in attendance.

Obviously, complications and deaths have been reported in association with MAC. Much of the following discussion is generic and applies to patients receiving intravenous sedation or analgesia whether or not an opioid was administered. The survey of the representative literature, results, and complications, however, includes only articles that state an opioid was used.

The House of Delegates of the American Society of Anesthesiologists,[5] on October 21, 1986, approved a statement on monitored anesthesia care in which the definition of services includes the following:

1. Performance of a preanesthetic examination and evaluation

2. Prescription of the anesthesia care required

3. Personal participation in, or medical direction of, the entire plan of care

4. Continuous physical presence of the anesthesiologist or, in the case of medical direction, of the resident or nurse anesthetist being medically directed

5. Proximate presence or, in the case of medical direction, availability of the anesthesiologist for diagnosis or treatment of emergencies

According to the statement, "all institutional regulations pertaining to anesthesia services shall be observed, and all the usual services performed by the anesthesiologist shall be furnished," including but not limited to the following:

1. Usual noninvasive cardiocirculatory and respiratory monitoring

2. Oxygen administration, when indicated

3. Intravenous administration of sedatives, tranquilizers, antiemetics, narcotics, other analgesics, β blockers, vasopressors, bronchodilators, antihypertensives, or other pharmacologic therapy as may be required in the judgment of the anesthesiologist

In this chapter, we briefly discuss preoperative evaluation, preparation, and monitoring and concentrate on patients in whose regimen an opioid has been included.

Our intent is to discuss our ideas on the subject of MAC based on our own experience and the literature available. Unfortunately, many of the well-designed studies that define the characteristics of opioids were performed with the subjects or patients during anesthesia rather than analgesia. Results collected during anesthesia are not always applicable to MAC, particularly when very large doses are used.

Also, the majority of studies and reports performed under MAC with opioids have been nonuniform in design and unclear in defining one or more critical areas. These include the state of sedation/analgesia desired and attained; doses of drugs used; complications observed; and criteria or time to discharge home or to the hospital room. We do not intend to be overly critical of these observations but merely to point out the difficulty in making comparisons and drawing conclusions from such data.

Thus, we focus on the definitions of MAC; the characteristics of an ideal narcotic in MAC; pharmacokinetics, pharmacodynamics, and complications associated with the use of opioids; a brief review of representative journal articles reported from a variety of settings; an overview of the status of the field; and a recommended approach to standardizing current and future studies so that observations may be made in a uniform manner.

DEFINITIONS

In 1988, the Joint Commission on Health Care Organizations (JCAHO) modified the application of its section on surgical and anesthesia services:[6] The chapter

applies to services for all patients who (1) receive general, spinal, or other major regional anesthesia or (2) undergo surgery or other invasive procedures when receiving general, spinal or other major regional anesthesia and/or intravenous, intramuscular, or inhalation sedation/analgesia that, in the manner used in the organization, may result in the loss of the patient's protective reflexes.

This statement implies that the description of characteristics required to provide safe anesthesia also applies to the provision of sedation/analgesia if loss of protective reflexes is possible. This suggests that the latter is a potentially dangerous complication. It also assumes that there may be other levels of sedation that are less hazardous. One of these is conscious sedation.

McCarthy et al.,[7] in definitions proposed by the American Dental Association Council on Dental Education, define conscious sedation as

minimally depressed level of consciousness that retains the patient's ability to independently and continuously maintain an airway and respond appropriately to physical stimulation and verbal command, produced by a pharmacologic or nonpharmacologic method, or a combination.

The Committee on Drugs, Section on Anesthesiology, American Academy of Pediatrics,[8] states:

For the very young or handicapped individual, incapable of the usually expected verbal response, a minimally depressed level on consciousness for that individual should be maintained. The caveat that loss of consciousness should be unlikely is a particularly important part of the definition of conscious sedation, and the drug and techniques should carry a margin of safety wide enough to render unintended loss of consciousness unlikely.

This definition draws our attention to the fact that patients could be incapable of responding appropriately. In this situation, a light level of sedation is especially important. In addition, the use of certain agents or dosages could unintentionally produce an undesired deeper state.

Shane,[9] a pioneer in the field of conscious sedation, emphasizes that somnolence or basal narcosis should not be produced. He highlights three equally important factors: amnesia, verbal rapport, and a profound local or regional block. The presumption is that the latter may not block the stress response of surgery without pharmacologic sedation/analgesia sup-

quired, with one "qualified person whose only responsibilities are observation and monitoring of the patient and who may administer drugs." These requirements emphasize two other important features of MAC:

1. Observation of the patient by a qualified individual who is not performing the procedure. This form of monitoring is required regardless of the type of equipment selected. As noted by Orkin,[14] "Newer monitors engender complacency with regard to direct observation of the patient. Less attention is directed to the patient, and we are lulled into believing that all is well if the monitors do not alarm."
2. Administration of agents must be done by an individual who is not performing the procedure. In addition to the efforts at monitoring during the operative phase, "risk management interest is now shifting appropriately to the postanesthetic recovery room."[14] As discussed later, because residual effects of sedative and opiate medication persist in the absence of painful stimuli, postoperative hypoventilation and hypoxia may ensue. The American Society of Anesthesiologists standards for postanesthesia care also address the issues of monitoring by methods appropriate to the patient's medical condition.[15]

THE OPIOIDS

Now that definitions, patient evaluation, and monitoring of the patients undergoing MAC have been discussed, we address the specific opioids. In this section, we examine opioids in the setting of MAC with respect to their ideal characteristics, untoward effects, specific pharmacokinetics and dynamics, and described use in the literature.

Characteristics and Effects

Listed in Table 16.3 are the ideal characteristics of intravenous analgesics used for mon-

TABLE 16.3 Ideal intravenous opioid characteristics for monitored anesthesia care

High therapeutic index (no respiratory or cardiovascular depression)
Water soluble, stable in solution and long shelf life
Nonirritating for intravenous administration
No hypersensitivity reactions
Rapid onset
Easily titrated in all patient populations
*Rapid return to baseline when effects no longer needed
*Analgesia persists after adverse side effects have dissipated[a]
*Amnesia for procedure but recall of discharge instructions[a]
*Ability to antagonize undesired effects

Source: Modified from White PF, Shafer A. Clinical pharmacology and uses of injectable anesthetic and analgesic drugs. In: Wetchler BV, ed. Problems in anesthesia: outpatient anesthesia. Philadelphia, Lippincott, 1988;2(1):37–54. Notable changes are marked with asterisks.
[a]Specifically relates to ambulatory patients.

itored anesthesia care, modified from White and Shafer[16] with notable changes marked by asterisks. Although most of the qualities on the list would be ideal for patients undergoing general anesthesia, many take on a different role during monitored anesthesia care. For example, during an open-heart operation the ability of high-dose narcotics to blunt sympathetic stimulation without causing injury to the heart is of prime importance. However, during monitored anesthesia care the ability to provide analgesia without adversely affecting ventilation is of paramount concern. Side effects such as nausea and vomiting, muscle rigidity, and histamine release can present a more difficult problem in the setting of monitored anesthesia care. In addition, since many of these patients are to undergo same-day surgery, the recovery period is of prime interest. Residual drug effects lead to increased recovery time and prolonged mental and psychomotor deficiencies. Unfortunately, most of the literature on opioids pertains to their use in anesthesia, with only a few articles relating to analgesia.

In order to focus on the aforementioned issues, we try to adapt the literature to the setting of monitored anesthesia care. In this section, we focus on the characteristics and effects of opioids as they may relate to MAC.

Respiratory Depression

Once a certain blood level is attained, all pure narcotics produce apnea. However, different narcotics have a different time course to reach maximal respiratory depression. In dogs given 0.3 mg/kg morphine intravenously, the peak respiratory depression was seen at 58 ± 9 minutes.[17] However after fentanyl (10 μg/kg, intravenous), decreased ventilation was seen within 30 seconds and apnea occurred at 1.5 minutes.[18] Sufentanil and alfentanil, similar to fentanyl, also exhibit their respiratory depressant effects shortly after injection.

After fentanyl, recovery of tidal volume, respiratory rate, and minute ventilation occur within 30 to 45 minutes, closely following the log concentration in cerebrospinal fluid (CSF) and plasma. With successive doses of fentanyl, the onset of apnea is the same, but the time to recovery of ventilation is longer.[18] The respiratory depressant effects of morphine do not correlate with either the plasma or CSF drug level. Ventilation can remain diminished for hours after plasma blood levels have fallen. This is thought to be secondary to morphine's low lipid solubility, which causes it to have a slow transit across the blood-brain barrier.[17]

Respiratory depression can be caused with doses of narcotics that are "too small to disturb consciousness and increases progressively as the dose is increased."[19] Opioids decrease minute volume mainly by decreasing respiratory rate to the point of complete apnea. They may also produce irregular and periodic breathing at doses that are considered therapeutic.[19]

Respiratory depression has been classically measured by a change in the carbon dioxide response curve. In 1956, Eckenhoff et al.[20] described a closed circuit system in which a patient could rebreathe CO_2. With $ETCO_2$ as the x axis and minute ventilation as the y axis, the curve produced represents the patient's respiratory drive. Later that same year, they looked at the effect of opiates on this curve.[21] In healthy adult human volunteers anesthetized with pentothal, the addition of either morphine or meperidine caused severe depression of respiration, as depicted as a rightward shift of the CO_2 response curve.

Sleep

It was soon noted that opiates shifted the curve but had only a small effect on its slope unless the volunteer fell asleep. Narcotics (morphine) combined with sleep caused a much greater depression in ventilation, which was reflected in a marked change in the slope of the CO_2 response curve in addition to the rightward shift. It was thought highly unlikely that respiratory sensitivity could change so dramatically with sleep, and it was postulated that, instead, sleep made certain feedback loops inoperative.[22] Sleep alone has been shown to cause respiratory depression. One study showed a decrease in CO_2 challenge to 28% of awake values during rapid eye movement (REM) sleep.[23] Recently, investigators have looked at the different stages of sleep and their additive effect on respiratory depression with morphine. Both REM and non-REM sleep were associated with a mild increase in resting transcutaneous CO_2. However, only non-REM sleep, when superimposed on respiratory depression caused by morphine, could produce a potentiated effect.[24] Not only is there a change in the response to CO_2 during sleep but the hypoxic ventilatory response also decreases to a level of 33% awake values during REM sleep.[25] Therefore, patients undergoing MAC who become somnolent will have less ventilatory drive reserve then if they were awake.

Continuous Infusions

The use of a continuous infusion allows less total drug to achieve the same effect during general anesthesia.[26,27] Bolus drug administration is associated with peaks and valleys.[28] Pathak et al.[27] showed that with an infusion technique of opioid during scoliosis surgery, less total narcotic was used, with fewer pa-

pression (μ_2). If this is true, an opioid might be developed in the future that is selective, providing profound analgesia without causing respiratory depression.

Agonists-Antagonists

Does the use of the agonists-antagonists prevent respiratory depression in monitored anesthesia care? Nalbuphine has been studied as compared to morphine in its ability to cause respiratory depression and analgesia. Gal et al.,[48] using a pain model (tourniquet ischemia) in healthy male volunteers, showed that 0.15 mg/kg nalbuphine caused a rightward shift of the CO_2 response curve. With additional doses there was no further shift or change of slope of the CO_2 response curve. This has been described as the ceiling of respiratory depression produced by nalbuphine.[16] This property would be optimal if the analgesic effects did not reach this ceiling, which was quantified by Gal et al.[48] as a maximum increase in pain tolerance of 40%.

The respiratory depressant effects of opioids can be summarized as follows:

1. Opioids produce dose-related depression of respiration, which may be aggravated by administration of more than one dose.
2. Sleep may also reduce response of ventilation to an increase in carbon dioxide or a reduction in oxygenation.
3. Continuous infusion decreases the total dose and eliminates the peaks and valleys of bolus administration.
4. Factors such as pre-existing respiratory problems, concurrent diseases, and increased age increase the potential for respiratory depression after opioids.
5. The addition of a benzodiazepine can attenuate or potentiate the respiratory depression of opioids depending on whether a lower narcotic dose is used and whether sleep is induced.
6. Biphasic respiratory depression is unlikely with alfentanil and probably with fentanyl in the dose customarily used for monitored anesthesia care.
7. Alfentanil may produce less sustained respiratory depression than fentanyl and also reduced total depression, since it is easier to titrate to its clinical endpoint.

Cardiovascular Effects

With the exception of meperidine, opioids produce a dose-dependent bradycardia. Direct depression of the myocardium does not occur unless large doses are used. Arteriolar and venous dilatation are primarily related to histamine release, which does not occur with the newer synthetic opioids. Cardiovascular instability in the setting of MAC is usually secondary to profound respiratory insufficiency.

Nausea and Vomiting

Nausea and vomiting are among the most common and undesired effects caused by opioid stimulation of the chemoreceptor trigger zone.[19] Also, opioids may increase vestibular sensitivity. It is for this reason that emetic effects are more often seen in ambulatory patients than in recumbent patients. With high-dose narcotics, this effect is attenuated. This is thought secondary to depression of the vomiting center.[49] Unfortunately, many of the patients under monitored anesthesia care are outpatients and are required to become ambulatory. The combination of low doses and increased vestibular sensitivity makes nausea and vomiting common problems, which require patients to remain in the ambulatory recovery room or to be admitted to the facility. Are these problems more frequent with any particular narcotic? When either fentanyl or alfentanil was used as an adjunct in general anesthesia for therapeutic abortions, both drugs produced a high incidence of nausea and vomiting (52 to 69%), with no statistical difference between them.[50] In comparing 3 μg/kg fentanyl to 15 μg/kg alfentanil in healthy volunteers, 7 of 8 patients in the fentanyl group were nauseated (4 vomited), and in the alfentanil group 4 of 8 were nauseated (1 vomited).[45] Kay and Venkataraman[51] found when comparing recovery between alfentanil and fentanyl supplemented anesthesia that 6 of 23 patients receiving alfentanil were nauseated (2 vomited) and 7 of 20 in the fentanyl group were nauseated (6 vomited).

Muscle Rigidity

Muscle rigidity is the phenomenon of abdominal and thoracic stiffness during the induction of anesthesia with an opioid. It is usually associated with high doses of narcotics,[52] rapid injection,[53] and the use of nitrous oxide.[54] The chest can become so stiff that it is impossible to ventilate the patient, and without prompt muscle relaxation it leads to hypercarbia and hypoxia.[55] Muscle rigidity has been reported during the recovery of both fentanyl and alfentanil anesthetics.[46,56] Although usually associated with large doses, rigidity has been reported with small intravenous doses of opioids.[57] This could have grave consequences for patients receiving small doses of opioids for monitored anesthetia care. White et al.[26] compared bolus to infusions with alfentanil and fentanyl. They found the highest incidence of chest wall rigidity in the fentanyl bolus group. Alfentanil and fentanyl were both associated with less chest wall rigidity when administered via an infusion. The cause of muscle rigidity now appears to be in a few discrete brain regions. Recently it was shown that the infusion of an opioid antagonist into the region of the nucleus raphe pontis and the nucleus reticularis pontis could attenuate muscle rigidity in rats induced with high-dose alfentanil.[58]

Histamine Release

Of the commonly used opioids, only meperidine and morphine are associated with histamine release.[59] Fentanyl, sufentanil, and alfentanil have not been reported to cause histamine release. It is postulated that the basic nature of morphine causes the displacement of histamine.[60]

Amnesia

Opioids alone have not been shown to produce amnesia. Scamman et al.[45] demonstrated in healthy volunteers that neither intravenous fentanyl (3.0 μg/kg) nor alfentanil (15 μg/kg) had any effect on a subject's immediate or delayed recall. In addition, Ochs et al.[61] showed in ASA I and II status patients that the addition of fentanyl (1.5 μg/kg) to midazolam (0.12 mg/kg) had no statistically significant difference in recall as compared to patients given midazolam (0.17 mg/kg) alone. With the same dose of fentanyl and diazepam (0.26 mg/kg), patients actually may have had increased recall as compared to diazepam (0.35 mg/kg) alone. This may be secondary to the decreased dose of diazepam in the patients who also received fentanyl, since a common clinical endpoint of slurred speech was used for dosing.

Pharmacokinetics and Dynamics

The purpose of using opioids during MAC is to modulate painful stimulation that cannot be controlled during the procedure. In order to accomplish this without adverse effects, it is important to understand the pharmacokinetics and dynamics of the different opioids. Table 16.4 shows some of these values for the most commonly used opioids.[52]

Onset

The onset of action of opioids occurs when they bind the opioid receptor. In order for an opioid molecule to bind its receptor it must cross a membrane from the plasma. There are three factors that are important. The first is size. With opioids this is of minor consequence, since all are relatively small molecules. Lipid solubility is a second factor, since biological membranes and the brain have a high lipid content. Of the commonly used opioids, only morphine has a very low lipid solubility, which gives it a relatively slow onset time. The third factor is the pKa and ionization at pH 7.4. Most opioids' pKa ranges from 7.9 to 8.5, with percent unionized ranging between 7 and 25%. The exception is alfentanil. By virtue of its low pKa (6.5), 89% of the injected drug remains unionized at normal physiologic

TABLE 16.4   Pharmacokinetic parameters

	Morphine	Meperidine	Fentanyl	Alfentanil	Sufentanil
pKa	7.9	8.5	8.4	6.5	8.0
% unionized of pH 7.4	23.0	7.4	8.5	89.0	19.7
Lipid solubility (octanol-water partition coefficient)	6.0	525.0	816.0	129.0	1,757.0
Protein binding (%)	63.0	82.0	84.0	92.0	93.0
Vd^{ss} (liters/kg)	3.4	4.4	4.0	0.7	1.7
Cl (ml/kg/min)	2.3	7.7	12.6	5.1	12.7
$T_{1/2}\beta$ (hr)	1.7	6.7	3.6	1.6	2.7

Source: Reprinted with permission from Sebel PS, Bovill JG. Opioid analgesics in cardiac anesthesia. In: Kaplan, JA, ed. *Cardiac anesthesia*. 2d ed. Orlando, Fla.: Grune & Stratton, 1987;1:67–123.

pH. Because only unionized molecules can cross biological membranes, this gives alfentanil a distinct edge. Alfentanil has an onset peak of 1 to 2 minutes, compared to 5 to 6 minutes for fentanyl and 20 minutes for morphine given via the intravenous route.[62] This makes alfentanil more easily titrated with less overshoot when given to a desired endpoint. This is one theory why alfentanil has been associated with less respiratory depression.[26]

Duration

For short procedures in the outpatient setting, duration of action is also an important consideration. As seen in Table 16.4, alfentanil has the shortest elimination half-life, an average of 94 minutes.[63] This short half-life is mainly a function of alfentanil's small volume of distribution, since its rate of clearance is less than half that of fentanyl and sufentanil. Morphine also has a short half-life, 104 minutes. In the case of morphine, however, the use of plasma parameters does not necessarily follow drug concentrations within the brain.[17] Many believe that morphine's clinical effect may last upwards of 4 to 5 hours.[49] Because of morphine's low lipid solubility, the blood-brain barrier is a major obstacle to its passage. It has been shown that the respiratory depressant effects do not parallel morphine serum levels.[17] This is in contrast to the more lipid-soluble drug fentanyl, for which plasma levels are a

good marker of the respiratory depressant effects.[18]

Effect of Dosage on Duration

Does dosage have an influence on the duration of action of the opioids? This question is related to the secondary question of which is more important for terminating the clinical effects of the narcotic: redistribution or metabolism. In this respect, fentanyl has been studied extensively. With small doses, because of fentanyl's large volume of distribution, clinical effects are short, and terminal half-life may be less than listed. However when large or repeated doses of fentanyl are used, the large volume of distribution acts as a storage depot (in poorly perfused tissues such as fat), prolonging fentanyl's clinical effects and terminal half-life.[18,64] In the setting of monitored anesthesia care, high doses would seem to be unlikely, so this prolongation of termination should not be significant. Hudson and Stanski,[65] with the aid of a model using pharmacokinetic data from the literature, compared alfentanil and fentanyl to see if there was a difference in the role of redistribution and metabolism in terminating their action. They did this by constructing a ratio, metabolism: total loss of drug, for different times after injection. They found that the termination of effects of alfentanil depended more on metabolism than on distribution. They felt this gave alfentanil more predictable kinetics and duration over a wide dose range.

Pre-Existing Conditions Affecting Duration

So far, the discussion of duration has concerned adult healthy patients. However, additional factors also are important. As the population becomes older, we see a preponderance of elderly patients presenting for monitored anesthesia care. Helmers et al.[66] compared alfentanil kinetics between young adults and elderly patients with a single 50 μg/kg bolus. They found that the rate of clearance was reduced, the elderly patients giving a half-life of 137 minutes, compared to 83 minutes in young adults. Scott and Stanski[32] also found the amount of fentanyl or alfentanil required by infusion in healthy elderly patients for elective surgery significantly decreased with age. They used power spectral analysis of electroencephalograms as a pharmacodynamic endpoint for dosing. In contrast to Helmers et al., they concluded that pharmacokinetics did not change but brain sensitivity increased with age. Children given a bolus of 20 μg/kg alfentanil have a lower clearance, but because of a decreased volume of distribution, the elimination half-life is reduced to 40 ± 3 minutes.[67] The presence of obesity may also prolong the elimination of alfentanil.[68] With a dose of 100 μg/kg using lean body weight, obese patients showed a terminal half-life for alfentanil of 172 minutes, while nonobese controls showed a half-life of 92 minutes. This, however, may not be the case when small doses are used. Cirrhosis of the liver has also been shown to prolong the elimination half-life of narcotics. Ferrier et al.[69] showed alfentanil half-life to be prolonged to 219 minutes in patients with cirrhosis. In addition, alcohol consumption has been shown to increase the terminal half-life of alfentanil.[70]

Potency

In order to arrive at the proper dosage for monitored anesthesia care, a careful look must be taken at relative potency. Using morphine for comparison, in dogs, de Castro et al.[71] found alfentanil, fentanyl, and sufentanil to be 31, 124, and 1240 times as potent as morphine, respectively (cited by Sebel and Bouill).[52]

Dosage in Monitored Anesthesia Care

What is the dosage of opioids in monitored anesthesia care? Most of the literature that tries to answer this question tells of the investigators' own combination of opioids, benzodiazapines, and other pharmaceuticals. Very few sources give analgesic dosages for narcotics; however, White has compared analgesic and anesthetic doses and potency ratios (Table 16.5).

Philip,[72] in describing supplemental medication for regional anesthesia, suggests a dose of 1 to 3 μg/kg fentanyl or 5 to 20 μg/kg alfentanil.

Recovery

Since monitored anesthesia care is performed in a large proportion of the patients having ambulatory surgery, length of recovery is very important. However, before discussing recovery, it is important to define it. Recovery has a spectrum, from early stages of being able to follow verbal commands (used as the definition in Gilbert et al.[73]) to the ability of performing cognitive and complex psychomotor functions such as driving a car.[74] Gelfman et al.[75] discuss recovery of their oral surgery patients by means of different psychomotor function tests (Trieger dot, perceptual speed, and flicker fusion). However, what stage of recovery does adequate performance of these tests represent? This is very important in deciding when patients can safely be discharged, or at what point they can make clear mental decisions or operate heavy machinery. Korttila[76] has compared the stages of recovery and the corresponding tests (Table 16.6).

To date no single clinically practical test is available to pinpoint a patient's stage of recovery. Recovery depends on the pharmacologic agents employed, their dosages, and the patient's response. Drugs with long terminal

TABLE 16.5 Therapeutic dosage ranges for the newer opioid compounds compared with the available analgesics

Drug (Trade Name)	Analgesic Dose[a]	"Anesthetic" Dose[b]	Potency Ratio[c]
Agonist			
Morphine sulfate	5–15 mg	1–6 mg/kg	1
Hydromorphine (Dilaudid)	1–2 mg	0.1–0.6 mg/kg	6–10
Methadone (Dolophine)	5–15 mg	NA	0.8–1.0
Meperidine (Demerol)	50–150 mg	5–20 mg/kg	0.08–0.1
Alphaprodine (Nisentil)	20–45 mg	NA	0.2–0.3
Fentanyl (Sublimaze)	100–200 μg	50–150 μg/kg	50–150
Sufentanil (Sufenta)	15–30 μg	5–20 μg/kg	400–1,000
Alfentanil (Alfenta)	500–1,000 μg	100–250 μg/kg	10–15
Agonist-antagonist			
Pentazocine (Talwin)	30–60 mg	NA	0.1–0.3
Butorphanol (Stadol)	1–3 mg	NA	4–6
Nalbuphine (Nubain)	5–15 mg	NA	0.8–1.0

Source: Reprinted with permission from White PF. Newer analgesic therapy. In: Hershey SG, ed. Refresher courses in anesthesiology. Philadelphia: Lippincott, 1984;12:211–224.

NA, Not available.

[a]Factors that alter the analgesic requirement include the patient's age, drug history, level of anxiety, type of operation, and presence of supplemental agents.

[b]High doses are used as sole anesthetics when combined with amnesic premedicants, relaxants, and vasodilating drugs. Although induction of anesthesia can be achieved with both fentanyl and sufentanil, alfentanil has the most rapid onset of action.

[c]Estimated potency ratios relative to morphine sulfate.

half-lives will retard recovery longer, as will larger doses of drugs with large volumes of distribution. Korttila,[74] in driving tests on adult human volunteers without surgery, has compiled recommended times of hospital stay and time before driving an automobile. For example, with fentanyl (100 μg, IV), the recommended discharge time is 1 to 2 hours, and with a dose of 200 μg it is 2 hours. Although this is not much of a difference, the recommendations for avoiding driving with 100 μg versus 200 μg are 2 hours and 8 hours, respectively. In other words, a twofold increase in dosage causes a fourfold increase in time till able to drive.[74]

Now that we have described the untoward effects (respiratory depression, nausea and vomiting, muscle rigidity, and histamine release), onset, duration, recommended dosages, and recovery characteristics of the commonly used narcotics, we look at the sedation recipes and studies in the literature. A compilation of the many drug combinations in the literature used for sedation, with results, complications, and recovery, are shown in Appendix 16.1.

As seen in Appendix 16.1, most sedation studies are from the dental literature. Many give the surgeon/operator's technique and recipe to provide "conscious sedation" for the patient while the procedure is performed. Most studies were performed in the surgeon's office on patients with health status that ranged from ASA I to III if it was noted. The intensity (degree) of sedation, when stated, had many different definitions. A multitude of combinations of agents were used, with some authors stating their endpoint of administration. In discussing results, most studies related the benefits of their regimens, how patients were satisfied, and whether patients would return for additional procedures. Few discussed any major complications, and only some discussed minor complications. In Appendix 16.1, Bennett[77] using fentanyl, diazepam, and methohexital, observed no complications, while

TABLE 16.6 The stages of recovery and the tests that correspond

Stage of Recovery	Test
Awakening	Patient can open eyes and answer questions
Immediate clinical recovery	Patient can sit up easily and steadily; Romberg test (negative); other clinical tests
Home-readiness[a]	Maddox wing test; patient can walk on a straight line
Street-fitness[a]	Flicker fusion test; psychomotor test batteries; electroencephalographic results
Full recovery (complete psychomotor recovery)[a]	Carefully selected psychomotor test batteries; real driving tests
Psychological recovery[a]	Psychological tests

Source: Adapted with permission from Korttila K. Postanesthetic cognitive and psychomotor impairment. Int Anesthesiol Clin 1986;24:59–74.
[a]More than a single test is needed.

in Campbell et al.[78] 85% of the patients receiving the same three drugs in smaller dosages had minor complications (delayed recovery, dizziness, gastrointestinal upset, drowsiness, muscular discomfort, and headache). The noting of complications appear to be related to how they are defined and accepted by the investigator. Recovery was discussed in many of the studies. Most listed the time the patient was discharged. Except for Gelfman et al.[75] none gave criteria for discharge.

RECOMMENDATION FOR FURTHER STUDY

It should be clear that much is known about the use of opioids in providing anesthesia. The literature surrounding their use in MAC is confusing and incomplete. Alfentanil has many potentially useful characteristics of an ideal opioid for MAC and needs further study. Appendix 16.2 contains some suggestions for uniform data collection when a clinical study is performed.

CONCLUSION

Monitored anesthesia care is gaining in popularity. Patients and physicians are finding it acceptable and desirable for use in many di-

agnostic procedures and for operations, particularly those performed under local or topical anesthesia. New agents have more predictable characteristics, a quicker onset, and a shorter duration than morphine or meperidine. They are potentially safer to administer to inpatients and outpatients.

Monitoring of oxygenation is rapidly becoming a standard. Anesthesia personnel are more cognizant of the risks of MAC, particularly those associated with reduced ventilation. Although we have learned much from the literature of the past 20 years, it is time to standardize our studies of new and old agents and combinations so that patient care can become more uniform and safe regardless of who is administering the agents or the location in which the procedure is performed.

REFERENCES

1. Campbell RL. Prevention of complications associated with intravenous sedation and general anesthesia. J Oral Maxillofac Surg 1986;44:289–301.
2. Midazolam: is antagonism justified. Lancet 1988;2:140–142. (Editorial)
3. Cohen MM, Duncan PG, Tate RB. Does anesthesia contribute to operative mortality? JAMA 1988;260:2859–2863.
4. Caplan RA, Ward RJ, Posner K, et al. Unexpected cardiac arrest during spinal anesthe-

sia: a closed claims analysis of predisposing factors. Anesthesiology 1988;68:5–11.

5. Position on monitored anesthesia care. Am Soc Anesthesiologists Dir Members 1989;606–607.

6. Joint Commission on Health Care Organizations. Surgical and anesthesia services (SA) accreditation manual for hospitals 1988;287.

7. McCarthy FM, Solomon AL, Jostak JT, et al. Conscious sedation: benefits and risks. J Am Dent Assoc 1984;109:545–557.

8. American Academy of Pediatrics. Guidelines for the elective use of conscious sedation, deep sedation, and general anesthesia in pediatric patients. Pediatrics 1985;76:317–321.

9. Shane SM. Conscious sedation for ambulatory surgery. Baltimore, Md.: University Park Press, 1983.

10. Bennett CR. Therapeutic goals of conscious sedation. In: Dionne RA, Laskin DM, eds. Anesthesia and sedation in the dental office. New York: Elsevier, 1986;39–45.

11. Bennett CR. The spectrum of pain control. In: Conscious sedation in dental practice. 2d ed. St. Louis: C.V. Mosby, 1978;10–23.

12. Kallar SK, Dunwiddie WC. Conscious sedation. In: Wetchler BV, ed. Problems in anesthesia: outpatient anesthesia. Philadelphia: Lippincott, 1988;2(1):93–100.

13. Standards for basic intraoperative monitoring. Am Soc Anesthesiologists Dir Members 1989; 609–610.

14. Orkin FK. Practice standards: the midas touch or the emperor's new clothes? Anesthesiology 1989;70:567–571.

15. Standards for postanesthesia care. Am Soc Anesthesiologists Dir Members 1989;613–614.

16. White PF, Shafer A. Clinical pharmacology and uses of injectable anesthetic and analgesic drugs. In: Wetchler BV, ed. Problems in anesthesia: outpatient anesthesia. Philadelphia: Lippincott, 1988;2(1):37–54.

17. Hug CC Jr, Murphy MR, Rigel EP, et al. Pharmacokinetics of morphine injected intravenously into the anesthetized dog. Anesthesiology 1981;54:38.

18. Hug CC Jr, Murphy MR. Fentanyl disposition in cerebrospinal fluid and plasma and its relationship to ventilatory depression in the dog. Anesthesiology 1979;50:342–349.

19. Jaffe JH, Martin WR. Opioid analgesics and antagonists. In: Goodman LS, Gilman A, eds. Pharmacological basis of therapeutics. 7th ed. New York: Macmillan, 1985;491–531.

20. Eckenhoff JE, Helrich M, Hege M. A method for studying respiratory functions in awake or anesthetized patients. Anesthesiology 1956; 17:66–72.

21. Helrich M, Eckenhoff JE, Jones RE, et al. Influence of opiates on the respiratory response of man to thiopental. Anesthesiology 1956;17:459–467.

22. Forrest WH, Bellville JW. The effect of sleep plus morphine on the respiratory response to carbon dioxide. Anesthesiology 1964;25:137–141.

23. Douglas NJ, White DP, Weil JV, et al. Hypercapnic ventilatory response in sleeping adults. Am Rev Respir Dis 1982;126:758–762.

24. Moote CA, Knill RL, Skinner MI, et al. Morphine produces a dose-dependent respiratory depression which is potentiated by non-REM sleep. Anesth Analg 1989;68:S201.

25. Douglas NJ, White DP, Weil C, et al. Hypoxic ventilatory response decreases during sleep in normal men. Am Rev Respir Dis 1982;125: 286–289.

26. White PF, Coe V, Schafer A, et al. Comparison of alfentanil with fentanyl for outpatient anesthesia. Anesthesiology 1986;64:99–106.

27. Pathak KS, Brown RH, Nash CL Jr, et al. Continuous opioid infusion for scoliosis surgery. Anesth Analg 1983;62:841–845.

28. White PF. Clinical uses of intravenous anesthetic and analgesic infusions. Anesth Analg 1989;68:161–171.

29. Kay B. Postoperative pain relief: use of an on-demand analgesia computer (ODAC) and a comparison of the rate of use of fentanyl and alfentanil. Anaesthesia 1981;36:949–951.

30. Mulroy MF, Coombs JHB, Isenberg MD, et al. Age, chronic obstructive pulmonary disease, and Innovar-induced ventilatory depression during regional anesthesia. Anesth Analg (Cleve) 1977;56:826–830.

31. Rozen P, Fireman Z, Gilat T. The causes of hypoxemia in elderly patients during endoscopy. Gastrointest Endosc 1982;28:243–246.

32. Scott JC, Stanski DR. Decreased fentanyl and alfentanil dose requirements with age: a simultaneous pharmacokinetic and pharmacodynamic evaluation. Pharmacol Exp Ther 1987;240:159–166.

33. Stone B, Barkin JS, Panullo W, et al. Hypercalcemia: a risk factor to patients undergoing gastrointestinal endoscopy. Am J Gastroenterol 1986;81:516–517.

34. Kissin I, Brown PT, Bradley EL Jr, et al. Diazepam: morphine hypnotic synergism in rats. Anesthesiology 1989;70:689–694.

35. Tucker MR, Ochs MW, White RP. Arterial blood gas levels after midazolam or diazepam administered with or without fentanyl as an intravenous sedative for outpatient surgical procedures. J Oral Maxillofac Surg 1986;44: 688–692.

36. Campbell RL, Dionne RA, Gregg JM. Respiratory effects of fentanyl, diazepam, and methohexital. J Oral Surg 1979;37:355.

37. Bailey PL, Moll JWB, Pace NL, et al. Respiratory effects of midazolam and fentanyl: potent interaction producing hypoxemia and apnea. Anesthesiology 1988;69:A813.

38. Tverskoy M, Fleyshman G, Ezry J, et al. Midazolam-morphine sedative interation in patients. Anesth Analg 1989;68:S297.

39. Becker LD, Paulson BA, Miller RD, et al. Biphasic respiratory depression after fentanyl-droperidol or fentanyl alone used to supplement nitrous oxide anesthesia. Anesthesiology 1976;44:291–296.

40. Hug CC Jr, Murphy MR. Tissue redistribution of fentanyl and termination of its effects in rats. Anesthesiology 1981;53:369.

41. McClain DA, Hug CC Jr. Pharmacodynamics of opiates. Int Anesthesiol Clin 1984;22(4):75–94.

42. Mahla ME, White SE, Moneta MD. Delayed respiratory depression after alfentanil. Anesthesiology 1988;69:593–595.

43. O'Connor M, Escarpa A, Prys-Roberts C. Ventilatory depression during and after infusion of alfentanil in man. Br J Anaesth 1983;55:217–222S.

44. Goldberg ME, Bartkowski RR, Seltzer JL, et al. The time course of respiratory depression after alfentanil anesthesia: a detailed evaluation. Anesthesiology 1988;69:A814.

45. Scamman FL, Ghoneim MM, Korttila K. Ventilatory and mental effects of alfentanil and fentanyl. Acta Anaesthesiol Scand 1984;28: 63–67.

46. Andrews CJH, Sinclair M, Pry-Roberts C, et al. Ventilatory effects during and after continuous infusion of fentanyl or alfentanil. Br J Anaesth 1983;55:211S–216S.

47. Bailey PL, Streisand JB, East KA, et al. Differences in magnitude and duration of opioid-induced respiratory depression and analgesia with fentanyl and sufentanil. Anesth Analg 1990;70:8–15.

48. Gal TJ, DiFazio CA, Moscicki J. Analgesic and respiratory depressant activity of nalbuphine: a comparison with morphine. Anesthesiology 1982;57:367–374.

49. Murphy MR. Opioids. In: Barash PG, Cullen BF, Stoelting RK, eds. Clinical anesthesia. Philadelphia: Lippincott, 1989;255–279.

50. Coe V, Shafer A, White PF. Techniques for administering alfentanil during outpatient anesthesia: a comparison with fentanyl. Anesthesiology 1983;59:A347.

51. Kay B, Venkataraman P. Recovery after fentanyl and alfentanil in anaesthesia for minor surgery. Br J Anaesth 1983;55:169S–171S.

52. Sebel PS, Bovill JG. Opioid analgesics in cardiac anesthesia. In: Kaplan JA, ed. Cardiac anesthesia. 2d ed. Orlando, Fla.: Grune & Stratton, 1987;1:67–123.

53. Scamman FL. Fentanyl-O_2-N_2O rigidity and pulmonary compliance. Anesth Analg 1983; 62:332–334.

54. Sokall MD, Hoyt JL, Georgis SD. Studies in muscle rigidity, nitrous oxide, and narcotic analgesic agents. Anesth Analg (Cleve) 1972; 51:16–20.

55. Comstock MK, Carter JG, Moyers JR, et al. Rigidity and hypercapnia associated with high-dose fentanyl induction of anesthesia. Anesth Analg 1981;60:362.

56. Christian CM, Waller JL, Moldenhauer CC. Postoperative rigidity following fentanyl anesthesia. Anesthesiology 1983;58:275.

57. Janis KM. Acute rigidity with small intravenous doses of Innovar: a case report. Anesth Analg (Cleve) 1972;51:375.

58. Weinger MB, Koob GF. Further elucidation of brain sites which mediate alfentanil-induced muscle rigidity in the rat. Anesthesiology 1988;69:A610.

59. Flacke JW, Flacke WE, Bloor BC, et al. Histamine release by four narcotics: a double-blind study in humans. Anesth Analg 1987; 66:723–730.

60. Rosow CE, Moss J, Philbin DM, et al. Histamine release during morphine and fentanyl anesthesia. Anesthesiology 1982;56:93–96.

61. Ochs MW, Tucker MR, White RP. A comparison of amnesia in outpatients sedated with midazolam or diazepam alone or in combination with fentanyl during oral surgery. J Am Dent Assoc 1986;113:894–897.

62. Stoelting R. Opioid agonists and antagonists. In: Pharmacology and physiolology in anesthetic practice. Philadelphia: Lippincott, 1987; 69–101.

63. Bovill JG, Sebel PS, Blackburn CL, et al. The pharmacokinetics of alfentanil (R39209): a new opioid analgesic. Anesthesiology 1982;57: 439–443.

64. Hug CC Jr. The pharmacokinetics of fentanyl. Piscataway, N.J.: Janssen Pharmaceutica, 1981.

65. Hudson RJ, Stanski DR. Metabolism versus redistribution of fentanyl and alfentanil. Anesthesiology 1983;59:A243.

66. Helmers H, Van Peer A, Woestenborghs R, et al. Alfentanil kinetics in the elderly. Clin Pharmacol Ther 1984;36:239–243.

67. Meistelman C, Sint-Maurice C, Loose JP, et al. Pharmacokinetics of alfentanil in children. Anesthesiology 1984;61:A443.

68. Bently JB, Finley JH, Humphrey LR, et al. Obesity and alfentanil pharmacokinetics. Anesth Analg 1983;62:245–292.

69. Ferrier C, Marty J, Bouffard Y, et al. Alfentanil pharmacokinetics in patients with cirrhosis. Anesthesiology 1985;62:480–484.

70. Rader JC, Nilsen OG. Pharmacokinetics of midazolam and alfentanil in outpatient anesthesia. Anesthesiology 1988;59:A465.

71. de Castro J, van de Water A, Wouters L, et al. Comparative study of cardiovascular, neurological, and metabolic side effects of eight narcotics in dogs. Acta Anaesthesiol Belg 1979;30:5–99.

72. Philip BK. Supplemental medication for ambulatory procedures under regional anesthesia. Anesth Analg 1985;64:1117–1125.

73. Gilbert J, Holt JE, Johnston J, et al. Intravenous sedation for cataract surgery. Anaesthesia 1987;42:1063–1069.

74. Korttila K. Recovery and driving after brief anaesthesia. Anaesthesist 1981;30:377–382.

75. Gelfman SS, Gracely RH, Driscoll EJ, et al. Recovery following intravenous sedation during dental surgery performed under local anesthesia. Anesth Analg (Cleve) 1980;59:775–781.

76. Korttila K. Postanesthetic cognitive and psychomotor impairment. Int Anesthesiol Clin 1986;24:59–74.

77. Bennett CR. A clinical evaluation of fentanyl for outpatient sedation in dentistry. Oral Surg 1972;34:882–885.

78. Campbell RL, Satterfield SD, Dionne RA, et al. Postanesthetic morbidity following fentanyl, diazepam, and methohexital sedation. Anesth Prog 1980;27:45–48.

APPENDIX 16.1 Sedation for procedures done under local/topical anesthesia (by surgeon)

Reference or Note No.	Procedure/ Demographics	Definition/Goal of Sedation	Sedation Agents (intravenous unless stated)	Results/Complications/ Recovery
a	Periodontal surgery (office) All ages ASA I 3,178 II 1,767 III 255 Total 5,200	"conscious sedation" "to alter the mood of the fearful, anxious patient so that a psychologically unacceptable procedure becomes acceptable" "rational response to command with all protective reflexes intact, yet calm, pleasantly relaxed"	Diazepam and methohexital (1,500) Above plus meperidine for surgery > 1.5 hrs (3,700)	Minor complications: 22 transient phlebitis 3 nausea and vomiting Satisfied patients
78	Extraction of third molars (office) All healthy Ages 18–28	"conscious sedation with Verrill's sign (ptosis of the lids) as the desired endpoint"	Fentanyl 100 μg Diazepam 5–10 mg Methohexital 15 mg in increments to endpoint	54% delayed recovery (?time) 49% dizziness 31% gastrointestinal upset 70% drowsiness 9% muscular discomfort 17% headache
77	Oral surgery (office) Ages 21–64 12 pts—4 groups		Group I: fentanyl < 200 μg Group II: fentanyl < 200 μg + diazepam 2.5 mg Group III: fentanyl unlimited diazepam 5 mg Group IV: fentanyl unlimited diazepam 10 mg methohexital 15–150 mg	All responded to questions All "relaxed" postdrugs No or mild subjective pain No major complications No nausea or vomiting No other side effects All discharged at 1 hr

APPENDIX 16.1 Continued

Reference or Note No.	Procedure/ Demographics	Definition/Goal of Sedation	Sedation Agents (intravenous unless stated)	Results/Complications/ Recovery
b	Oral surgery All healthy Ages 6–11 (25) 12–20 (25) 21–30 (25) 31–45 (25)		"Shane's method"c Alphaprodine 30 mg (adult) Hydroxyzine 50 mg (adult) Atropine 0.6 mg (adult) Methohexital 30–60 mg (adult)	"patient's great enthusiasm and lack of recall the day following the procedure"
d	ENT surgery (Hospital office) ASA I, II, III	"conscious sedation" goals: 1. sedate with minimal risk 2. relieve anxiety and fear 3. supplement analgesia of local Never lose communication with pt	Diazepam 1–2 mg doses until "Verrill's sign" or horizontal nystagmus; speech is slurred at endpoint Fentanyl 1 cc increments until control of pain or RR < 12	Feel pts need to be observed 30 minutes or longer
45	No surgery Paid volunteers Mean age 22.8 40 Total ASA I Sedation only	Fixed doses given to study the ventilatory and mental effects of alfentanil and fentanyl	Scopolamine 0.25 mg Group I: placebo Group II: fentanyl 1.5 µg/kg Group III: fentanyl 3.0 µg/kg Group IV: alfentanil 7.5 µg/kg Group V: alfentanil 15 µg/kg	CO_2 response least affected in IV; most in III No difference in groups with symbol cancellation, delayed or immediate recall Group III had significant difference in tapping skills
e	Plastic surgery (office) 814 patients	"patient awake or easily arousable"	Lorazepam 0.04 mg/kg 20 min prior to the procedure Fentanyl 25 µg before local 25 µg/30 min 100–300 µg total	1.5 hrs to discharge No major complications 6% nausea
f	Repair hand deformities (local) Inpatients Ages 14–68 100 pts	"in dosages which cause general quiescence and a state of indifference to environmental stimuli while allowing the patient to remain arousable in surgery"	Premedication: two-thirds usual dose Droperidol/fentanyl (Innovar) 0.5 cc/10 kg	5 pts required general anesthesia No major complications Somnolence for 24 hrs

	Population	Definition	Drugs	Results
g	Elective diag. Laparoscopy, Ages 20–35, ASA I, II, Outpatients	"conscious sedation" "patient reacts to commands, breathes spontaneously and, in fact, cooperates with the anesthesiologist without later being fully aware of the procedure."	Premed: hydroxyzine 1.5 mg/kg; In OR: flunitrazepam 0.01 mg/kg, fentanyl 1 μg/kg	End tidal CO_2 after sedation from 4.6 to 5.9%; Increase in mean BP 10%; All discharged 6–8 hrs after procedure; No major complications
73	Cataracts, Ages 18–90, Mean age 67, ASA I 7%, II 83%, III 9%, Total 60 pts, Outpatients, Retrobulbar and local	"The degree of sedation was evaluated at the time of insertion of the nerve blocks, on the basis of the patient's response to the injections, persistence of lid reflex, ability to obey simple commands and awareness of surroundings."	Group I: fentanyl mean dose 71 μg, diazepam mean dose 4.7 mg; Group II: nalbuphine 7.3 mg, methohexital 36 mg	Group II 81% markedly drowsy or unarousable as judged by investigator and surgeon; Vomiting 4% I & II; Excitation 7% I & II; Dysphoria 4% I only; Minor snoring 15% I & II
75	Third molar extractions (office), Ages 18–35, ASA I, Total 94		Group I: fentanyl 100 μg, diazepam 12.5 mg, methohexital 20–40 mg, naloxone 0.4 mg at end; Group II: diazepam 15 mg, methohexital 20–40 mg; Placebo saline group in double cross-over	All pts able to walk to RR and perform testing at 10 min; Trieger dot test abn to 3 hr postop; Perceptual speed and flicker fusion test abn at 3 hr; These changes seen with both groups but not with control
35	Third molar extractions (office), ASA I, II, Total 40	"achieve mood alteration and an increase in pain threshold in a conscious and cooperative patient while maintaining stable vital signs."	Group I: midazolam (total 0.2 mg/kg); Group II: fentanyl 1.5 μg/kg midazolam (total 0.125 mg/kg); Group III: diazepam (0.446 mg/kg) total; Group IV: fentanyl 1.5 μg/kg diazepam (total 0.31 mg/kg)	Sedation endpoint reached faster in midazolam groups; ABG's: groups with fentanyl had lower PO_2, pH, O_2 Sat, and higher PCO_2

APPENDIX 16.1 Continued

Reference or Note No.	Procedure/ Demographics	Definition/Goal of Sedation	Sedation Agents (intravenous unless stated)	Results/Complications/ Recovery
h	Periodontal surgery (office) 10,000 pts Ages 9–78 ASA I (6,322) II (3,057) III (621)	"conscious sedation" "to alter the mood of the fearful, anxious patient so that a psychologically unacceptable procedure becomes readily accepted."	Drugs given until pt had slurred speech Diazepam, meperidine, methohexital (7,443) Diazepam, methohexital (2,557)	No major complications Minor complications transient phlebitis (4.1%) nausea, vomiting (0.37%) dysphoria or excitation (0.42%)
i	Dental extractions (office) 50 pts ASA I, II (per description) Ages 13–36	Endpoint of sedation half-lid sign (Verrill's sign) Sedation assessed on 1–5 scale by surgeon	Group I (25): butorphanol 1 mg diazepam to endpoint (12.5 mg median) Group II (25): meperidine 50 mg diazepam to endpoint (15.0 mg median)	Sedation better in group I More patients in group I felt operative sleepiness, relaxation and lack of awareness was complete Although not stated, sig. no. group I pts were sleepy at time of discharge (1) nausea, (1) dizziness, (1) pruritus group I
j	Plastic surgery Outpatients Total 211	"patient should experience minimal anxiety and pain, remain calm, quiet, and comfortable. A restless, anxious patient may disrupt the surgeon's equanimity and concentration."	Premed (45 min): morphine (10 mg) IM promethazine (50 mg) triaxolam (0.5 mg) PO OR: diazepam 2.5 mg/min till speech incoherent or deep sleep Group I (112): no additional MSO_4	Fewer pts receiving OR MSO_4 had pain on local injection Less total diazepam needed when MSO_4 used No major complications Nausea group I 14%; II 23% Pain on injection I 13%; II 18%

k	Periodontal surgery Review 1,708 pts Ages 15–69 Mean age 44 ASA I, II, III Retrospective	"alter the patient's mood, elevate the pain threshold, keep the protective reflexes active, have only minor deviations in the patient's vital signs, and achieve a degree of amnesia."	Group II (99): MSO$_4$ 2 mg/ 2–3 min, until undefined endpoint "operators had little experience in periodontal surgery and sedation" Pentobarbital, meperidine, scopolamine (1,063) Pentobarbital, meperidine (59) Diazepam, meperidine, scopolamine (140) Diazepam, meperidine (162) Diazepam alone (35) Diazepam, nalbuphine (249)	"episodes of transient hypo- and hypertension, one suspected anginal attack" 1 case of laryngospasm 2 pts resp. depression Rx with naloxone 1 pt becoming belligerent Rx with naloxone Constant communication to take deep breath
l	Upper GI endoscopy Ages 19–87 Mean age 56 Total 90 pts Inpatients and outpatients	"The endpoint of sedation is to have a calm, rousable patient."	Groups A, B, C: all meperidine (mean 48.88 mg; all but 5 pt 50 mg); diazepam (mean 9.2 mg) 1–20 + mg) A: placebo gargle B: no gargle C: lidocaine gargle	No difference between groups in sore throats, gagging, dysphagia, and unpleasant experience "variable sedation"
31	Upper and lower endoscopy Mean age 66.2 114 pts		Group A: diazepam 10 mg, atropine 0.5 Group B: A + meperidine 50 mg Group C: A + fentanyl 50 μg	All patients had a fall in PaO$_2$ on ABG but only sig. in groups B and C at 2 min With adult scope B&C had a sig. decrease in PaO$_2$ With pediatric scope only group C had sig. PaO$_2$ change

APPENDIX 16.1 Continued

Reference or Note No.	Procedure/ Demographics	Definition/Goal of Sedation	Sedation Agents (intravenous unless stated)	Results/Complications/ Recovery
m	Upper endoscopy Ages 17–84 Mean age 48 100 pts		Group A: diazepam until dysarthric no mean dose given Group B: diazepam 10 mg pethidine 50 mg < 70 kg 75 mg > 70 kg naloxone 0.4 mg at completion	No difference between groups in recovery as measured by p performance test before endoscopy and 2 hrs after Cooperation better and retching less in group B

All relevant factors stated in original sources are listed here; if factors are not listed here, they were not stated in original sources.

[a]Ceravolo FJ, Meyers H, Baraff LS, et al. Full dentition periodontal surgery utilizing intravenous conscious sedation: a report of 5,200 cases. J Periodontol 1986;57:383.

[b]Miller A. Administration of the Shane technique of intravenous amnesia. Pa Dent J 1971;38:10–14.

[c]Shane SM. Intravenous amnesia to obliterate fear, anxiety, and pain in ambulatory dental patients. J Md State Dent Assoc 1966;9:94.

[d]Scamman FL, Klein SL, Choi WW. Conscious sedation for procedures under local or topical anesthesia. Ann Otol Rhinol Laryngol 1985;94:21–24.

[e]Colon GA, Gubert N. Lorazepam (Ativan) and fentanyl (Sublimase) for outpatient office plastic surgical anesthesia. Plast Reconstr Surg 1986;78:486–488.

[f]Hunter JM, Schneider LH, Dumont J, et al. A dynamic approach to problems of hand function. Clin Orthop 1974;1C4:112–115.

[g]Beilin B, Vatashsky E, Aronson HB. "Conscious sedation" for laparoscopy. Isr J Med Sci 1986;22:346–349.

[h]Ceravolo FJ, Meyers HE, Michael JJ, et al. Full dentition periodontal surgery using intravenous conscious sedation: a report of 10,000 cases. J Periodontol 1986;57:383–384.

[i]Zallen RD, Cobetto GA, Bohmfalk C, et al. Butorphanol/diazepam compared to meperidine/diazepam for sedation in oral, maxillofacial surgery: a double-blind evaluation. Oral Surg 1987;64:395–401.

[j]Riefkohl R, Cole NM, Cox EB. The effectiveness of benzodiazepines and narcotics in outpatient surgery. Aesth Plast Surg 1984;8:227–230.

[k]Daniel SR, Fry HR, Savord EG. Intravenous "conscious sedation" in periodontal surgery: a selective review and report of 1,708 cases. J West Soc Periodontol 1984;32:133–146.

[l]Cantor DS, Baldridge ET. Premedication with meperidine and diazepam for upper gastrointestinal endoscopy precludes the need for topical anesthesia. Gastrointest Endosc 1986;32:339–341.

[m]Boldy DAR, English JSC, Lang GS, et al. Sedation for endoscopy: a comparison between diazepam, and diazepam plus pethidine with naloxone reversal. Br J Anaesth 1984;56:1109–1112.

APPENDIX 16.2   Suggestions for uniform data collection

Define patient population
  Physical status[a]
  Age (in geriatric population, evaluate mental
    status pre- and post-operatively)[b]
  Associated conditions: pulmonary, cardiac,
    liver, kidney, obesity
Define and standardize operative procedure
  Setting: office, clinic, hospital
  Operator: specialty, experience
Define and standardize anesthetic technique(s)
  Regional, local, topical
  Conscious sedation, deep sedation
  Confirm state of alertness or sedation with time
Use a single agent or as few as possible
  Indication
  How dosage was derived
Record position of patient
  Sitting/prone
Record results of monitoring
  Vital signs
  Oxygen saturation, blood gases
  If supplemental oxygen was administered,
    route, amount, effect
Define and describe phases of recovery
  Immediate, delayed

Criteria for discharge home, to hospital room
Time to meet discharge criteria home:[c] sits in
  chair, stands with support, stands without
  support, walks with support, walks without
  support, negative Romberg sign
Amnesia and recall
Cognitive and motor testing: digit symbol
  substitution; Trieger; Flicker Fusion
Define and describe complications
Nausea, vomiting: frequency, severity (scoring
  system:[c] 0 absent; 1 one to two times;
  2 moderate—more than two times;
  3 severe—requires treatment; 4 persistent
  vomiting even with treatment)
Prolonged drowsiness
Respiratory, circulatory depression
Dizziness
Unanticipated hospital admission (outpatient):
  medical, surgical, social, anesthetic
Severity: major, minor, grave (paraplegia, brain
  damage, lifelong care or fatal prognosis),[d]
  death
Define anesthesiologist's global assessment of
anesthetic

[a]Cohen MM, Duncan PG, Physical status score and trends in anesthetic complications. J Clin Epidemiol 1988;41:83–90.

[b]Folstein MF, Folstein SE, McHugh PR. "Mini–mental state": a practical method for grading the cognitive state of patients for the clinician. J Psychiatr Res 1975;12:189–198.

[c]Epstein BS, Levy ML, Thein M, et al. Evaluation of fentanyl as an adjunct to thiopental–nitrous oxide oxygen anesthesia for short surgical procedures. Anesthesiol Rev 1975;2:24–29.

[d]Brunner E. The national association of insurance commissioners' closed claim study. Int Anesthesiol Clin 1984;22:17–30.

Chapter 16 Discussion

JEAN M. MILLAR: The authors draw long overdue attention to the dangers of procedures under sedation or local anesthesia.

Monitored anesthesia care (MAC) is not recognized specifically in the United Kingdom, although informally anesthesiologists frequently attend local anesthesia patients who are at risk. However, there seems to be a general failure of those carrying out such procedures to appreciate the dangers to patients of inadequate analgesia and respiratory and cardiovascular depression. Most are not monitored at all, and suggestions that this might be advisable are met with bland assurances that problems are never encountered.

The problems may be summarized as follows:

1. The difference between light and deep sedation may be very slight. The potential for partial or complete loss of reflexes and respiratory depression exists in virtually every case, and particularly where a sedation technique has been selected because of the patient's physical status.
2. Many of those administering local anesthesia are not trained in monitoring level of consciousness and adequacy of reflexes and respiration, nor in resuscitation.
3. The single-handed operator/sedationist is accepted as common practice where the operator/anesthesiologist would be condemned as unsafe practice.
4. The dangers of inadequate analgesia particularly in patients with angina or inadequately controlled hypertension are underestimated. Tachycardia due to anxiety or adrenaline in local infiltration solutions may be dangerous, and Gravenstein and colleagues[1] found desaturation in unsedated patients having local infiltration for oral surgery procedures, which they attributed to breath holding in response to fear or discomfort. General anesthesia may be a better option here.
5. The same level of monitoring is required as for general anesthesia. This is rarely achieved.
6. The recovery time after sedation is frequently longer than after light general anesthesia, particularly using propofol. The same postoperative restrictions exist, but patients are frequently not fully informed of these. While simulated driving tests[2] would suggest that driving skills are impaired for up to 2 hours after local anesthetics and 8 hours after benzodiazepine sedation, patients should not drive for at least 24 hours.

In the light of these problems, the setting out of guidelines for MAC is most welcome.

Definitive studies of the use of opioids in sedation are scarce, and there is little hard evidence as to which opioid is the best, particularly in ambulatory cases. Most of the data given in this presentation relate to general anesthesia with inference by extrapolation as to which opioid is the ideal. The concept of alfentanil infusion is an appealing one but more information is needed about dosage.

In a study by Milligan and others[3] of sedation for outpatient fiber optic endoscopy, the addition of bolus alfentanil 5 μg/kg to basal midazolam sedation 0.05 mg/kg improved operating conditions and clinical and psychomotor recovery over maintenance with increments of midazolam. No respiratory depression or desaturation below 91% was detected.

The suggested standardized study would help clarify some of the problems outlined.

REFERENCES

1. Gravenstein N, Paulus DA, Dowlick MF, et al. Pulse oximetry monitoring during oral surgery outpatient procedures. Anesthesiology 1986;65: A167.
2. Korttila K. Recovery and driving after brief anaesthesia. Anaesthesist 1981;30:377–382.
3. Milligan KR, Howe JP, McLoughlin J, et al. Midazolam sedation for outpatient fibreoptic endoscopy: evaluation of alfentanil supplementation. Ann R Coll Surg Engl 1988;70:303–306.

BEVERLY K. PHILIP: The administration of opioids by infusion is an appropriate technique to provide analgesia and sedation during monitored anesthesia care. Alfentanil infusions for this application have several potential advantages outlined by the authors, including more stability of effect and less total dose allowing more rapid recovery. At Brigham and Women's Hospital, we use alfentanil infusions in a technique consisting of a 5 μg/kg initial bolus followed by an initial infusion rate of 0.5 μg/kg/min (Table 16.7). Incremental boluses of

TABLE 16.7 Dosage of alfentanil by infusion for monitored anesthesia care

Initial bolus	5 μg/kg
Initial infusion	0.5 μg/kg/min
Incremental bolus	2.5–5 μg/kg
Incremental infusion	0.25–0.5 μg/kg/min

2.5 to 5 μg/kg may be accompanied by a change in the infusion rate of 0.25 to 0.5 μg/kg/min. These doses can be compared with those reported with the use of alfentanil infusions for analgesia and sedation outside the operating room. Cohen et al.[1] describe a regimen for the intensive care unit that consists of an initial rate of 0.5 μg/kg/min; for longer-term sedation in patients breathing spontaneously, a rate of 0.2 μg/kg/min was administered. The use of alfentanil infusions for postsurgical patients has been reported by Andrews and colleagues.[2] Spontaneously breathing patients were given 10 to 20 μg/kg alfentanil until pain-free, followed by an infusion of 0.17 to 0.33 μg/kg/min. Alfentanil was continued in these patients after discharge from the recovery ward for up to 130 hours, at a lower infusion rate averaging 0.14 ± 0.04 μg/kg/min. There were no respiratory complications.

Delayed respiratory depression after intraoperative alfentanil infusions does, however, occur. In an earlier report, Sebel et al.[3] described two patients who developed respiratory arrest requiring reintubation 50 and 70 minutes after the cessation of intraoperative alfentanil infusions. Plasma alfentanil concentration at the time of the respiratory arrest in the former patient was 95 ng/ml. The plasma alfentanil level during one of the arrests reported by Mahla et al.[4] was 87 ng/ml. Blood levels at which spontaneous ventilation resumes postoperatively have been determined, and that alfentanil concentration is 226 ± 10 ng/ml, with 95% confidence limits of 246 to 205.[5] Significant respiratory depression after apparent recovery from alfentanil infusion does occur at concentrations well below those expected to allow spontaneous ventilation, and therefore at times after a patient would be expected to be safely recovered. The low alfentanil concentrations obtained during the reported respiratory arrests indicate that a secondary peak in alfentanil blood level is not the cause. More likely, decreased stimulation in the recovery room as well as the development of sleep per se are contributory factors.[6] An adequate period of postoperative observation and monitoring is mandatory for patients who have received prolonged alfentanil infusions for monitored anesthesia care.

A brief comment should also be made concerning rigidity with low-dose opioid. In the reference cited,[7] the drug actually given was 2 ml Innovar. This dose would consist of 5 mg droperidol in addition to 100 μg fentanyl. The patient experienced uncontrollable facial grimace, neck and back stiffness, and anxiety; no chest wall rigidity or impairment of ventilation occurred. This episode has the hallmarks of an acute extrapyramidal reaction due to droperidol, rather than opioid rigidity. Rigidity has frequently been reported in association with general anesthesia; however, rigidity in the awake, sedated patient receiving monitored anesthesia has not been observed.

Opioid κ receptor agonists are characterized by analgesia, sedation, and limited respiratory depression. These characteristics suggest their use as a component of monitored anesthesia care for ambulatory patients. Butorphanol is the most useful of the clinically available κ agonists because of its pronounced, pleasant sedation and its mild μ antagonist activity.[8] Butorphanol enjoys high patient acceptance. Premedication and sedation with butorphanol should be titrated in 0.005 to 0.01 mg/kg increments, to approximately 0.04 mg/kg. Choice of dose limits should include the long duration of butorphanol action, which is comparable to morphine, in order to avoid prolonged recovery.

Opioids such as fentanyl and alfentanil are often used in conjunction with benzodiazepines for monitored anesthesia care to provide increased sedation. The effects and side effects of the opioid-benzodiazepine combinations warrant further discussion. The authors have presented data on the increased respiratory depression seen during sedation with benzodiazepine-fentanyl combinations. Enhanced and prolonged sedation has also been seen. The concomitant administration of opioid and benzodiazepine reduces the doses needed to achieve a given sedative endpoint. Premedication with fentanyl 100 μg reduced the midazolam needed for sedation for oral surgery from 0.17 mg/kg to 0.12 mg/kg.[9] A similar effect has been shown with alfentanil. The coadministration of alfentanil with midazolam for total intravenous anesthesia resulted in a shift to the left in the plasma concentration-effect curve for midazolam;[10] in other words, patients were equally sedated at lower midazolam concentrations if they had also received alfentanil (Figure 16.1).

Benzodiazepines also interact with opioids to augment their hypnotic effect. Dundee and colleagues[11] gave fentanyl or alfentanil before a midazolam induction using 0.3 mg/kg. Opioid premedication decreased the time to midazolam induction and increased the effectiveness of the induction, measured as percent of patients asleep at 3 minutes. When benzodiazepines are given before the opioids, anesthesia induction is also facilitated. Patients were premedicated with diazepam (0.125 mg/kg, intravenous) before a 100-μg/kg alfentanil infusion.[12] Significantly fewer patients who received diazepam plus alfentanil, rather than alfentanil alone,

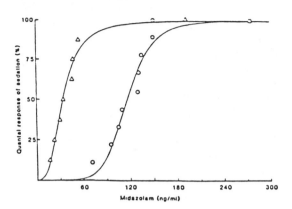

FIGURE 16.1 Evaluation of sedation during infusions of midazolam alone (○) and midazolam plus alfentanil (△). (Adapted with permission from Persson MP, Nilsson A, Hartvig P. Relation of sedation and amnesia to plasma concentrations of midazolam in surgical patients. Clin Pharmacol Ther 1988;43:324–331.)

were able to respond to verbal commands at 90 seconds after completion of the infusion. Vinik and colleagues[13] showed that midazolam, the other commonly used benzodiazepine, also can augment anesthesia induction with opioid. A dose of alfentanil sufficient to prevent response to verbal command was 0.13 mg/kg in that study; the induction dose for midazolam was 0.22 mg/kg. When alfentanil was given with midazolam, anesthesia induction was achieved with doses of 0.028 mg/kg (21% of the individual dose) plus 0.07 mg/kg (33%), respectively. This interaction is synergistic (Figure 16.2).

The ability of benzodiazepines to enhance the hypnotic effect of opioids such as alfentanil is of particular concern if the anesthetic plan is monitored care. The change from conscious to unconscious sedation carries with it increased risk of the loss of protective reflexes and the inability to maintain a patent airway. When benzodiazepines are given in combination with opioids as part of monitored anesthesia care, particular attention must be given to administering the medication doses in small, titrated increments and allowing time to observe effects that may develop.[14]

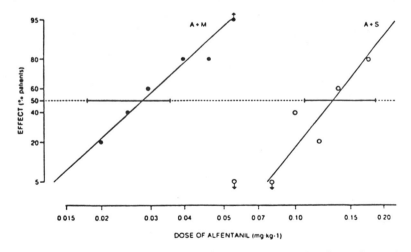

FIGURE 16.2 Dose of alfentanil needed for sleep induction when given with saline (A + S) and with 0.07 mg/kg midazolam (A + M). (Reprinted with permission of the authors and publisher from Vinik HR, Bradley EL, Kissin I. Midazolam-alfentanil synergism for anesthetic induction in patients. Anesth Analg 1989;69:312–317.)

REFERENCES

1. Cohen AT, Kelly DR. Assessment of alfentanil by infusion as long-term sedation in intensive care. Anaesthesia 1987;42:545–548.
2. Andrews CJH, Robertson JA, Chapman JM. Postoperative analgesia with intravenous infusion of alfentanil. Lancet 1985;2:671.
3. Sebel PS, Lalor JM, Flynn PJ, et al. Respiratory depression after alfentanil infusion. Br Med J 1984;289:1581–1582.
4. Mahla ME, White SE, Moneta MD. Delayed respiratory depression after alfentanil. Anesthesiology 1988;69:593–595.
5. Ausems ME, Vuyk J, Hug CC Jr, et al. Comparison of a computer-assisted infusion versus intermittent bolus administration of alfentanil as a supplement to nitrous oxide for lower abdominal surgery. Anesthesiology 1988;68:851–861.
6. Jaffe RS, Coalson D. Recurrent respiratory depression after alfentanil administration. Anesthesiology 1989;70:151–153.
7. Janis KM. Acute rigidity with small intravenous dose of Innovar. Anesth Analg (Cleve) 1972;51:375–376.
8. Rosow CE. Butorphanol in perspective. Acute Care 1988;12(suppl 1):2–7.
9. Ochs MW, Tucker MR, White RP. A comparison of amnesia in outpatients sedated with midazolam or diazepam alone or in combination with fentanyl during oral surgery. J Am Dent Assoc 1986;113:894–897.
10. Persson MP, Nilsson A, Hartvig P. Relation of sedation and amnesia to plasma concentrations of midazolam in surgical patients. Clin Pharmacol Ther 1988;43:324–331.
11. Dundee JW, Halliday NJ, McMurray TJ, et al. Pretreatment with opioids: the effect on the onset of action of midazolam. Anaesthesia 1986;41:159–161.
12. Silbert BS, Rosow CE, Keegan CR, et al. The effect of diazepam on induction of anesthesia with alfentanil. Anesth Analg 1986;65:71–77.
13. Vinik HR, Bradley EL, Kissin I. Midazolam-alfentanil synergism for anesthetic induction in patients. Anesth Analg 1989;69:312–317.
14. Philip BK. Supplemental medication for ambulatory procedures under regional anesthesia. Anesth Analg 1985;64:1117–1125.

17 PALLIATIVE THERAPY FOR CANCER

F.P. Boersma, G. Vanden Bussche, and H. Noorduin

Every year nearly 6 million new cancer patients are diagnosed and more than 4 million die.[1] Pain is one of the most dreaded consequences for patients with cancer. Studies suggest that moderate to severe pain is experienced by one-third of cancer patients receiving active therapy and by 60 to 90% of patients with advanced cancer.[2] Analgesic drug therapy is the mainstay of cancer pain management.[3-5] Drugs can be effective in a high percentage of patients, but only if used correctly, i.e., the right drug in the right dose at the right intervals.[6] These restrictions often come down to a compromise between the effectiveness of pain control and the prevention of serious side effects. Therefore, pain control is often deficient even when applied in hospitals and still more when patients are treated at home, causing serious domestic problems.

Epidural pain control can be applied clinically to selected patients who have reached the terminal phase of a metastasized malign process, for whom pain treatment with conventional analgesics is either inadequate or accompanied by too many disagreeable side effects. Opioids injected near the spinal cord produce analgesia without concomitant sensory, motor, or autonomic blockade.[7-9] After spinal subarachnoid or epidural administration, narcotic analgesics and endogenous opioid peptides interact with opiate receptors in the superficial layers of the dorsal horn to suppress transmission of nociceptive impulses.[7-11] Opioids reach their sites of action in the dorsal horn of the spinal cord either by diffusion from the cerebrospinal fluid (CSF) or by uptake into the posterior radicular artery.[10] Most active are agonists with a high affinity for opioid receptors.[12] Two recent developments improve epidural cancer pain control on an outpatient basis: the use of the opioid sufentanil and the continuous infusion technique with a portable pump to a subcutaneously implanted reservoir connected with an epidural catheter. The aim of this chapter is to investigate the usefulness of continuous epidural infusion of sufentanil for control of cancer pain in the home situation.

PATIENTS AND METHODS

The study protocol was approved by the ethics committee of the Refaja Hospital, and all patients gave informed consent. Only those patients qualified for the study who were in the terminal phase of their disease and for whom conventional oral analgesic therapy had not been sufficiently effective or had given rise to too many disagreeable side effects. All patients described their pain as very severe or unbearable. In all cases, the pain was chronic, sometimes with acute exacerbations. This investigation included 35 patients, 18 females and 17 males, who suffered from different types of cancer (Table 17.1).

Pain control began with a short stay (3 to 4 days) in the hospital. On the first day an epidural catheter and injection reservoir with a silicone rubber septum were implanted under local anaesthesia. The implantation was carried out under intravenous antibiotic prophylaxis. Pain control began during surgery in the operating room. Immediately after insertion of the epidural catheter, a loading dose of 30 to 50 μg sufentanil in 10 ml saline 0.9% was administered.[13] When the patient reported that the pain had disappeared, the catheter was tunneled subcutaneously and connected to the outlet tube of the portal. A small subcutaneous pocket was constructed in order to accommodate the reservoir. The fixation points on the base of the reservoir were then sutured to the fascial floor of the pocket with nonabsorbable suture, and the subcutaneous pocket was closed in layers. In 33 patients a portal was implanted. In two patients who suffered from severe diabetes, which is considered a contraindication for portal implantation, the catheter was tunneled subcutaneously, approximately 20 cm toward the flank of the patient.[14] In 29 patients insertion of the epidural catheter was performed in the lumbar region, and in the other 6, in the cervical region.

In the intensive care unit, immediately after the operation, continuous sufentanil infusion was

started. The sufentanil was delivered to the portal with the Pharmacia Deltec CADD 1 pump by puncturing the subcutaneous reservoir through the skin with a 90°-bend Huber-point needle, which was connected via an extension tube to the medication cassette of the pump.

The administration of oral narcotic analgesics was stopped, but non-narcotic analgesics were given to control wound pain, when present.

The patients remained another 2 to 3 days in the hospital in order to titrate the infusion rate and to monitor possible side effects. In the observation period, the following parameters were monitored during 48 hours:

1. Pain relief
2. Consciousness
3. Further side effects
4. Electrocardiogram (continuously) and blood pressure (noninvasively)
5. Rectal temperature (continuously)
6. Percutaneous oxygen saturation (continuously)

Sufentanil plasma and sufentanil CSF levels were determined in 15 patients. Venous blood samples of 10 ml were taken 24 hours after surgery and on the day of discharge from the hospital. Concomitant with the first blood sample, 5 ml CSF was drawn by a single lumbar puncture, irrespective of the location of the catheter tip. After extraction, all samples were subjected to duplicate radio-immunoassay, with a detection limit of 0.01 ng/ml⁻¹.[15] Further blood samples were taken by the general practitioner 2 and 6 weeks after discharge. The sufentanil infusion rate could be changed after consultation between the general practitioner and the anesthesiologist.

TABLE 17.1   Patient data

Number of females	18
Number of males	17
Mean age (range)	64 (28–86) years
Type of cancer	
Gastrointestinal tract	15
Lung	5
Gynecological	6
Urogenital	6
Breast	3

RESULTS

After insertion of the epidural catheter and administration of the loading dose of sufentanil, the pain always disappeared very rapidly, usually within 3 to 4 minutes. No complica-

TABLE 17.4 Sufentanil cerebrospinal fluid levels

Patient	Sex	Infusion Level	Sufentanil (ng/ml)
1	F	L2–L1	0.950
2	M	C6–C7	ND
3	M	L2–L1	ND
4	M	C6–C7	ND
5	M	L1–T12	0.027
6	M	T1–C7	0.038
7	M	L2–L1	0.900
8	F	C6–C7	0.011
9	M	C6–C7	ND
10	F	L2–L1	0.565
11	M	C6–C7	ND
12	F	L1–T12	0.040
13	F	L1–T12	ND
14	F	L2–L1	0.090
15	M	T12–T11	0.430

ND, nondetectable.

TABLE 17.5 Results, (mean, range)

Number of patients	35
Mean infusion rate/patient	359 (150–800) μg/24 hr
Mean infusion days/patient	91 (7–413)
Total period of infusion days	3,193

tribution. At autopsy, metastases of a primary rectum carcinoma were found in the epidural space, resulting in mechanical obstruction and ingrow into central nervous tissue. Invasion of the bladder by cervical cancer in a female patient evoked extremely painful cramps. There was no point in raising the dose of sufentanil. The administration of an oral spasmolytic, propantheline bromide, while maintaining the sufentanil dose, resulted in adequate analgesia. Metastasized pancreatic cancer led to a similar decision in another patient. Here it was preferable to simultaneously administer oral diclophenac sodium while keeping the epidural sufentanil infusion unchanged. This combination of drugs resulted in adequate analgesia. Finally, one patient developed decubitus and later necrosis of the skin overlying

the portal, because of a loss of body weight of 40 kg. This complication necessitated portal reimplant at the other side of the body.

Three patients, 7, 12, and 15, and their relatives had given permission for postmortem studies, which concentrated in particular on the examination of the spinal cord (Table 17.6). A final blood sample for sufentanil level determination was taken 1 to 3 days before death with the infusion rate at a constant level. After death, the bodies were transported to the hospital for autopsy. The spinal cords were removed 4 to 6 hours after death and frozen to a temperature of $-70°C$. Autopsy was performed as described by Ludwig.[16]

Sufentanil tissue concentrations were determined in the epidural fat and in the white and grey matter of the spinal cord near the tip of the epidural catheter. After extraction, all samples were subjected to duplicate radioimmunoassay, with a detection limit of 0.02 ng/ml^{-1}.[15]

Sufentanil plasma concentrations ranged from 0.32 to 0.84 ng/ml^{-1}. In the epidural fat, the highest sufentanil concentrations were measured in subjects 12 and 15. Sufentanil concentrations in the epidural fat were many times higher than in the white and grey matter of the spinal cord. Subject 7 was highly cachectic, and at autopsy no epidural fat was found. The biopsy from the epidural space consisted

TABLE 17.6 Patient data

Patient	Sex	Age (years)	Weight (kg)	Sufentanil (μg/24 hr)	Infusion Period (days)
7	F	45	45	600	97
12	F	70	51	800	57
15	M	55	69	750	24

of connective tissue and blood vessels. The sufentanil concentration in this sample was several times smaller than in the white matter of the spinal cord (Table 17.7).

DISCUSSION

Continuous epidural sufentanil infusion to combat cancer pain has both advantages and limitations. Major advantages of a continuous infusion by means of the Port-a-Cath system were that the epidural catheter did not have to be removed or replaced because injection pain (even in the long term) did not occur. Patients could take baths or showers whenever they wished, as temporary withdrawal and reinsertion of the needle was a simple matter and patients were far less dependent on the services of health care staff. The application of epidural cancer pain management using sufentanil was determined by the segmental analgesia.[17] Terminal cancer patients with pain in a limited number of connected dermatomes were the main indication. The loading dose, 50 μg sufentanil at lumbar level and 30 μg sufentanil at cervical level, produced a rapid and effective analgesia. Side effects such as pruritus and urinary retention were relatively rare, since all the patients had been pretreated with oral opioids. Late respiratory depression, which may be seen with epidural morphine, did not occur. Early respiratory depression was observed in all patients during the first hour after the administration of the loading dose of sufentanil and the start of the epidural infusion. The temporary decrease in oxygen saturation is probably attributable to rapid vascular absorption. The levels of sufentanil in serum and CSF were no help for the determination of the ideal dosage of sufentanil, as no correlation was found between analgesia and sufentanil plasma concentration after long-term epidural infusion. At the autopsies, no epidural fat was found at high thoracic and cervical level, which contrasts with the findings at the lumbar level. The absence of epidural fat in subject 7 led to a greater vascular resorption, resulting in higher plasma concentrations, and to a higher concentration in the white matter of the spinal cord. In subjects 12 and 16, the epidural fat probably acted as a depot, leading to lower sufentanil concentrations in the white and grey matter of the spinal cord. It is likely that the nutritional condition of the patients and the amount of epidural fat play a role in epidural analgesia with lipophilic opioids.

In a few patients, increasing the dose of epidural sufentanil infusion because of waning analgesia did not have the desired better analgesic effect. The system should be checked for integrity. Minor technical faults could always be easily corrected. The epidurogram should be inspected for deviations. For the diagnosis of obstructing metastases, an epidurogram proved to be an effective aid. In the course of cervical epidural sufentanil infusion, new pain complaints, entirely unrelated to tolerance but related to the segmental analgesia, could develop at the lumbar level. These examples show that patients themselves must not be able to increase the dosage of the epidural infusion. In view of the pathophysiological diversity of the origins of cancer pain and the spread and the growth of cancer, it is fre-

TABLE 17.7 Sufentanil concentrations in plasma and tissue

		Tissue (ng/g⁻¹)		
Subject	Plasma (ng/ml⁻¹)	Epidural Fat	Spinal Cord White Matter	Spinal Cord Grey Matter
7	0.84	558	1,534	379
12	0.71	5,562	498	130
15	0.32	4,979	962	527

TABLE 18.1 Novel routes of administration: advantages and disadvantages in comparison to oral route

Route of Administration	Comment
Subcutaneous infusion	Currently preferred for prolonged parenteral administration
Intravenous infusion	Useful to rapidly titrate analgesic for severe pain; requires maintenance of intravenous line
Spinal epidural and intrathecal	May avoid some adverse effects of systemic opioid administration; requires surgery to implant continuous infusion pump
Intraventricular	Requires surgery to implant catheter and reservoir; may not avoid systemic side effects of opioids
Sublingual	Available for buprenorphine (morphine also used by this route); avoids gastrointestinal tract
Intranasal	Under development; noninvasive; potentially convenient mode of administration with rapid onset of action
Buccal	Under development; same as sublingual and transmucosal
Transmucosal	Under development for fentanyl; rapid onset of action; convenience and ease of use make suitable for children; useful as means to supplement transdermal fentanyl?
Transdermal	Under development for fentanyl; convenient method for long-term parenteral administration; useful for children

fluctuations in opioid concentrations in the blood (and also presumably at spinal cord and brain receptor sites), and this may be associated with short-lived analgesia and sedation followed by rapid return of pain. These bolus effects may be minimized by the oral administration of slow-release morphine preparations,[7] but nausea, vomiting, and bowel obstruction may contraindicate this method of morphine administration. One may be further limited in this approach if the patient has rapidly escalating pain, so that a fast onset of action and relatively large dose of morphine are required for optimum pain control. In these circumstances, parenteral opioids are often useful. In fact, a recent study of cancer patients notes that 46 of 91 patients (51%) required more than one route of opioid administration at some time during the last month of life.[8] For these reasons, newer methods of opioid delivery have been growing in popularity recently.[9] These newer routes include (1) contin-

uous intravenous and subcutaneous infusion, (2) continuous and intermittent spinal epidural and intrathecal administration, (3) intermittent intraventricular, (4) intranasal, (5) sublingual and buccal, (6) transmucosal,[10] and (7) transdermal administration (Table 18.1). The continuous modes of administration often allow the attainment of sustained blood and cerebrospinal fluid (CSF) opioid concentrations so that peak-and-trough bolus effects are minimized. However, most of these modes of administration require an implanted or portable drug infusion pump.

Recently a transdermal therapeutic system (TTS—Alza Corporation) has been developed that allows the continuous administration of a potent opioid agonist (fentanyl) through the skin in the absence of a drug delivery pump. This transdermal system includes a drug reservoir and a rate-controlling membrane, which allows a constant rate of diffusion of drug through the skin. From this system, fentanyl is released at a rate of 25 μg/hr/10cm². The amount of drug administered can be varied by changing the surface area of the patch; 10, 20, 30, and 40 cm² size patches will deliver 25, 50, 75, and 100 μg/hr, respectively. The 40-cm² patch contains a total of 10 mg fentanyl.

This chapter summarizes existing knowledge relating to the use of transdermally administered fentanyl (TTS fentanyl) in the management of cancer pain and includes a discussion of comparative pharmacokinetic data available in cancer and postoperative patients when fentanyl is used by this route. In addition, the limited information relating to its safety, clinical usefulness, and side effect profiles is reviewed.

CLINICAL STUDIES OF TRANSDERMAL FENTANYL IN CANCER PAIN

Two studies have examined the clinical usefulness of TTS fentanyl in the long-term management of cancer pain. These studies, summarized here, support the claim that transdermal administration of fentanyl is useful and safe in cancer patients. Furthermore, the available pharmacokinetic data indicate sustained blood levels of fentanyl are achieved during serial patch changes over several weeks, supporting the concept of continuous transdermal absorption and a constant drug infusion through the skin by this mode of drug administration.

Miser et al.[11] studied five patients with cancer pain in whom oral administration of opioids were either ineffective or not possible. The patients ranged in age from 16 to 68 years and wore fentanyl patches from 3 to 156 days. The transdermal dose was selected after intravenous fentanyl infusions (0.5 to 1.0 μg/kg/hr) were titrated to achieve satisfactory pain relief as judged by a score of < 35 mm on a visual analog scale of pain intensity. A transdermal dose was then selected that would deliver the same microgram dose per hour, and the intravenous infusion was tapered and discontinued over 6 hours. The patients changed their patches every 24 hours.

The range of transdermal fentanyl doses required to achieve good to excellent pain relief in the five patients studied was 75 to 305 μg/hr. The median effective dose was 225 μg/hr. It is important to note that steady-state blood concentrations of fentanyl were linearly related to the transdermal fentanyl dose in the 75 to 305 μg/hr dose range studied (Figure 18.1). This linearity, even at the higher dose ranges, suggests that the therapeutic (and toxic) effects of transdermal fentanyl may be more easily predictable as the dose is titrated upward or downward.

Serial plasma fentanyl determinations in one patient measured from 0 to 1,200 hours following daily 125 μg/hr patch changes documented that plasma fentanyl concentrations plateaued in the range of 2.5 to 3.5 ng/ml, starting at 200 hours after patch application (Figure 18.2). This patient obtained adequate pain relief while fentanyl blood concentrations were maintained in this range and did not

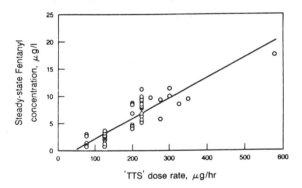

FIGURE 18.1 Linear relationship of fentanyl dose and blood concentrations. Graph of steady-state fentanyl blood concentrations versus dose administered by transdermal patch shows that as the dose is increased, there is a linear increase in blood concentration. This suggests that one can predict therapeutic and toxic effects related to dosage changes if they are correlated with blood concentrations. (Reprinted with permission from Miser AW, Narang PK, Dothage JA, Young RC, Sindelar W, Miser JS. Transdermal fentanyl for pain control in patients with cancer. Pain 1989;37:15–21.)

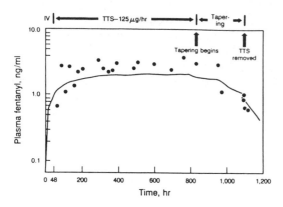

FIGURE 18.2 Blood concentration–time profile in a cancer patient wearing transdermal fentanyl for many days. Graph showing blood concentration–time profile in one patient wearing serial 125 μg/hr TTS (fentanyl) patches over 800 hours, which were then tapered by 25 μg/hr decrements after 800 hours. Note that a constant or steady-state blood concentration is not obtained for almost 200 hours, even after an intravenous bolus of fentanyl is given as a loading dose. Also note that the half-life of elimination was about 34 hours. (Reprinted with permission from Miser AW, Narang PK, Dothage JA, Young RC, Sindelar W, Miser JS. Transdermal fentanyl for pain control in patients with cancer. Pain 1989;37:15–21.)

require any additional analgesics, suggesting that these blood levels represent therapeutically effective concentrations for this patient. These concentrations differ from those determined to be "minimally effective" (MEC) in postoperative patients.[12] Higher fentanyl blood concentrations may be required in cancer patients compared to postoperative patients due to greater severity of pain or the presence of tolerance that may accompany chronic opioid administration.

Miser et al.[11] tapered transdermal fentanyl doses over a 12-day period with relatively little decrement in plasma concentrations. Upon removal of the fentanyl patch, plasma concentrations declined relatively slowly, with an estimated terminal elimination half-life of approximately 34 hours. In a second patient the

estimated elimination half-life was 11.5 hours. The calculated half-life of elimination for fentanyl after removal of transdermal patches in post-operative patients was determined to be 16 to 17 hours.[13] (Further discussion of the comparative pharmacokinetics of transdermal and intravenous fentanyl in postoperative and cancer pain follows.) Miser et al.[11] concluded that transdermal fentanyl was an effective alternative for cancer patients who could not take oral opioids.

Simmons et al.[14] evaluated the potential usefulness and safety of transdermal fentanyl in 39 cancer patients in a multi-institutional study. Patients ranged in age from 37 to 78 years, with the median age of 61 years, and included 16 males and 23 females. Transdermal administration of fentanyl was indicated if patients reported moderate to severe pain and their pain could be relieved satisfactorily with oral or parenteral doses of morphine during a prestudy "stabilization" period.

The doses of morphine required to control pain in the prestudy stabilization phase ranged from 60 to 790 mg/day (mean dose = 120 mg/day). Starting doses of transdermal fentanyl were estimated based on estimates of the relative potency of morphine and fentanyl. For purposes of the study, 10 mg intramuscular (IM) morphine was assumed to be equivalent to 100 μg intravenous (IV) fentanyl. Furthermore, the relative potency of oral to parenteral morphine was taken to be 6:1, as determined by Houde et al.[15] Therefore, 360 mg/day oral morphine was estimated to be approximately equivalent to 100 μg/hr fentanyl delivered transdermally. Using these somewhat arbitrary estimates, the median starting dose of transdermal fentanyl in the 39 patients studied was 50 μg/hr, with the range being 25 to 250 μg/hr. Using this methodology no patients were overdosed, and titration to analgesic doses could be undertaken as is customary when switching patients from one analgesic to another. Patients were allowed to self-administer oral morphine on an as-needed basis for pain that was not satisfactorily controlled by transdermal fentanyl alone. The range of these so-called "morphine rescue doses" was from 0 to

720 mg/day (median dose = 105 mg/day). Transdermal fentanyl doses were adjusted on the basis of daily morphine rescue doses required over the 3-day period. The patches were changed every 3 days.

Transdermal fentanyl patches were worn from 5 to 365 days in the study, with the median being 84 days. Patients reported improved pain relief in comparison to their prestudy pain intensity while wearing transdermal fentanyl patches as indicated by a (modest) decrease in the mean visual analog pain scores at 1 month into the study.

Twenty-three of 39 patients (59%) increased their fentanyl dose by more than 50% while on the study. This rate of dose increase is within the range of that seen in continuous infusion of morphine by both intravenous and subcutaneous administration.[16,17]

Based on the available data from the studies cited, it would appear that transdermal fentanyl is useful and safe in all stages of cancer pain management. Furthermore, patient compliance with and acceptance of this mode of therapy was excellent.

COMPARATIVE FENTANYL PHARMACOKINETICS FOLLOWING TRANSDERMAL AND INTRAVENOUS ADMINISTRATION IN POSTOPERATIVE PAIN

Transdermal drug absorption is complicated (Figure 18.3). Normally, when drugs are applied to the skin, the rate-limiting step in their absorption into the systemic circulation is the passive diffusion of drug through the keratinatous stratum corneum. Drug is absorbed from the skin via its uptake into the cutaneous microcirculation. However, the permeability of the stratum corneum is variable and is affected by skin temperature, body site, skin blood flow, suntanning, and a host of other factors.[18] The rate controlling membrane in the TTS fentanyl system allows drug to be released at a constant rate, and more slowly than the slowest rate of absorption through the stratum corneum, so that the rate of drug entry into the

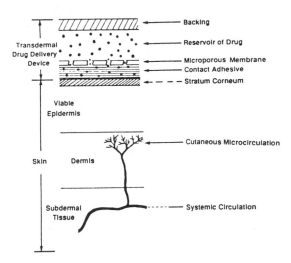

FIGURE 18.3 Schematic illustrating steps of absorption of transdermally administered drugs. Fentanyl delivered from the drug reservoir through the polymeric control membrane must diffuse through the lipophilic stratum corneum and through the epidermis to reach the microcirculation in the dermis. Diffusion through the stratum corneum is the rate-limiting step, but is also influenced by many variables. The function of the microporous membrane is to release drug at a slower rate than can be diffused through the stratum corneum and epidermis, and removed by the microcirculation. In this way, the drug delivery device, through this control membrane, allows constant rate of delivery of drug into the systemic circulation. (Reprinted with permission from Varvel JR, Shafer SL, Hwang SS, Coen PA, Stanski DR. Absorption characteristics of transdermally administered fentanyl. Anesthesiology 1989;70:928–934.)

circulation is determined by the properties of the drug delivery system rather than by the variability of absorption through the stratum corneum.

Pharmacokinetic observations of transdermal fentanyl in cancer pain patients are limited to those reported by Miser et al.[11] However, evaluation of the pharmacokinetics of fentanyl when administered transdermally in the postoperative setting[13,19,20] may provide information pertinent to devising optimal dosing regimens for short-term (i.e., postoperative) and long-term (i.e., chronic cancer pain) dosing.

Varvel et al.[13] studied 8 postoperative patients managed with 100 μg/hr transdermal fentanyl patch systems and compared the pharmacokinetics of transdermal to intravenous fentanyl in the same patients. Blood samples were drawn at various intervals (between 2 and 1,440 minutes) after the start of the intravenous fentanyl infusion, which was administered at a rate of 150 μg/min for 5 minutes in 7 patients, and for 6.5 minutes in an additional patient. The transdermal system was placed 24 hours after the administration of the intravenous infusion (on the first postoperative day). Subsequent blood samples were taken at various intervals from 2 to 72 hours after the transdermal system placement.

The rate of absorption of fentanyl was constant, beginning 4 to 8 hours after placement of the patch, and continued until the patch was removed at 24 hours. Serum fentanyl concentrations plateaued at 14 hours and remained relatively constant until the patch was removed. The terminal half-life of elimination was calculated to be 17 hours with the transdermal system as compared to 6 hours after the termination of the 5-minute intravenous infusion. The bioavailability of transdermal fentanyl was calculated to be about 92%. Mean serum concentrations with TTS (fentanyl) were 1.8 ± 0.8 ng/ml during the period 14 to 24 hours after TTS application. Determination of peak serum concentrations demonstrated that there was a fourfold interindividual variation among the 8 patients at 24 hours following transdermal application (Figure 18.4). It was apparent that absorption continued after patch removal (from a cutaneous depot), and this accounted for the longer half-life observed after transdermal administration in comparison to intravenous administration.

The relatively long half-life of transdermal fentanyl suggests potential problems in the clinical management of cancer pain. For example, if patients experienced a significant adverse effect that required discontinuation of

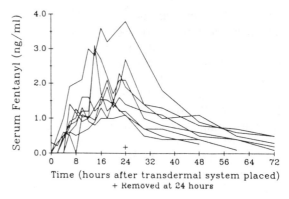

FIGURE 18.4 Interindividual variation in transdermal fentanyl serum levels. Graph of serum fentanyl concentration versus time in eight postoperative patients in which 100 μg/hr patch systems were placed. This demonstrates the wide interindividual variations in peak serum fentanyl concentrations. (Reprinted with permission from Varvel JR, Shafer SL, Hwang SS, Coen PA, Stanski DR. Absorption characteristics of transdermally administered fentanyl. Anesthesiology 1989; 70:928–934.)

fentanyl, one would require from 16 to 24 hours before half the drug was eliminated.[19,20] Therefore, the occurrence of respiratory depression or unacceptable levels of sedation could necessitate the repetitive administration or continuous intravenous infusion of naloxone in addition to discontinuation of transdermal fentanyl. This was required in only one patient (reported by Simmons et al.[14]), who became somnolent and demonstrated bradypnea after wearing transdermal fentanyl patches for several months for the management of severe pain from metastatic carcinoid tumor. The somnolence and respiratory depression were reversed with an intravenous naloxone infusion administered over several hours. However, equally important, in other patients transdermal fentanyl was continued during many concomitant events in which sedative-hypnotic drugs were coadministered for the management of complications occurring in advanced cancer. These included abdominal surgical procedures, herpes zoster eruptions, and chemotherapy infusions. Thus, it appears that the transdermal admin-

TABLE 18.2   Transdermal fentanyl: advantages and disadvantages in comparison to other routes

Advantages	Disadvantages
Easy to place patch	Easy to remove patch[a]
Convenient to use (3-day drug reservoir)	Long elimination half-life (difficult to reverse toxicity)
High patient acceptance (ideal for children?)	Potent opioid available outside hospital (problematic if drug diversion occurs)
Inexpensive compared to surgically implanted and external pump systems	Slow attainment of steady-state blood levels (cannot rapidly titrate to rapidly increasing pain intensities)

[a]Could be problematic if patch is removed inadvertently with clothing or while asleep, or if it is deliberately removed by a child or confused adult.

istration of fentanyl is a useful and very convenient method of administration of this potent opioid for prolonged use.

CONCLUSION

Transdermal administration of fentanyl provides a convenient method of continuous drug administration (Table 18.2). As such, it is comparable to other continuous methods of opioid delivery, although much less invasive (and perhaps less expensive), since it does not require needles, IV tubing, and expensive external pumps, or the surgical implantation of infusion pumps. Hence, it would appear to provide an obvious advantage over subcutaneous opioid infusion systems, which are often used when prolonged parenteral administration of opioids are required, and spinal opioid infusions systems.[17,21] Furthermore, the simplicity of this mode of drug delivery makes it a potentially ideal method for providing long-term analgesia in children. The possible disadvantages relate to (1) the relatively long half-life of fentanyl when administered by this route, and hence the potential difficulty of reversing toxicity, and (2) the requirement for systemic absorption, so that supraspinally medicated therapeutic and toxic effects are experienced. However early clinical studies in cancer patients appear to show the relative safety of this approach.

Future studies are needed to define the role of transdermal fentanyl in cancer pain management with respect to other available treatments. For example, comparisons of the efficacy and safety of transdermal fentanyl in relation to oral sustained-released opioid preparations and continuous subcutaneous and patient-controlled infusion paradigms, would be useful. The convenience of this route of administration, coupled with its apparent safety and effectiveness, provides great promise for the usefulness of transdermal fentanyl in the management of cancer pain.

REFERENCES

1. Foley KM, Arbit E. The management of cancer pain. In: DeVita VT, Hellman S, Rosenberg SA, eds. Cancer: principles and practice of oncology. 3d ed. Philadelphia: Lippincott, 1989;2064–2087.
2. Foley KM. The treatment of cancer pain. N Engl J Med 1985;31:84–95.
3. Twycross RG. Choice of strong analgesic in terminal cancer: diamorphine or morphine? Pain 1977;3:93–104.
4. Walsh TD. Oral morphine in chronic cancer pain. Pain 1984;18:1–11.
5. Houde RW. Analgesic effectiveness of the narcotic agonist-antagonists. Br J Clin Pharmacol 1979;7:S297–S308.
6. Jaffee JH, Martin WR. Opioid analgesics and

recovery. During the operation, with excessive anesthetic one sees signs of overdose, which for opioids such as alfentanil are respiratory depression, rigidity, and bradycardia.

An inadequate dose of opioid contributes to an uneven anesthetic course, with hemodynamic and autonomic instability. Here we see a charting of a bolus alfentanil anesthetic where the patient was given repeated boluses of 2 mg/kg alfentanil to suppress movement and reduce systolic blood pressure and pulse responses. The systolic blood pressure frequently ran below and above repeatedly normal levels ± 15, and there was also some variability in pulse rate, particularly on the high end.

After the operation, excessive opioids, which are the excessive opioid boluses given in response to variable patient responses, will cause a prolongation of side effects. Here you run into problems for ambulatory patients. We need an opioid administration method that will optimize the anesthetic dose for ambulatory surgery patients by a variable continuous infusion technique.

For outpatients, variable continuous infusion has an added convenience factor: the administration technique, for anything other than the briefest procedure, is simplified by using an infusion pump rather than administering repeated boluses at frequent intervals.

The theoretical advantages of alfentanil by infusion rather than by bolus have been borne out in patient studies. Dr. Kallar presented the data from White, showing decreased dosing and side effects. This has also been shown in other general surgical patients, where the patients who received alfentanil by infusion rather than by bolus had fewer total response episodes, fewer episodes of hypertension and tachycardia.

What is equally interesting is the end of the case. The alfentanil concentrations were lower, and when measured 10 minutes after discontinuation of nitrous oxide, the infusion technique allowed the anesthesiologists to use less naloxone to reverse respiratory depression. At Brigham and Women's Hospital, we primarily give alfentanil before surgery by variable continuous infusion, and we mainly use the Bard pump.

A protocol at our hospital for the day surgery patient is the following. Use mild premedication. If benzodiazepine is used, the dose should be reduced so as not to compound the postoperative situation. Begin alfentanil early, during the application of monitoring devices, starting with a bolus of 10 µg/

kg and continuing with an infusion rate of half, up to 1 µg/kg/min. To this anesthetic, we add an induction agent, barbiturate or another agent, such as nitrous oxide. This is sufficient for the anesthetic unless a neuromuscular agent is desired for intubation. During the operation, if there are signs of light anesthesia, incremental boluses can be given, and if the higher level of stimulus is anticipated to continue, an increase in the infusion rate as well. If the patient exhibits no response to intraoperative stimuli, we decrease the infusion rate until a minimum effective dose is reached.

DR. BEVAN: Dr. Robert Miller, just a few points on neuroanesthesia.

DR. ROBERT MILLER: Which narcotic you employ mainly depends on the pharmacodynamics of the individual case of neurological surgery. The longer the case, the longer-acting drug you can use. If one desires to talk to patients immediately or soon after surgery, one must use a drug with a shorter tail of sedation. In that context, Ira Isaacson was most helpful to us in pointing out that 0.4 µg/kg/hr was an adequate background dose, and when we stopped the anesthetic 20 minutes prior to the end of the surgical procedure, we could then extubate our patients and talk to them.

Second, when using evoked potentials, higher doses of fentanyl and sufentanil, in our experience, have minimal side effects on conduction delay time. This is in contradistinction to both flurane and enflurane. High-dose fentanyl, industrial concentrations using 100 µg/kg, might be considered excessive for a neurological surgery in all but exceptional circumstances.

Third, blood flow to the spinal cord must be maintained. The use of the narcotic supplementation should allow for lesser concentrations of volatile anesthetics, which should take less effect in inhibiting autoregulation. Intrathecal injections of opioids, as we use them, give prolonged pain relief in the postoperative, postanesthetia period. We have found this technique extremely valuable when laminectomy is combined with fusion of the back. We then employ a patient-controlled analgesic pump, with patients having "the best of all possible worlds." In other words, they like the system.

DR. FAWZY G. ESTAFANOUS: Now Dr. Mekhail from the Cleveland Clinic has a discussion to present.

DR. NAGY MEKHAIL: At the Cleveland Clinic, we are interested in the interaction between opioids and the adrenergic system at the level of myocardium. We studied the effects of fentanyl and sufentanil on tissue-culture-grown neonatal rat cardiomyocytes. The addition of 50 ng/ml fentanyl to the tissue culture medium stimulated protein biosynthesis significantly. At the same time, it stimulated the spontaneous beating rate of the cardiomyocytes in the culture. For comparative purposes, a similar dose of 50 ng/ml sufentanil was added to other sets of cultured myocytes. Sufentanil stimulated protein biosynthesis and beating rate as fentanyl did.

The incubation of tissue cultures with naloxone at a concentration of 10^{-6} M did not block the protein synthesis or beating rate stimulation induced by fentanyl or sufentanil. We investigated these observations on the whole organ level using the isolated, perfused isovolumic Langendorff preparation of rat hearts. Fentanyl and sufentanil had comparatively equal positive inotropic responses. They increased left ventricular pressure and left ventricular dP/dt more than 50% above the control. These effects were not blocked by naloxone (10^{-6} M) infusion but by infusion of propranolol (10^{-7} M) in the case of fentanyl and a 15-fold higher dose (5×10^{-6} M) of propranolol in the case of sufentanil.

These preliminary data show that such fentanyl and sufentanil action on the isolated cells or whole organ might be mediated through the adrenergic system. The exact mechanism underlying these actions is currently being investigated.

DR. LOWENSTEIN: Could you tell us how you might reconcile this with the prevailing literature?

DR. MEKHAIL: Epinephrine and norepinephrine were shown to have trophic and chronotropic effects on the isolated cardiomyocytes of rat. Moreover, recent research on the interaction between the opioid and adrenergic systems showed that opioid-induced vasoconstriction was successfully blocked by α-adrenergic blocking agents on several animal models.

DR. CARL E. ROSOW: I don't know that anyone has ever tested fentanyl or sufentanil in skeletal muscle. I know the older narcotics produced depression of metabolic rate. But I think that we're still getting up at least an order of magnitude or two higher than what we see here.

DR. LOWENSTEIN: Dr. Mekhail, I think you gave a number of preparations, but I think I understood that this was a saline-perfused Langendorff preparation.

DR. MEKHAIL: The Langendorff preparations were perfused with Krebs buffer gased with 95% O_2 and 5% CO_2. The doses used were injected as boluses, diluted by the myocardial flow, which averaged 15 to 20 ml/min. The time of injection was just a few seconds.

DR. DANIEL B. CARR: These are very interesting data. Many others have found that the apparent cardiovascular effects of opioids may be diametrically opposed, depending upon the level studies. Your findings echo what Dr. Thomas Smith and others have found in isolated myocytes; yet Clo, Eiden, Liang, and others have found anti-inotropic and anti-chronotropic actions of opioids in vivo or upon innervated myocardium. Possibly, if one were to look at opioid actions on innervated myocardium in an anesthetized animal, that would be another story still. If one looks at basal state versus stressed state, opioid neuroendocrine effects are frequently opposite. While yours is a very interesting finding, it is necessary to exercise caution because at each level the physiological controls probed by opioids can be widely disparate. The controls can be widely disparate in terms of physiology.

DR. LOWENSTEIN: We will certainly look forward to hearing more of that.

DR. MICHAEL B. HOWIE: I'd like to get back to Simon de Lange's comment that a lot of his staff are reluctant to use sufentanil in a difficult case. He seemed to suggest that there was something especially difficult about using sufentanil in a sick case as opposed to just reducing the dose compared to a fentanyl induction dose.

DR. DE LANGE: This is what my colleagues have found. Even though they have tried giving sufentanil much more slowly, and at a much lower rate, they still prefer to use fentanyl under these circumstances. There's much more hemodynamic instability in the bad valve with sufentanil than with fentanyl.

DR. HOWIE: Have you ever compared actual volume for volume, put the same amount of sufentanil in the same volume as you would a fentanyl syringe? Giving it at the same rate? I think that often people tend to be very fast with the 10-cc syringe as compared to the large syringe, and that's where the difference lies in the dropping blood pressure, rapid change in systemic vascular resistance. That's sometimes where it comes, because people just push the thumb a little faster on the small syringe.

DR. JAMES HART: I'd like to say that pharmaco-dynamics is when pharmacokinetics doesn't work. If we had a good endpoint of anesthesia, we wouldn't need more pharmacokinetics than we do for inhalation agents. We can certainly go into the operating room and anesthetize somebody with halothane without detailed information about uptake but with some understanding of what's going on. It's the same sort of thing with intravenous agents. I really think, Mike, you've got the correct answer about the supposed differences between fentanyl and sufentanil as reported in the literature: first, the equivalency of dose and second, equivalency of dose rate.

Don Stanski isn't here but, I know they have data in their laboratory to show that what we predicted earlier based on ability to reverse membranes—lipid solubility, protein binding, ionization, and so forth—is, in fact, holding up. They usually give the low-rate infusion, and they look at the EEG chains and speculate shift. Sufentanil and fentanyl are absolutely superimposable in terms of onset of effect.

What's more interesting is the kinetics of these drugs in the brain; some of our earlier assumptions about this are not proving out. These drugs have a much longer time course within the central nervous system than we had thought. Even though blood levels are falling off progressively, the brain levels are not falling off quite at the same rate.

People may get a confused message from some of the other work that has been done. Dr. Lowenstein showed a slide from Earl Wynands' work where the fentanyl concentrations range all the way up the screen and you have a few responses at the top and more at the bottom. I think it shows that with an opioid, even in the presence of substantial premedication, you may not be able to achieve all the characteristics you'd like in an anesthetic. But it also tells you something about what kind of concentration you need to supplement rationally with other drugs.

DR. LOWENSTEIN: Dr. Philbin has just done a double-blind study comparing fentanyl and sufentanil administered at an equirapid or equislow rate. He has gone up to 40 µg/kg of sufentanil followed by an infusion, and he is not able to distinguish the fentanyl from the sufentanil.

DR. HART: You take sufentanil out to the equivalent of 5,000 ng/ml in plasma to test something that Ted Eger suggested to us, that this is such a highly lipid-soluble drug it might start to act like an anesthetic agent. There's some evidence in bacteria—not bacteria, what's those little things that float around?—that it might be in terms of membranes. But we can't get any further MAC reduction.

DR. LOWENSTEIN: Dr. Rosow is one of the investigators of this study. So he has this slide legitimately.

DR. ROSOW: It isn't all on this slide. We did start comparing fentanyl with sufentanil, the reason being that implicit in all this talk about infusions and doses is that the suppression of response is related to the opioid dose. This is the assumption in dose recommendations in the package insert, isn't it? But we tried a blind trial comparing the usual clinical dose range of fentanyl and sufentanil to find a hemodynamic responder. It happened to be a 20% increase in systolic blood pressure, and we also had hormonal response. We couldn't find any difference. Everybody responded, so we thought that what we might be doing wrong is not giving enough drug or giving it by infusion. Maybe the levels were dropping. So we tried a study with a wide range of sufentanil doses, and as you heard, the highest-dose group got up to really astronomical sufentanil plasma levels. Then we simply looked for the responders.

This confirms what Earl saw: with oxygen alone, without nitrous oxide and a lot of other adjuvants, the opioid isn't a complete anesthetic nor should it be expected to be.

DR. ESTAFANOUS: Those using sufentanil almost every day can confirm that the speed of induction—beginning sufentanil slowly—is really not accompanied by any hemodynamic differences between sufentanil and fentanyl. It is the 10-cc syringe versus the 50- or 75-cc syringe.

DR. LOWENSTEIN: It's one of the things that makes it easy to study blindly. All you have to do is dilute.

DR. HOWIE: I'm just amazed that a lot of people who have anecdotal comments about sufentanil will quite calmly give midazolam combined with fentanyl or propofol or anything else. If there is a difference (of times) it is in the calcium channel blockers that the patient receives pre-op. I think there is, in fact, more vasodilation with drugs like diltiazem, but actually sometimes the patients' volume is stabilized because they have been pretreated for so many days with a vasodilator and probably have a higher volume than other patients who have been on simply β blockade.

DR. H. RONALD VINIK: My bias relates to one's need to know the endpoint one is dealing with in anesthesia. Obviously, in the cardiac milieu, one is very concerned with the hemodynamic response. One looks for an endpoint to titrate a drug to, and decides on its effectiveness, decides whether it will be hemodynamic, hypnotic, analgesic, amnesic; then one looks at the drugs needed to get to that endpoint. My bias comes from the fact that we have now shown quite definitively that the addition of 0.07 mg midazolam to 60 μg/kg of alfentanil given within a 3-minute period, relatively fast, is a total intravenous anesthetic and patients are totally unconscious. If you give sufentanil, not at 10 or 15 μg/kg but 0.5 μg/kg, you can have total unconsciousness with less than 0.1 mg/kg of midazolam. We have a very potent synergistic interaction for at least one component of that combination, which is hypnosis. Whether it applies to the hemodynamic concentration or other effects individually or combined of those drugs, and with it the relationship of those potencies of 5 to 10 times of fentanyl versus alfentanil—whether it also holds when you combine it with another drug—is completely unknown and still needs to be found out.

DR. LOWENSTEIN: How do you define unconsciousness?

DR. VINIK: Unconsciousness, in our studies, was defined as failure to respond to command spoken in a loud clear voice on two consecutive occasions.

DR. LOWENSTEIN: Thank you. Dr. Rosow, I think we have time for one more comment.

DR. ROSOW: In patients who are not deaf.

I feel I have to answer Peter. We have to address the issue of potency. We didn't get any dose response, so we can't measure relative potency. That was the whole point. We have a literature filled with people making assumptions that 50 μg/kg of fentanyl is or isn't equal to however many μg/kg of sufentanil. There is no parallel dose response curve in the literature. I'm sure that it exists at some lower level.

DR. VINIK: Or it exists in the presence of another drug. And that is absolutely key. For example, Dr. de Lange made a crucial observation. With alfentanil they could titrate anesthesia to the patient's need, control hemodynamics, and do all of that with a certain dose of lorazepam. And on that background, you could titrate, you could define the dose response curve or concentration response curve. But once you lower the dose of lorazepam to a less than satisfactory level, you could anesthetize any patient with alfentanil. So that becomes a crucial

issue. The opioids are not total anesthetics, but if you use a background drug, be it nitrous oxide or lorazepam, at a stable but substantial level, you can begin to define concentration responses in terms of most criteria of anesthesia.

DR. DAN FOLEY: In your study of the fentanyl patch, have you noticed any problems if someone takes a hot shower?

DR. RICHARD PAYNE: The question is, were there any problems with patients doing routine daily activities like taking hot showers. No. The adhesive is remarkably adhesive. And although there were problems occasionally with the patches becoming dislodged, particularly in a defective batch, patients generally were able to take showers with no problems. Ours was not a pharmacokinetic study, so we didn't measure blood levels with changing conditions like vasodilation, but the patients didn't report anything that would make us think there would be an alteration in kinetics on that basis.

SPEAKER FROM THE FLOOR: Dr. Coombs reported that very low doses and lots of them are extremely effective in counteracting the side effects.

DR. DENNIS COOMBS: Yes, it's a possible solution. When we try to do this, the difficulty is compounding management. It's not that it can't be done, even with nalbuphine, to some extent. There is an abstract at the ASA this year looking at that issue from a number of directions. If you have given naloxone, you can antagonize the analgesia as well. The difficulty is having an infusion attached and not being absolutely certain the patient isn't going to lose the infusion or that it's going to be adequately monitored. On the other hand, some of these complications really are less frequent than it seems. At least in the continuous infusion studies with fentanyl, nausea and pruritis seem to be less common, although they still occur.

DR. FOLEY: One of our problems has been trying to titrate patients effectively with naloxone and the complicating issues thereof.

DR. COOMBS: There is a nice review in a Canadian journal just this last year on the subject; this is a difficult area because epidural and intrathecal narcotics are widely projected in clinical management today, largely without continuous monitoring. Most of our studies have been done on a continuous monitoring basis, and that's probably what happens at most institutions. That's what the publications come from, and those patients become, as you say, more stimulated. I don't think there is necessarily a relation between an excessive narcotic effect and respiratory rate. That alone is not an adequate monitor. You can get adequate analgesia or superb analgesia, but the price you pay is monitoring, and it doesn't really seem to matter which narcotic you use. Many of us probably thought that Theresa Bood's study was surprising, that butorphenol is known to be very sedative, that it's not a major problem in epidural administration and would probably not leave too much respiratory depression. In fact, it wasn't all that different from morphine. So we don't have a good answer to this. No matter what you do, whether it's naloxone infusion or nalbuphine administration, the issues don't completely go away.

DR. PAUL F. WHITE: I agree with your criticism of studies that have failed to adequately assess the respiratory depressive effects of these modalities. But I think in the future, with the availability of telemetry pulse oximetry studies will have more relevant information about ventilatory depression. That's not as good as CO_2, perhaps, but at least it's very accessible. At our institution, all study patients are monitored at least while they are at bed rest, which I think is when they are at highest risk. There are virtually no studies looking at intramuscular or intravenous opioids that give us good solid information.

DR. FOLEY: Nor do we have relative potencies for those drugs.

DR. BRACE NATCHER: Basically, our acute pain service follows Dr. Reddy's suggestion to look at the increasing level of sedation rather than merely concentrate on respiratory rate. We have some data showing a very close correlation to rising CO_2 and depth of respiration. Our nurses are really trained in that. Until more sophisticated monitoring comes along, I suggest you look at that.

DR. COOMBS: Of course, the patient who has had major abdominal or thoracic surgery is going to have a 70% reduction in vital capacity and changes in many other parameters, so that hypoxia is likely to occur more rapidly.

DR. ROBERT MILLER: In all the studies that we have read, almost none has studied these patients in the preanesthetic, preoperative period to find out if they are subject to sleep apnea.

DR. MICHAEL STANTON-HICKS: This doesn't rule out sleep apnea altogether. In the last couple of years, I've been involved with two cases in which there were deaths postoperatively. The narcotic levels found in these patients, who had received narcotics by intramuscular injection, was below what is regarded as an analgesic dose. Both patients were within the seventy-fifth percentile of the mesomorphic statistical probability of falling into the sleep apnea range. They were both nonabdominal operations. They were orthopedic surgeries where the patients were required to lie on their backs. And the hypoxic event occurred, in one case, 8 hours after the surgery, after the patient had already called home (he was a 17-year-old), and in the other, 13 hours after surgery. So I think other factors, purely serendipitous unfortunately, are involved.

QUESTION FROM THE FLOOR: There is a question of apnea as related to a large number of factors particular to our patients. There is a lot involved in this for a 17-year-old to die. "Lying on his back" would indicate to me that he had an obstructed episode, which may have been compounded by a small amount of narcotic in his body.

DR. STANTON-HICKS: Yes. In fact, that was the case. It is interesting that in the circadian cycle it occurred during that period of increased REM sleep which is full of activity.

QUESTION FROM THE FLOOR: When you replace the patch, do you replace it in the same position?

DR. STANTON-HICKS: In fact, the patches were changed every three days, and the cutaneous site was rotated. But the patches do stay on for three days, and it is clear from the Stanski studies that there is a cutaneous depot of drug that can be seen even after 24 hours of application. But we did rotate the patch sites.

DR. CARL C. HUG, JR: For 20 or 30 years it was commonplace knowledge that if you wanted to make an animal tolerant, the way to do it was to put pellets of morphine under the skin. I'm fascinated by the fact that we put patches of morphine on people, in some cases for hundreds of days, and we don't get tolerance, at least not a lot.

DR. FOLEY: I think this is an argument that we continually have. I know that you've given a talk on that issue. I've recently reviewed all the clinical data that address this issue, because if one looks at the historic aspects of tolerance, tolerance was only of interest in its relation to physical dependence and the appearance of physical dependence. Historically, in the literature, it was a sign that an animal, and more important, a human being, was physically dependent. It was not looked at from the perspective of tolerance to analgesics, but because tolerance occurred in a variety of animal studies that induced pain, it was assumed that tolerance would therefore develop in the same way to clinical pain. I think for cancer patients, our best example from a group of patients who take analgesics over a period of time, there is very good evidence that demonstrates a shift in the dose response curve in patients tested two weeks apart when given chronic administration of morphine, as an example, or Medipan.

There is evidence that tolerance develops, but a second, more complicated component is that many patients have stable pain and seem to be able to obtain stable relief of pain. As their pain escalates with the progression of disease—that is Frans Boersma's experience—they begin escalating doses. So there is a clue to tolerance developing. It's the extent to which tolerance develops, the limit to which tolerance develops. I think there is very good clinical evidence to suggest that there is no limit to tolerance. The construct in animal literature indicated the cross-tolerance was complete. Now there is very good evidence in humans and in animals to show that cross-tolerance is incomplete.

The phenomenon initially recognized as an outgrowth of the physical dependence field is changing because of this opportunity to look at it, making it more complicated. I think Frans's data and Richard's data suggest this and support it. We don't understand its mechanisms. I would like to ask whether Paul White thinks that he's seeing the acute tolerance in some of his data when he shows us rapid changes in levels.

DR. PAUL F. WHITE: Whether the tolerance is acute or subacute, there is plenty of evidence that it is developing, even in the chronic model. I'm surprised that you comment, Carl, because in fact Richard showed evidence that with a transdermal patch there was only a 10% dose sparing over the morphine requirement prior to the application of the patch. So you could say that the pain was getting worse, but presumably it's pretty stable. The application of fentanyl transdermally had some spectacular results in certain patients; if you look at the rescue requirement, it was 10 to 15% less.

DR. FOLEY: What do you think about acute tolerance?

DR. WHITE: I think tolerance does develop rapidly, whether you define it as acute or subacute. It

develops at a very rapid rate, whether in a couple of hours or a few days.

QUESTION FROM THE FLOOR: We have seen some evidence of what I believe is acute tolerance occurring with a single dose of epidural fentanyl, just 50 μg, in measured patient-controlled anesthesia requirements at 24 or 48 hours afterwards. Just a single application of fentanyl given to a patient who is not experiencing pain at the time can increase the PCA requirements. I believe it does occur. We also see it with our continuous infusion PCA patients.

DR. HUG: I don't remember the dosage but that is, of course, where Bill Martin started. He was looking at spinally transected animals and developing acute tolerance in the spinal dog. My recollection is that it was days, but I don't remember the dosage.

DR. FOLEY: In that model it was, in fact, days. He demonstrated that chronic tolerance develops to all the parameters, except he did not study pain. He looked at endocrine, blood pressure, and heart rate. I think the literature we have, at least on humans, except for this clinical experience, has not looked at pain, and its dimensions, and whether it is physiologic or psychological in that dimension.

DR. HUG: Dr. White's comments are, in fact, correct, but I still think transdermal fentanyl may be very useful in these patients, even though the morphine requirements pre- and postfentanyl patches didn't change much. I think the dimension here, which we were not able to study directly given our study design, was that those patients who were on mean taking rescue doses of 110 ml/day morphine appeared to have good pain relief. I suspect that without the fentanyl patch their morphine doses would have been much higher and their side effects would have been much greater. But, given our study design, we really couldn't address that issue adequately.

This brings up the issue as to what else we need to know about how to use transdermal fentanyl. One thing we need is further studies in which we can directly assess transdermal fentanyl in relation to slow-release morphine, subcutaneous infusion, and so on.

DR. TONY L. YAKSH: When we ask if tolerance develops, we are faced with a moving target. There is no question that in the animal models such changes in dose response exist. In the chronic pain patient, however, the question is less clear. The pain state is changing; the kinetics of the drug may be altered (increasing or decreasing clearance). However the fact that the clinician can point to long intervals of little change in drug dosing suggests that the pain state in humans may differ. My own thinking is that the degree of tolerance is related to drug occupancy. Occupancy must rise with stronger stimuli. It may be simplistic, but I think that failure of drug dosing to rise in man relates to the comparatively less pain in the cancer patient, as compared to an acute animal model (such as the 53°C hot plate). Clearly other variables could be relevant.

DR. FOLEY: Tony, do you think that the changes on the dinorphenergic systems that Albert Hertz and other people are talking about, and these chronic arthritic models, are relevant?

DR. YAKSH: Five years ago I would have said that biochemical explanations on this matter were untenable. Now I believe that there are pharmacodynamic explanations for changes in response following drug exposure, i.e., a change in receptor number or coupling. It is clear from work done by Allen Basbaum, Gary Bennett, and the Hertz group, among others, that neurotransmitters evoke tonic changes in a variety of oncogenes and nuclear promoters. Corticosteroids will alter receptor expression, and so on. These events all coalesce to suggest that biochemical discriminable events exist which might alter the manifestation of the drug receptor interaction in the face of chronic pain.

DR. ESTAFANOUS: Dennis Mangano, in 1973, published a paper about how electrocardiographic signs of ischemia disappear or decrease after induction of anesthesia. So we agree that sedating the patient and decreasing the metabolic rate can improve signs of ischemia. Until about ten years ago, it was the practice in many institutions to keep patients heavily sedated and ventilated over 24 hours, and we did use a regimen of morphine sedation. In the last few years we have started extubation earlier. We are also aware that postoperative hypertension may be a cause of ischemia, and controlling postoperative hypertension is a routine now in many places.

How much of that is related to your study? Are you controlling postoperative hypertension, or are you extending sedation and anesthesia, and if the latter, eventually the patients have to wake up.

DR. DENNIS T. MANGANO: Yes, we are controlling postoperative hemodynamics. I think you can maintain anesthesia in patients and decrease oxygen requirements. If so, the ischemia probably should decrease in incidence and severity unless you have untoward hemodynamic changes, which may even increase ischemia with stress. We are controlling postoperative hypertension and hemodynamics.

DR. ESTAFANOUS: Eventually you are going to let the patient recover from anesthesia, so are we talking about anesthesia, or heavy sedation and gradual withdrawal from heavy sedation?

DR. MANGANO: In the previous studies we found that the incidence of ischemia seems to decrease over the first 15 hours after bypass; ischemia continued in only about 10% of patients. So there seems to be a pattern of acute ischemia occurring over a 15-hour period, at least over the first 48 hours after surgery. This seems to be the highest risk period.

DR. ESTAFANOUS: You may be advocating going to prolonged sedation and prolonged postoperative ventilation for these patients.

DR. MANGANO: Over the first 15 hours following bypass.

DR. ESTAFANOUS: We are looking at the incidence of perioperative myocardial ischemia for the last 15 years. Many changes have been introduced intraoperatively, such as myocardial protection, changes in our techniques, etc. In spite of changing our techniques and waking patients up earlier, the incidence of perioperative ischemia did go down about 50% over the last 15 years. The point I am trying to make here is that there are many variables we have to consider to validate all of this.

DR. MANGANO: In cardiac surgery patients, there are many factors, including thrombosis and spasm. But this is and will be a problem. What we are starting to see is a change in the mortality statistics. The number of angioplasties is increasing, and we have older and sicker patients coming to cardiac surgery. I think there is a trend toward increasing mortality in patients over the next decade.

DR. HEXSON: I see a trend toward increased focus on the postoperative period. The French group, Ecofee and St. Maurice, have made very interesting observations, and it would appear that maintaining analgesia after surgery by epidural analgesia or by opioids is something that we need to focus on much more.

QUESTION FROM THE FLOOR: I think that is a very important area. I drew my ideas from the study that Henrik Elit and his colleagues did on patients undergoing hysterectomy. They maintained epidural analgesia for up to 24 hours postop, yet they found that the cumulative nitrogen balance was much better over the week following surgery just from the initial 24 hours of continued analgesia postop. I certainly agree with your comments.

DR. MICHAEL NUGENT: Studies involving outcomes of vascular surgery have one major advantage over outcome studies in patients having cardiac surgery. The results of the latter are clouded, because the patients have undergone surgery on the heart with varying degrees of technical success. For example, Slogoff has reported in coronary artery bypass patients that the surgeon's assessment of adequacy of coronary artery grafts and the aortic cross-clamp time are more predictive of perioperative myocardial infarction than perioperative ischemia or the quality of the anesthesiologist. The best-quality studies will therefore probably involve patients having major vascular surgery, because it is easier to define the results of experimental interventions in this high-risk group of patients.

The question of narcotics of β blockers has not been resolved. In a study by Pasternak that looks at β blockers in patients with abdominal aortic aneurysm, the group with no β blockers had a 20% incidence of CKMB elevation and the β blocker group had a lower incidence. We are getting to the same point with narcotics as with β blockers.

DR. STEVE SLOGOFF: There are some questions I would ask before being convinced that either the administration of postoperative analgesia or the use of sufentanil versus halothane is going to improve outcome.

The Benefiel-Roizen study is a fine one, but I think it has a flaw. Dr. Benefiel described their null hypothesis before he described their study. He said they had administered isoflurane and sufentanil to about 100 patients and the study was stopped by the statisticians because there was a significant difference in outcomes. Because of that significant difference, they have concluded that sufentanil is better than isoflurane for these patients. The problem is with the null hypothesis that was proposed—the effect of either sufentanil or isoflurane on myocardial stress.

In the study, one patient—Dr. Benefiel said two, but his data sheet shows one patient—had an infarction, and that was the patient who had received sufentanil. The null patient who had received isoflurane had an infarction, and in the data subsequently presented, the incidence of ischemia was identical in both groups. So the null hypothesis came out to be validated; that is, there was no difference in the cardiac effects in the two groups.

Their data, however, have no question. Why should patients who receive sufentanil have fewer strokes than patients who receive isoflurane, or why should patients who receive sufentanil have more renal disease or congestive heart failure? Dr.

Benefiel's point about congestive heart failure and isoflurane with rebound vasoconstriction and hypertension does not rest on hard data that support that position. The major problem with this study is that they have an answer but they don't have the question. I don't think we can say that they were able to reject the null hypothesis based on the data in that study.

DR. DAVID J. BENEFIEL: Many of your points are valid, and I am certain you would feel a lot better about our study if there had been a large incidence of myocardial infarction. The focus of Dr. Slogoff's studies in coronary artery surgery is the single outcome of myocardial infarction. Unfortunately, vascular surgery is not so simple. The kidney is at risk for ischemic injury during suprarenal cross-clamp. There are many mechanisms whereby an anesthetic might influence the vulnerability of the kidney to that ischemic insult. We showed catecholamines were higher in the renal insufficiency group. The anesthetic itself may also exert an influence on the incidence of postoperative renal insufficiency.

Our null hypothesis was not that there might be a difference in myocardial stress but that there might be a difference in outcome as defined prospectively, and if there was a difference in outcome, it might be attributable to myocardial stress. One of the problems with my presentation was the use of the word stress to define several different phenomena. Pain associated with surgery is a stress that produces cardiovascular and neuroendocrine responses, including changes in blood pressure and pulse with an increase in catecholamine levels. Myocardial stress can mean anything that increases myocardial oxygen consumption, or in a more narrow and precise sense, stress is the force per unit area experienced by the myocardium. The anesthetics we chose to compare each reduce myocardial stress in their own way. Isoflurane is a vasodilator and reduces the force per unit area (wall stress) experienced by the left ventricular myocardium. Sufentanil reduces catecholamine secretion during surgery and will reduce myocardial oxygen consumption by preventing an increase in the inotropic state of the heart.

I do not think the results in our study are in dispute, only their interpretation and significance. The fact remains that there was a difference in the outcome between groups, given the way the anesthetics were administered.

Dr. Slogoff is skeptical about an anesthetic's influence on strokes. It is known that the cerebral circulation responds to catecholamines, and there was a difference in the levels of catecholamines between those patients who suffered complications and those who did not. There may be other humoral responses affecting coagulation that we did not measure. Our study should raise a question about possible mechanisms of intraoperative stroke.

There may be some phenomena related to cardiac ischemia, but we certainly didn't see them. Clearly, we didn't see them intraoperatively in terms of the echo. What we were looking for was differences in outcome, and we found differences, but unfortunately we didn't find a clear explanation as to why, and I agree that we were somewhat disappointed. However, it is not uncommon in any study that for the first time demonstrates a significant new finding not to give a simple explanation as to why. It is natural to speculate; subsequent studies may prove or disprove the speculations.

DR. NUGENT: If one is going to study the incidence of perioperative myocardial infarctions in patients having major vascular surgery and an estimated incidence of perioperative infarction of 5% is used, then one will have to have a study group of more than 1,500 patients to show that a given intervention has decreased the perioperative infarction rate to less than 1%. Until you design a multicenter randomized perspective study, which is not easy to do, you are going to have to look at more subtle and less definitive outcome results, such as congestive heart failure, myocardial ischemia, or other markers such as CKMB elevation.

DR. NORMAN STARR: On the Siliciano-Mangano study, are they going to continue this research to include major catecholamine levels or responses that reflect stress, because when you select a period of time, do you know that catecholamines or stress responses have been reduced or gone away after this time?

DR. MANGANO: No, we don't know. Measuring catecholamines is necessarily intermittent. The intermittent measurements can never be correlated with an ischemic episode, because you cannot time the measurements with spontaneously occurring ischemia, so you'll never find the causal relationship between acute catecholamine changes and ischemic changes.

Previous studies using this dose of sufentanil and morphine have demonstrated that catecholamines can be suppressed. Thus, we are looking for hemodynamic markers or endpoints, and we see from these results that they are approximately the same.

DR. K.J.S. ANAND: Can I just comment on the Benefiel-Roizen study? I think we are limited by our ability to study one tiny portion of physiology and then relate that to what happens in the entire body. This ties in with the ultimate outcome studies that can be done. For example, we've concentrated in our studies on hormonal and metabolic changes. But those are not the only changes occurring. For example, changes in acute phase reactions: these go up quite markedly at about 24 hours following surgery. One of those acute phase reactions is fibrinogen, and it has been that blood viscosity changes following increases in fibrinogen. We haven't even mentioned the effects of surgical stress on the immune system, and there are other things that change at those points. In trying to relate the observations we've made to ultimate patient outcome, there will always be limitations on investigators who perform such studies.

DR. J. F. VILJOEN: We've seen these patients being studied. All the variables have been introduced: their ages, their demographic data, and so on. But what about the anesthesiologists? Were these patient data assembled, one group by a first-year resident, another group by a fellow, another by a professor and yet another by someone else?

DR. SLOGOFF: Hemodynamics can be just as well controlled by a second-year anesthesia resident as by a professor of anesthesia. If we can establish that the researchers are reasonably similar with respect to hemodynamic control, it doesn't matter, and you can always do multivariate analysis and exclude one group versus another. So I don't think it makes a difference, if you can achieve the same hemodynamic control.

DR. BENEFIEL: We did look at the anesthesiologists. It was a small group of anesthesiologists whose primary duty is cardiovascular anesthesia. No outcome differences could be attributed to the various anesthesia attendings.

DR. ROBERT MERIN: The most striking observation from that study was the different incidences of renal failure. I don't necessarily accept the congestive heart failure; that was pretty subjective. But there certainly was a difference in renal failure. Twenty-five years ago, several investigators demonstrated that if you diurese patients, preferably with mannitol, and control hemodynamics, preferably with vasodilator or ganglion blocker, then you can markedly decrease the incidence of postoperative renal complications after aortic cross-clamp surgery. I've heard no mention of an attempt at doing any of that on a controlled basis in this study, and perhaps that's because the study wasn't designed to investigate the effect of anesthetics on renal function.

But it may be a big flaw to stop the study because of a difference in renal outcome related to the anesthetic when, in fact, the problem wasn't addressed, that is, the problem of renal failure after aortic cross-clamping.

DR. BENEFIEL: The renal failure incidence was low. The incidence of renal insufficiency is perhaps what you were seeing, which was defined by a rise in creatinine of 1.0.

DR. SLOGOFF: I'm finishing up a paper that deals with renal failure after cardiopulmonary bypass, so I am familiar with the approach they used.

The only paper that I know that has documented the levels of creatinine changes Dr. Benefiel mentions is the Charleson paper, which looks at patients similar to this having major vascular surgery. It said a creatinine elevation of this magnitude 24 hours after surgery represented a significant reduction in creatinine clearance. But I am not sure that a creatinine that goes up half a milligram percent into the range of above 1.5 at six days postop can be attributed to isoflurane or sufentanil. I have a problem with that, since that constituted the largest objective difference other than the subjective diagnosis of congestive heart failure.

DR. BENEFIEL: Most patients have a decrease in BUN and creatinine after aortic surgery. When the creatinine stays the same or increases, it is a distinctly abnormal situation. As I have already mentioned, it is possible that the anesthetic or the way it modifies the patient's response may influence the incidence of renal insufficiency.

As for congestive heart failure, it is of interest that in the study by Yeager et al., they found that congestive heart failure was higher in the high-stress group, the same finding as we had. Further studies should probably address the question of why CHF increases with higher stress even though, as in our study, the incidence of intraoperative myocardial ischemia, hemodynamics, and the volume of fluid administered were not different.

Let me remind Dr. Slogoff and Dr. Merin that the definition of CHF was rales at least one-third up the back or a chest X-ray demonstrating pulmonary edema. The diagnosis also required acute intervention with intravenous diuretics. The diagnostic criteria were applied by a blinded observer. The diagnosis of CHF is always subjective, but the diagnosis was made in a consistent manner and there was a difference between groups.

The regimen to decrease the incidence of renal failure, mannitol and fluid administration prior to aortic cross-clamp, was routine except in patients already in renal failure.

DR. IRA ISAACSON: I think Dr. Mangano very eloquently showed the importance of the postoperative period, yet Dr. Benefiel did mention the postoperative management of these patients, and I think we would all agree that patients who were given 10 to 15 μg/kg sufentanil for a 3-hour aortic procedure wake up or, in that case, don't wake up. Similarly for the patients who had primarily an isoflurane anesthetic at the end of a 3-hour operation. Unless your operating rooms are different than my operating rooms at Emory, if I tried to do a primary inhalation anesthetic in my operating room, patients would wake up hypothermic, tachycardic, hypertensive, and hypercarbic. That issue is never addressed. When did the patients in the sufentanil group get weaned and extubated? When did the patients in the isoflurane group get weaned and extubated? Some of the isoflurane group had intraspinal opioids. Was there a difference among those groups within the isoflurane group that had intraspinal opioids versus intermittent intravenous medication? There are so many flaws to this study. Another question was, "What about the anesthesiologists?" Well, what about the surgeons? I look at these data and say, "You don't need isoflurane or sufentanil, you need a new vascular surgeon."

DR. BENEFIEL: Dr. Isaacson has brought up several good points. First, he commented about the procedure taking 3 hours at Emory and that at the end of surgery his patients wake up and are hypothermic, tachycardic, and hypercarbic. Most of the procedures in this study took longer than 3 hours. Let me describe a typical procedure and you will see why. For a thoracoabdominal aneurysmectomy, the patient is placed in a right lateral semidecubitus position. An incision is carried from the midleft chest to the pubis, traversing the costal cartilages and diaphragm. An extrapleural and retroperitoneal dissection is carried out exposing the descending aorta from near the left atrial appendage to the bifurcation below the renal arteries. Then the aorta is clamped above the celiac axis and a graft is sewn in and carried down to the celiac. The celiac is detached from the aorta and connected to the graft. The clamp is then moved to below the celiac on the graft. Then the superior mesenteric artery is attached in a similar fashion and the clamp is moved below it. Then the renal arteries are attached and perfused. Finally, an infrarenal anastomosis is made. Throughout the repair, the lumbar arteries are back-bleeding and must be ligated. After hemostasis is complete, the closure includes repair of the diaphragm and the thoracoabdominal incision. Because of the extensive dissection and blood loss, extubation is done only when respiratory mechanics are demonstrably satisfactory. Despite the respiratory depression attributable to sufentanil, more patients in the isoflurane group required mechanical ventilation. Blood pressure, temperature, and heart rate are all controlled before extubation.

Dr. Isaacson also asked about spinal opiates. This subgroup was examined, and no outcome differences could be attributed to the spinal opiates.

As for his comment that we need a new vascular surgeon, I am afraid I do not have a response for that. We did, however, look at the four surgeons in the study as a variable, and no outcome difference could be attributed to them.

DR. SLOGOFF: I compliment Dr. Hickey on a wonderful study. I know how difficult that type of research is. One of the most striking things about it is, in the preemies one of the worst complications you saw was intracranial hemorrhage, and we do have a hypothesis in the study to explain that. Not the epinephrine or the norepinephrine or any other thing, but the glucose can explain that. The significant rise in glucose as a consequence of the stress response, and its affect on osmolality, may be indictable in the increased incidence of intracranial hemorrhage. I think his particular study in that particular group of patients shows something important. The one flaw in this study is that, particularly as it relates to the cardiac, he states he compared halothane to sufentanil. I'm not sure that is what he really compared. He compared sufentanil to halothane to tolerance. Is that correct? And there were times when the halothane wasn't on during the operation. Is that correct?

DR. ANAND: The group received halothane induction and maintenance up to the start of bypass and then was given supplements of morphine before, during, and after bypass.

DR. SLOGOFF: I understand that. But did you maintain a constant alveolar concentration of halothane, or if patients became hypotensive, did you back off on the halothane or sometimes turn it off?

DR. ANAND: Yes.

DR. SLOGOFF: So you are possibly comparing not sufentanil to halothane, but sufentanil anesthesia to sometimes no anesthesia. That is a major issue. The beauty of sufentanil is that patients can tolerate it hemodynamically, but it may not be sufentanil versus halothane.

DR. AMIRA SAFWAT: I have a question for Dr. Mangano relating to epidural narcotics for postoperative tachycardia and hypertension.

DR. MANGANO: The study has never been done, and it is a difficult problem. People have used thoracic epidural analgesia to control hypertension. There are also studies under way addressing patients undergoing noncardiac surgery, looking at the incidence of ischemia postoperatively.

DR. MERIN: There is a Japanese group that has done 200 various open-heart procedures under continuous thoracic epidural anesthesia with catheter placement 24 hours preoperatively. The problem is the systemic anticoagulation used in patients with epidural catheters. Most investigators are not willing to take that risk. We are involved in a study now where we are looking at intrathecal opiates given just preoperatively in patients for coronary bypass grafting. We're not willing to take the risk of an epidural catheter. I think there may be some other groups doing that, but that's the problem with an epidural for cardiac surgery, systemic anticoagulation.

DR SAFWAT: It is related to the state-of-the-art monitoring intraoperative ischemia.

DR. MANGANO: That is true. Afterload increases can cause regional wall motion abnormalities. Even with preload/afterload conditions fixed, and temperature of the myocardium unchanged, wall motion abnormalities represent regional ventricular dysfunction or stunning state, versus ischemia. It is very hard to differentiate. But when regional wall motion abnormalities occur without substantial change in loading conditions intraoperatively, they're probably indicative of ischemia.

DR. SLOGOFF: Dr. Mangano's argument that the ischemia in the postpump period after coronary bypass is highly predictive of adverse outcome has to be responded to in the following way.

To my way of thinking, most, perhaps 95 to 98% of myocardial infarctions associated with coronary artery bypass grafting are intraoperative events. The systolic wall motion abnormalities that he says predict infarctions I contend actually are infarctions when he sees them. That's why they are so predictive. The ones that go away and get better were, in fact, ischemia. The ones that don't go away and don't get better are infarctions. Smith had the same observation—when they don't go away, they are infarctions. It isn't that there was intermittent ischemia by systolic wall motion and then three days later there was an infarction. It was just infarction from the start.

DR. MANGANO: First of all, I did not say that there are any data substantiating that postoperative ischemia predicts infarction in patients undergoing coronary surgery. That's still unknown. The data from Leung that we just published show that when you look at ischemic changes by segmental wall motion immediately following bypass, they are most predictive in that small group of patients. It is true that when you get a wall motion change intraoperatively, it could be part of the infarction process itself, and therefore it is obvious that it predicts infarction. Outcome predicts outcome. It is a very difficult proposition. All we're left with is to find an early marker—a predictor or an early marker of the outcome process itself—that will enable us to detect outcomes early and treat them aggressively. Perhaps early treatment may blunt the severity of the outcome.

DR. SLOGOFF: And I agree with that entirely. In your continued anesthesia study, what was the incidence of perioperative infarction in the two groups?

DR. MANGANO: They're about the same: three and four in each group.

DR. SLOGOFF: So your incidence in infarction is . . .

DR. MANGANO: About 10%.

DR. MERIN: I would like to ask Mike Nugent if he has any further information on a particularly intriguing study that he coauthored in *Anesthesiology* this year,[3] on the effects of halothane versus isoflurane and enflurane on the thrombotic process that may be responsible for myocardial infarction.

DR. NUGENT: Cardiologists have used thrombolytic therapy in the setting of acute myocardial infarction for several years. The final common pathway of a perioperative myocardial infarction commonly involves thrombus formation in a coronary artery. It also recently has been reported that unstable angina is usually characterized by ruptured atheromata with attached thrombus, while stable angina is characterized by smooth atheromata. Therefore, both unstable angina and perioperative myocardial infarction frequently involve platelet aggregation and intracoronary thrombus formation. Cycloxygenase inhibitors, such as aspirin, that inhibit platelet function, were given to patients after suspected

---

[3]Bertha BG, Folts JD, Nugent M, Rusy BF. Halothane but not isoflurane or enflurane protects against spontaneous and epinephrine-exacerbated acute thrombus formation in stenosed dog coronary arteries. *Anesthesiology* 1989;71:96–102.

myocardial infarction, reduced coronary and cerebral vascular mortality. Aspirin is known to increase coronary artery graft patency rates from 85 to 92% after coronary bypass graft surgery. Unfortunately, the same intervention resulted in an increased incidence of postoperative bleeding.

A model developed by John Folts in Madison, Wisconsin, involves a stenosed dog coronary artery in which thrombi form, break off, and reform in a cyclical fusion. We found that halothane blocks thrombus formation, while isoflurane and enflurane did not decrease the frequency of thrombus formation. These results were not too surprising because in platelet aggregometric studies halothane inhibits platelet function to a greater extent than isoflurane or enflurane. Thorazine and droperidol also inhibit thrombus formation, probably by blocking the α_2-adrenergic receptor on platelets. Epinephrine classically has been known to increase the frequency of formation of thrombus in this model. This fact could be significant when deciding what inotropic agent to use for coming cardiopulmonary bypass after coronary artery surgery. In our model, epinephrine increased the rate of thrombus formation by 50%, while dopamine decreased the frequency of thrombus formation by 50%. Amrinone completely eliminated the formation of thrombi, probably because of phosphodiesterase inhibition, which increased intraplatelet cyclic AMP stabilizer platelets.

DR. MERIN: You didn't answer my question. No more data except that study published in *Anesthesiology*?

DR. NUGENT: You mean in terms of outcome on people with halothane? A recent review of this model of intracoronary thrombus formations appears in *Circulation*, July 1989, by Willison. Over eight studies using this model have appeared in *Circulation* and *Circulation Research*, as discussed in the review article.

DR. MERIN: A lot of things were inconclusive about that particular study.

DR. CARL C. HUG, JR.:   I am not familiar enough with your model but, for example, in your dog model, what is the coagulation state of that preparation? Is it equivalent to our patients' if they are into bypass and heparinized and have probably had a coagulopathy in most cases for some period of time thereafter? I wouldn't indict epinephrine unless you have similar coagulopathy.

I don't think it matters if it's 20 or 22. I just can't believe that the situation is a setup for thrombosis in that period of time for the first 24 hours.

DR. NUGENT: That's why you look at models at the molecular level; you look at them at the tissue level; you look at them in dogs; and then you bring them back to people.

SPEAKER FROM THE FLOOR: In science and medicine, we all need to work with models. But is it an extrapolation when somebody says, "Don't use epinephrine from a bypass because you are going to thrombose somebody"? I don't think so, because I don't think the data are complete yet and epinephrine is one of the most versatile drugs that we've got.

DR. ESTAFANOUS: But do we have information that epinephrine after bypass in a patient who was heparinized, and probably stayed partly heparinized, will cause thrombosis in this particular subset of patients?

QUESTION FROM THE FLOOR: Dr. Nugent referred twice to the need for larger studies. We do over 100,000 aortic procedures annually in this country, and we don't have any outcome data of any epidemiologic significance whatsoever. The only way we are going to get them is through a national data bank multicenter type of study. Ten years ago we discussed this, five years ago we discussed it. Are we going to discuss this again in five years and still

not be able to tell patients or colleagues, "We're going to do a triple A, and this is the approach we should take because in 50,000 patients last year in the United States, this is the approach that was taken from preoperative assessment to postoperative management. We have the data to support our decisions."

DR. NUGENT: The only way it is going to happen is if the National Institute of Health funds it. Big money.

SPEAKER FROM THE FLOOR: The cost of initial setup of a data bank was estimated to be $17 million. The ASA asked, "Where is the $17 million going to come from?" We do 25 million anesthetics per year in the United States; it would cost 70 cents per patient.

DR. MANGANO: I think your point is very well taken, and I am all for outcome studies, but the closer you get to outcome in epidemiologic studies, the further away you get from mechanisms. And it has to be both. We need detailed, precise, small studies in 50 patients, 20 patients, even 5 patients, that try to get at the underlying mechanisms, which are extremely complex—the interaction of thrombosis and supply-demand indices.

III DELIVERY METHODS

19 OPIOID ADMINISTRATION BY CONTINUOUS INFUSION

James R. Jacobs, Peter S.A. Glass, and J.G. Reves

The physics of volatile gases, the physiology of the pulmonary circulation, and the technology of the calibrated vaporizer make it possible to continuously deliver the potent inhalation anesthetic drugs at an inspired gas concentration that is easily and efficiently manipulated. These drugs are only moderately soluble in blood, so that the partial pressure of the agent in the blood equilibrates with the alveolar drug concentration quickly and roughly parallels changes in the inspired gas concentration. Additionally, the concept of MAC (minimum steady-state alveolar concentration of anesthetic at 1 atmosphere required to abolish movement in 50% of patients in response to a noxious stimulus) has for 25 years provided not only a measure of relative potency between the inhaled anesthetics but also a guide to anesthetic dosing. With a knowledge of MAC and with the availability of the vaporizer, delivery of the potent inhalation agents is based not on drug dosage, which has a time-varying influence on drug effect secondary to pharmacokinetic processes, but rather on the partial pressure of the drug in the blood, which is presumably acting as the driving force in determining the concentration of drug at its site of action and hence the magnitude of drug effect.

In contrast, the most common method of administering intravenous anesthetic drugs, the opioid analgesics in particular, is by intermittent bolus injection. Only recently has there been a groundswell of interest in continuous infusion of opioid anesthetic drugs and in determining the plasma concentrations of these agents required to provide adequate anesthetic conditions during various surgical stimuli. Much of this enthusiasm was initiated by the introduction of alfentanil, for which continuous infusion is the most convenient means of administration for other than the briefest of procedures. Techniques and instrumentation for implementing continuous drug infusions are now undergoing rapid development and are becoming increasingly important. In this chapter, we discuss some of the theoretical and practical implications of continuous opioid infusions in anesthesia, with emphasis of pharmacokinetic model-driven drug delivery.

RATIONALE FOR ADMINISTERING OPIOIDS BY CONTINUOUS INFUSION

Variable-rate continuous infusions are an intuitively reasonable mode of administering in-

241

travenous anesthetic drugs.[1,2] After all, no one today would contemplate intermittent open-drop administration of a volatile anesthetic drug onto a Schimmelbusch mask. This can presumably be attributed to factors other than the sheer convenience of the anesthetic vaporizer, factors such as the continuous requirement for anesthesia during the surgical procedure and the continuously varying magnitude of surgical stimulation.

The opioids in clinical use can be assumed to follow linear first-order pharmacokinetics following intravenous infusion. It is a curious result of first-order kinetics that, for example, 40 μg/kg fentanyl given over 1 hour using a pharmacokinetically oriented continuous infusion continuously maintains a plasma fentanyl concentration of 10 ng/ml, whereas the plasma level 1 hour following a 50 μg/kg bolus will be less than 10 ng/ml (based on a typical set of kinetic parameters[3] for fentanyl). Reiterating, less drug given as an infusion maintains a particular plasma drug concentration over a period of time more efficiently than more drug given as a bolus. Here, then, is theoretical support for continuous infusion techniques in that it is possible that a titrated infusion will result in lower total drug dosages than intermittent bolus dosing.

From a clinical perspective, it is frequently conjectured that administering opioids by continuous infusion avoids the peaks and valleys in plasma drug concentration that result from intermittent bolus dosing (Figure 19.1). It is suggested that avoiding the peaks will prevent some of the adverse effects, such as rigidity, that may manifest themselves when an opioid is present in the plasma at an excessively high concentration. Avoiding the valleys should forestall the hemodynamic, autonomic, or other signs of responsiveness to surgical stimulation that may occur when the plasma opioid concentration falls below a threshold level. If fentanyl and its analogues were not as hemodynamically benign as they are, it is likely that continuous infusion paradigms would have evolved sooner.

Using a titrated continuous infusion of fentanyl, sufentanil, or alfentanil as part of a balanced anesthetic technique, it is possible in

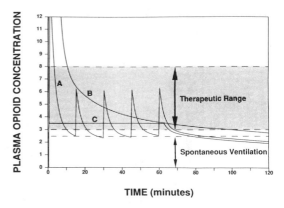

FIGURE 19.1 Simulation of plasma drug concentrations resulting from three dosing schemes for administration of a hypothetical opioid (kinetics[3] of fentanyl were used in constructing the graph) during a surgical procedure lasting 70 minutes. Curve A results from a loading bolus of 8 μg/kg followed by boluses of 1.5 μg/kg every 15 minutes. This dosing scheme results in the classic peaks and valleys, where the plasma opioid concentration alternately swings between subtherapeutic and supratherapeutic levels. Curve B results from a single bolus of 20 μg/kg. Curve C results from a pharmacokinetic model-based continuous infusion scheme designed to maintain a constant therapeutic plasma opioid concentration. Note that at 65 minutes the plasma opioid concentration resulting from all three schemes is approximately equal but that recovery occurs most rapidly with the infusion technique, with the intermittent bolus method following close behind. When the therapeutic threshold is variable, as it is during the variable stresses of surgery, or when the surgical procedure is completed sooner than expected, a continuous infusion will be far superior to the intermittent technique, both in maintaining a therapeutic concentration and in providing the potential for rapid recovery most consistently.

most cases to continuously maintain a plasma opioid concentration just above the therapeutic threshold. In so doing, excessive concentrations are avoided, and the concentration will quickly fall below the threshold for respiratory depression when the infusion is terminated near the end of surgery. Accordingly, Sebel and Bovill[4] have stated that "[t]he most efficient manner of fentanyl administration, both in terms of total drug needed and hemodynamic stability, is by continuous infusion with the infusion rate adjusted according to variations in patient requirements." This situation is precisely analogous to routine delivery of the potent inhalation anesthetics, where the depth of anesthesia is best controlled by continuous administration and careful titration. Opioid effect is related to the plasma opioid concentration, and the plasma opioid concentration is controlled better by continuous infusion techniques than by intermittent dosing.

The expected advantages of continuous infusion have been documented under the conditions of a variety of research protocols. In direct comparisons with intermittent bolus administration, continuous opioid infusions have been shown to result in (1) greater hemodynamic stability,[5-7] (2) fewer incidences of hemodynamic breakthrough and other signs of patient responsiveness,[5,6,8] (3) decreased incidence of requirement for naloxone,[6] (4) decreased incidence of side effects,[6] (5) suppression of the cortisol and vasopressin responses to cardiopulmonary bypass,[9] (6) reduced need for supplemental anesthetics or vasoactive drugs,[5,6] (7) decreased total drug dosages,[8,10] (8) more rapid recovery,[8] (9) more predictable suppression of somatosensory cortical-evoked potentials and repeatable wake-up tests in patients undergoing spinal surgery,[10] and (10) reduced need for postoperative ventilatory support.[10] In addition to studies directly comparing bolus and continuous administration, there have been many describing the use of continuous opioid infusions in noncomparative investigations or simply as the primary anesthetic. Continuous infusions have consistently been found to be an efficacious and clinically attractive mode of administering the opioid. The logistical, medical, and economic significance of these results remains to be elucidated, but it has been our observation that most of our colleagues who have tried continuous infusion techniques have gone on to adopt

them as standard practice. This, more so than any statistically significant investigation, has impressed us as compelling support for opioid administration by continuous infusion.

POSTULATES TO CONTINUOUS OPIOID INFUSIONS

Before discussing the practical implementation of continuous opioid infusions, it is useful to consider several accepted principles related to continuous infusion practices in general and to continuous opioid infusions in particular. Infusion concepts are still evolving; it is likely that these postulates will be better defined by future research.

First, use of a continuous infusion does not imply total intravenous anesthesia. Early experience with continuous infusions in Europe was often obtained in the context of studies with total intravenous anesthesia where potent inhalation agents and nitrous oxide were excluded, but this need not be the case. Continuous infusion of a drug is simply an attractive means of administration whenever the agent would otherwise be delivered by intermittent boluses.

Second, continuous infusion does not mean constant infusion. This comment is based on both pharmacodynamic and pharmacokinetic considerations. Considering the former, just as one would not choose a single vaporizer setting for use throughout an anesthetic with isoflurane, it is critical that continuous intravenous infusions be titrated according to patient responsiveness. With regard to opioid infusions, this is particularly significant with respect to the common requirement that patients be oriented and breathing spontaneously before leaving the operating room. Therefore, a continuous infusion technique will require variable-rate infusions if the plasma opioid concentration is to be titrated to match patient's pharmacodynamic needs. In fact, it has been demonstrated[11] that there are no inherent advantages in giving fentanyl by infusion compared to intermittent bolusing when the infusion is not titrated. Recalling that a constant-rate infusion requires 4 to 5 elimination half-lives to obtain a steady-state plasma concentration, efficient titration of the infusion requires quantitative consideration of the drug's pharmacokinetics, and here is where the issue of continuous infusions becomes somewhat more complicated. Even in the most simple scheme, increasing the plasma drug concentration requires a loading dose in addition to an increase in the infusion rate. Since drug cannot be forcibly removed from the blood, deciding when and by how much to decrease the infusion rate to lower the plasma drug concentration will ideally be based on an appreciation for the rate at which drug will be eliminated or redistributed from the blood. The pharmacokinetic basis for variable-rate infusions is discussed in greater detail in the next section.

Third, use of a continuous infusion technique does not preclude the use of periodic bolus doses. As just mentioned, boluses are used throughout the anesthetic as loading doses to increase the plasma opioid concentration. Miniature boluses can also be used independently of an increase in the infusion rate to blunt isolated, short-lived, intense stimuli; this approach is particularly valuable when using alfentanil, since the plasma alfentanil concentration will quickly return to its prebolus level.

Finally, continuous infusion of an opioid alone is not ideal in many situations. Even with the very high plasma opioid concentrations that have been used in cardiac anesthesia, it has not been possible to reliably obtund responses to surgical stimulation in the absence of a hypnotic agent.[12,13] In the presence of 66 to 70% nitrous oxide it is possible to induce and maintain acceptable anesthetic conditions with a continuous opioid infusion, but doing so requires that the opioid infusion be painstakingly titrated if the patient is expected to be capable of breathing spontaneously at the end of operation. We have done this with fentanyl, sufentanil, and alfentanil in general surgical patients, but administering anesthesia in this way is a nerve-racking experience for the anesthesiologist, since the rigid titration tends to result in periods of very light anesthesia (which stems from concern to have

the opioid concentration as low as possible to ensure spontaneous ventilation at the end). We have found instead that addition of a hypnotic (e.g., midazolam) in combination with the opioid infusion to be a preferable technique. Addition of a hypnotic drug with amnestic properties generally provides a smoother induction of anesthesia, ensures lack of recall, and allows much lower plasma opioid concentrations to be used. High opioid concentrations and a hyperdynamic myocardium are avoided, and concerns about spontaneous ventilation at the end of surgery are lessened. However, just as the opioid and hypnotic can act together to provide excellent hypnosis and analgesia, they can also act synergistically to produce undesirable effects when the plasma concentration of one or both agents is unnecessarily high. When used appropriately, continuous infusions of an opioid and a hypnotic (with or without nitrous oxide) are an attractive alternative to infusion of an opioid alone, and in combination with a muscle relaxant they have become a popular anesthetic technique in our department.

IMPLEMENTING CONTINUOUS INFUSIONS

Researchers and clinicians have been talking about continuous infusions for a long time. Much has been written about the theory and practice of infusing many different classes of drugs, including the opioids and other anesthetic drugs.[1,2,14-16] For a drug such as sodium nitroprusside, with evanescent pharmacokinetics and an effect that is immediate and readily measured, implementing an infusion is reasonably straightforward; the immediacy between a change in infusion rate and the resulting change in steady-stage drug effect makes the dose-response curve immediately tangible. However, when a drug's pharmacokinetics are significantly multicompartmental, as is true of fentanyl and its analogues, there is a contorted relationship between infusion rate and drug effect. Since the opioids exert their effects through specific opioid receptors, and since the occupation of these receptors is related to the opioid concentration in the plasma, it is more logical to control the plasma opioid concentration than to control the opioid infusion rate. To do so requires a quantitative or at least intuitive appreciation for the pharmacokinetics of the drug being infused.

In 1968, Kruger-Thiemer[17] presented analytical equations giving the time-varying infusion rate required to achieve and maintain a specified plasma drug concentration based on a compartmental pharmacokinetic model of the drug being infused. Schwilden[18] elaborated on this method for the two-compartment model. As is now well known, maintaining a specified plasma concentration of a drug with kinetics described by a two-compartment model requires a bolus (B) to fill the central compartment to the desired concentration, a constant infusion to replace drug being eliminated (E) from the central compartment by excretion or metabolism, and superimposed on this an exponentially declining infusion to replace drug being transferred (T) into the peripheral compartment. This is the BET scheme. Implementation of the BET scheme requires a computerized infusion pump programmed with the appropriate equations and the drug's kinetic parameters,[19,20] and even then the implementation is only approximate, since the equations specify infusion rates with infinite resolution that vary continuously as a function of time.

As a more practical alternative, intravenous infusion schemes are generally based on the idea of a loading dose (slow bolus or brief high-rate infusion) followed by a constant infusion. To subsequently raise the plasma drug concentration, another small loading dose is given and the infusion rate is increased. This practice has been discussed at length in the classic paper by Wagner[21] and by many other authors. The challenge is to use a loading dose that is (1) not so large or rapidly administered that the plasma opioid concentration ends up being almost as high as it would be in a standard bolus administration scheme, and (2) large enough to ensure that the plasma drug concentration does not dip below the therapeutic level during the interval until the continuous infusion provides an effective plasma concentration.

tration. The clinician must know the loading dose and infusion rate required to effect proportional changes in the plasma drug concentration, appreciate that redistribution is likely to be more prominent at the beginning of an anesthetic than towards the end, and consider the rate of drug elimination and the potential for redistribution when deciding when to terminate the opioid infusion.

Continuous intravenous infusions of anesthetic drugs have not been widely accepted. Their popularity has waxed and waned throughout the history of modern anesthesia. Twenty years ago, induction of anesthesia with sodium thiopental and maintenance with continuous infusion of thiopental and succinylcholine was common practice. Infusions of ketamine or Innovar were used in the late 1970s. An infusion technique for fentanyl was first reported in 1980,[22] but it has taken almost a decade for opioid infusions to start gaining popularity. The introduction of alfentanil in the United States in 1987 and the coincident release of the Bard Alfentanil Infuser were major contributors to the present interest in continuous opioid infusions. Early clinical experience with alfentanil demonstrated that it was most conveniently administered by continuous intravenous infusion. This can be attributed to alfentanil's relatively brief elimination half-life and to the large doses required to maintain therapeutic plasma concentrations. The Bard infusion pump greatly simplified administration of alfentanil by providing the clinician with a small, light-weight syringe pump with controls specifically designed to administer boluses and infusions of alfentanil on a body weight–adjusted basis. That this device was capable of administering a loading dose followed immediately by a continuous infusion made implementation of a Wagner-type approach to continuous infusions reasonably straightforward. It was soon realized that the Bard device, later named the MiniInfuser and now the InfusOR, could equally well be used to administer other drugs packaged in a concentration of 500 µg/ml (like alfentanil) and a drug in any concentration if appropriate scaling factors were considered. The convenience

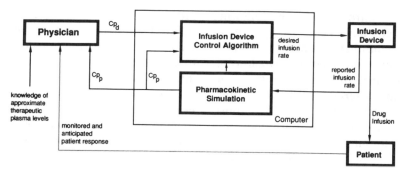

FIGURE 19.2 Schematic illustration of the authors' approach to pharmacokinetic model-driven drug delivery. In this computer-assisted continuous infusion (CACI) device, the physician enters the desired plasma drug concentration (Cp_d). An infusion device control algorithm uses a pharmacokinetic model for the drug being infused to determine what the infusion rate should be for the next infusion interval (e.g., 9 seconds). The infusion device delivers drug to the patient, and the infusion rate is fed into a simulation of the pharmacokinetic model to compute the current predicted plasma drug concentration (Cp_p). The quantities computed in the simulation are available to the algorithm. On the basis of monitored and anticipated patient response, knowledge of approximate therapeutic plasma drug concentrations (e.g., Cp_{50}), and on Cp_p, the physician can alter Cp_d as necessary.

fentanil, alfentanil, midazolam, thiopental, and propofol alone or in combinations. During the past three years, we have used our CACI device as a clinical instrument or research tool to administer the primary or adjuvant anesthetic drug(s) to more than 500 patients of all ages undergoing cardiac or noncardiac surgery. Clinically, CACI has been adopted as the preferred means of delivering continuous intravenous infusions of these drugs. Our clinical use of CACI most commonly involves the administration of an opioid with midazolam or propofol (Table 19.2). Typically, the midazolam is used to induce anesthesia and the plasma level is not altered significantly throughout the remainder of the anesthetic. The opioid is added prior to intubation of the trachea and is titrated using the same criteria that are used to titrate a manual infusion. As a research tool, CACI has been useful in that it facilitates the attainment of relatively steady-state plasma drug concentrations, which is a requirement in many research protocols.

In spite of this advanced technology, or by some points of view because of it, drug administration using CACI still must be guided by two fundamental tenets of pharmacotherapy: pharmacokinetic variability and pharmacodynamic variability. With regard to the former, any linear

TABLE 19.2 Common opioid infusion schemes: typical plasma concentrations

	Induction and Maintenance (ng/ml)
Fentanyl concentrations	
+ oxygen	20–50
+ N$_2$O:O$_2$	2–8
+ midazolam[a] ± N$_2$O	2–8
Sufentanil concentrations	
+ oxygen	Undetermined
+ N$_2$O:O$_2$	1–5
+ midazolam[a] ± N$_2$O	0.5–4
Alfentanil concentrations	
+ oxygen	500–1,500
+ N$_2$O:O$_2$	100–500
+ midazolam[a] ± N$_2$O	50–500

[a]Midazolam concentrations: patient premedicated, induction 100–200 ng/ml; patient not premedicated, induction 75–125 ng/ml; maintenance 50–100 ng/ml.

time-invariant two- or three-compartment pharm-cokinetic model is a gross simplification of the complex processes determining the plasma drug concentration output resulting from a drug dos-age input and thus should be expected to provide only an approximate prediction of the plasma concentrations. In addition to this fundamental limitation, pharmacokinetic identification exper-iments are typically fraught with measurement (e.g., blood sampling, sample processing, and assay variability) errors and methodological (e.g., bolus versus infusion input) errors. Thus, the most contentious aspect of pharmacokinetic model-driven drug delivery is the accuracy of the pharmacokinetic model. Remarkably, most in-vestigators have found that plasma drug levels measured during CACI administration are typ-ically within about ±30% of those predicted.[2] This degree of accuracy has been clinically ac-ceptable and should improve further as phar-macokinetic data for specific patient populations (i.e., population kinetics) become available.[32]

Shown in Figure 19.3 are measured and predicted plasma fentanyl concentrations from two typical patients from one of our clinical studies in which the accuracy with which our CACI device could deliver fentanyl was as-sessed. These graphs provide a visual impres-sion of the accuracy with which the measured fentanyl levels followed those predicted by the instrument. Shown in Figure 19.4 are box-and-whisker plots summarizing some of our expe-rience with CACI administration of fentanyl, sufentanil, and alfentanil. The measure of ac-curacy given is the percent absolute prediction error, calculated as the absolute value of 100·(predicted-measured)/predicted for each mea-sured and CACI-predicted plasma drug sam-ple. The fentanyl data represent 391 measured and CACI-predicted plasma samples from 24 patients[33] using the kinetic parameters pub-lished by McClain and Hug.[3] The sufentanil data represent 182 samples from 39 patients using the kinetic parameters published by Bov-ill et al.[34] The alfentanil data represent 140 samples from 26 patients using the pharma-cokinetic parameters published by Bovill et al.[35] Notice that the median absolute predic-tion error for fentanyl and alfentanil is well

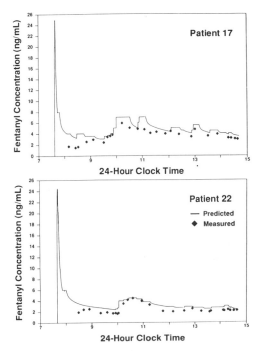

FIGURE 19.3 Measured and CACI-pre-dicted plasma fentanyl concentrations ob-tained in two patients receiving fentanyl administered by the authors' CACI device. The anesthesiologist used CACI to titrate the fen-tanyl infusion in combination with nitrous ox-ide to provide anesthesia for an orthopedic surgical procedure. The solid line represents the plasma fentanyl concentration predicted by the CACI device intraoperatively. The dots show the measured fentanyl concentration in samples taken at various times throughout the fentanyl infusion and subsequently assayed by a radio-immunoassay technique.

below 30% and that for sufentanil is about 35%. Many factors influence accuracy but foremost among them are the robustness and applicability of the pharmacokinetic model used to program the CACI device. We are now using population kinetics[36] to further improve our accuracy with alfentanil and are hoping to determine a pharmacokinetic model that bet-ter describes the kinetics of sufentanil in our patient population.

Pharmacodynamic variability can generally be defined as differences in pharmacological

CONCLUSION

There was a time when intermittent administration using a Schimmelbusch mask was the preferred means of delivering volatile anesthetics. Today, continuous delivery using a calibrated vaporizer is the only acceptable method of administering these drugs. Although an analogy can be drawn between the Schimmelbusch mask and a syringe, we do not wish to suggest that infusion pumps or CACI devices will supplant the syringe in the delivery of intravenous drugs. We do suggest that titrated, continuous infusions are an efficient and efficacious means of administering opioids in many situations. We expect that continuous opioid infusions will be adopted by ever-increasing numbers of anesthesiologists. With pragmatic efforts to determine opioid pharmacokinetics and concentration-effect relations for a wide spectrum of clinical circumstances, and with the introduction of better infusion devices, including CACI, techniques for the administration of opioids by continuous intravenous infusion will be permanently established in anesthesia and are likely to improve patient care.

REFERENCES

1. White PF. Clinical uses of intravenous anesthetic and analgesic infusions. Anesth Analg 1989;68:161–171.
2. Glass PSA, Jacobs JR, Reves JG. Intravenous drug delivery systems. In: Miller RD, ed. Anesthesia. 3d ed. New York: Churchill Livingstone, 1990.
3. McClain DA, Hug CC Jr. Intravenous fentanyl kinetics. Clin Pharmacol Ther 1980;28:106–114.
4. Sebel PS, Bovill JG. Opioid analgesics in cardiac anesthesia. In: Kaplan JA, ed. Cardiac anesthesia. 2d ed. Orlando, Fla.: Grune & Stratton, 1987; 91.
5. Alvis JM, Reves JG, Govier AV, et al. Computer-assisted continuous infusions of fentanyl during cardiac anesthesia: comparison with a manual method. Anesthesiology 1985;63:41–49.
6. Ausems ME, Vuyk J, Hug CC Jr, et al. Comparison of a computer-assisted infusion versus intermittent bolus administration of alfentanil as a supplement to nitrous oxide for lower abdominal surgery. Anesthesiology 1988;68:851–861.
7. de Lange S, de Bruijn N, Stanley TH, et al. Alfentanil-oxygen anesthesia: comparison of continuous infusion and frequent bolus techniques for coronary artery surgery. Anesthesiology 1981;55:A42. (Abstr.)
8. White PF. Use of continuous infusion versus intermittent bolus administration of fentanyl or ketamine during outpatient anesthesia. Anesthesiology 1983;59:294–300.
9. Hynynen M, Lehtinen A-M, Salmenpera M, et al. Continuous infusion of fentanyl or alfentanil for coronary artery surgery. Br J Anaesth 1986;58:1260–1266.
10. Pathak KS, Brown RH, Nash CL, et al. Continuous opioid infusion for scoliosis fusion surgery. Anesth Analg 1983;62:841–845.
11. Sladen RN, de Bruijn N, Stanski D, et al. A clinical comparison of bolus versus continuous infusion of fentanyl for coronary artery bypass surgery. Anesthesiology 1986;65:A9. (Abstr.)
12. Wynands JE, Wong P, Townsend GE, et al. Narcotic requirements for intravenous anesthesia. Anesth Analg 1984;63:101–105.
13. Sonntag H, Stephan H, Lange H, et al. Sufentanil does not block sympathetic responses to surgical stimuli in patients having coronary artery revascularization surgery. Anesth Analg 1989;68:584–592.
14. Stanski DR. The role of pharmacokinetics in anaesthesia: application to intravenous infusions. Anaesth Intensive Care 1987;15:7–14.
15. Stanski DR. Narcotic pharmacokinetics and dynamics: the basis of infusion applications. Anaesth Intensive Care 1987;15:23–26.
16. Schwilden H, Stoeckel H, Schuttler J, et al. Pharmacological models and their use in clinical anaesthesia. Eur J Anaesth 1986;3:175–203.
17. Kruger-Thiemer E. Continuous intravenous infusion and multicompartment accumulation. Eur J Pharmacol 1968;4:317–324.
18. Schwilden H. A general method for calculating the dosage scheme in linear pharmacokinetics. Eur J Clin Pharmacol 1981;20:379–386.
19. Schwilden H, Schuttler J, Stoekel H. Pharmacokinetics as applied to total intravenous

anaesthesia: theoretical considerations. Anaesthesia 1983;38(suppl):51–52.

20. Schuttler J, Schwilden H, Stoekel H. Pharmacokinetics as applied to total intravenous anaesthesia: practical implications. Anaesthesia 1983;38(suppl):53–56.

21. Wagner JG. A safe method for rapidly achieving plasma concentration plateaus. Clin Pharmacol Ther 1974;16:691–700.

22. Hengstmann JH, Stoeckel H, Schuttler J. Infusion model for fentanyl based on pharmacokinetic analysis. Br J Anaesth 1980;52:1021–1024.

23. Crankshaw DP, Boyd MD, Bjorksten AR. Plasma drug efflux: a new approach to optimization of drug infusion for constant blood concentration of thiopental and methohexital. Anesthesiology 1987;67:32–41.

24. Reves JG, Glass P, Jacobs JR. Alfentanil and midazolam: new anesthetic drugs for continuous infusion and an automated method of administration. Mt. Sinai J Med (NY) 1989; 56:99–107.

25. Martin RW, Hill HF, Yee HC, et al. An open-loop computer-based drug infusion system. IEEE Trans Biomed Eng 1987;BME34:642–649.

26. Schuttler J, Kloos S, Schwilden H, et al. Total intravenous anaesthesia with propofol and alfentanil by computer-assisted infusion. Anaesthesia 1988;43(suppl):2–7.

27. Shafer SL, Siegel LC, Cooke JE, et al. Testing computer-controlled infusion pumps by simulation. Anesthesiology 1988;68:261–266.

28. Tackley RM, Lewis GTR, Prys-Roberts C, et al. Computer-controlled infusion of propofol. Br J Anaesth 1989;62:46–53.

29. Tavernier A, Coussaert E, D'Hollander A, et al. Model-based pharmacokinetic regulation in computer-assisted anesthesia: an interactive system, CARIN. Acta Anaesthesiol Belg 1987; 38:63–68.

30. Jacobs JR. Algorithm for optimal linear model-based control with application to pharmacokinetic model-driven drug delivery. IEEE Trans Biomed Eng 1990;37:107–109.

31. Jacobs JR, Glass PSA, Reves JG. Computer-assisted continuous infusion (CACI): a new concept in intravenous drug delivery. Clin Res 1989;37:338A. (Abstr.)

32. Maitre PO, Ausems ME, Vozeh S, et al. Evaluating the accuracy of using population pharmacokinetic data to predict plasma concentrations of alfentanil. Anesthesiology 1988;68: 59–67.

33. Glass PSA, Jacobs JR, Smith LR, et al. Pharmacokinetic model-driven infusion of fentanyl: assessment of accuracy. Anesthesiology 1990. (Under revision.)

34. Bovill JG, Sebel PS, Blackburn CL, et al. The pharmacokinetics of sufentanil in surgical patients. Anesthesiology 1984;61:502–506.

35. Bovill JG, Sebel PS, Blackburn CL, et al. The pharmacokinetics of alfentanil (R39209): a new opioid analgesic. Anesthesiology 1982;57:439–443.

36. Maitre PO, Vozeh S, Heykants J. Population pharmacokinetics of alfentanil: the average dose–plasma concentration relationship and interindividual variability in patients. Anesthesiology 1987;66:3–12.

37. Ausems ME, Hug CC Jr, Stanski DR, et al. Plasma concentrations of alfentanil required to supplement nitrous oxide anesthesia for general surgery. Anesthesiology 1986;65:362–373.

38. Gourlay GK, Kowalski SR, Plummer JL, et al. Fentanyl blood concentration–analgesic response relationship in the treatment of postoperative pain. Anesth Analg 1988;67:329–337.

39. Sebel PS, Barrett CW, Kirk CJC, et al. Transdermal absorption of fentanyl and sufentanil in man. Eur J Clin Pharmacol 1987;32:529–531.

Chapter 19 Discussion

JOHN H. PETRE: The authors present information regarding the development of an intelligent, user-programmable infusion device to administer by continuous infusion opioids during surgical procedures. Reasons for applying this technique and the benefits realized are summarized.

During the past decade, the efficacy of automated anesthesia delivery systems has been developed and clinically investigated.[1-4] These specially designed systems regulate the administration of inhalation agents using concepts consistent with the theory of closed-loop control.[5-9] Widespread clinical acceptance of these methods did not materialize, primarily because of the complexity of the systems, the lack of consistently accurate feedback control information, and the costs associated with such technically sophisticated devices.

In recent years, the routine use of opioids has gained popularity during surgical procedures, replacing inhalation anesthetics as the primary anesthetizing agent.[10,11] At this time, in conjunction with such changes in practice, it seems appropriate to examine the possibility of developing an automated anesthesia delivery system that could continuously administer opioids.

As the authors demonstrate, improvements in technology have permitted the development of complex delivery instruments. These operator-programmable devices are capable of simplifying complex delivery interactions and minimizing the possibility of inappropriate drug delivery. Coupled with new monitoring approaches, which appear to predict more accurately the state of patient anesthesia, closed-loop control systems for the delivery of opioids may soon become a reality. However, many problems inherent in closed-loop control must first be examined before automated systems can be designed. These include the following:

1. The ability to monitor accurately the state of patient anesthesia during all phases of the surgical procedure
2. The ability to predict patient response characteristics to adjustments in opioid delivery
3. The need to determine the appropriate and most effective mode of control for the feedback system (overdamped, underdamped, a combination, etc.)
4. The need to investigate interactive and outside effects such as those associated with drug interactions and external stimuli
5. The ability to adjust control for patient variability, either individually or among groups (an adaptive control system)

Naturally, the process of commercialization of closed-loop opioid delivery systems will be slow to materialize. Government approval of automated patient-controlled systems has been historically slow, and significant clinical data must be obtained prior to serious FDA consideration. However, despite these obstacles, there is no doubt that in the future, control instruments to deliver opioid infusions will be developed and commercialized.

REFERENCES

1. Smith NT, Quinn ML, Flick J, Fukui Y, Fleming R, Coles JR. Automatic control in anesthesia: a comparison in performance between the anesthetist and the machine. Anesth Analg 1984;63:715–722.

2. Kraft HH, Lees DE. Closing the loop: how near is automated anesthesia? South Med J 1984;77:7–12.

3. Jewett WR. The Arizona program: development of a modular, interactive anesthesia delivery system. Contemp Anesth Pract 1984; 8:185–206.

4. Spain JA, Jannett TC, Ernst EA. The Alabama automated closed-circuit anesthesia project. Contemp Anesth Pract 1984;8:177–183.

5. Zagorchev P, Kirova K, Kozhukharov R. Dynamic control of anesthesiologic protection by automated analysis of cardiac rhythm. Khirurgiia (Sofiia) 1986;39:34–39.

6. Jordan WS, Jaklitch RR, Heining MP. Computer applications in intravenous anaesthetic administration. Int J Clin Monit Comput 1986; 3:269–278.

7. Sugg BR, Palayiwa E, Davies WL, Jackson R, McGraghan T, Shadbolt P, Weller SJ, Hahn CE. An automated interferometer for the analysis of anaesthetic gas mixtures. Br J Anaesth 1988;61:484–491.

8. Lorino AM, Cigarini I, Benichou M, Bonnet F, Lorino H, Harf A. Automated monitoring of respiratory parameters in the anesthetized patient in mechanical respiration. Ann Fr Anesth Reanim 1988;7:479–485.

9. Wallroth CF. Technical conception for an anesthesia system with electronic metering of gases and vapors. Acta Anaesthesiol Belg 1984;35:279–293.

10. Reves JG, Glass P, Jacobs JR. Alfentanil and midazolam: new anesthetic drugs for continuous infusion and an automated method of administration. Mt Sinai J Med (NY) 1989; 56(2):99–107.

11. Alvis JM, Reves JG, Govier AV, Menkhaus PG, Henling CE, Spain JA, Bradley E. Computer-assisted continuous infusions of fentanyl during cardiac anesthesia: comparison with a manual method. Anesthesiology 1985;63(1):41–49.

20 TRANSMUCOSAL NARCOTIC DELIVERY

James B. Streisand and Theodore H. Stanley

The administration of drugs by application to the mucous membranes of the nose and mouth has been practiced by humans for centuries. The widespread use of cocaine confirms the efficacy and potential of the nasal mucous membranes for systemic drug delivery. Murrell,[1] in 1879, and Fantus,[2] in 1926, noted the absorptive power of the mucous membranes under the tongue when nitroglycerin drops were administered for treatment of angina pectoris. At present, a variety of drugs, including isoproterenol, isosorbide dinitrate, ergonovine, testosterone proionate, desmopressin, and oxytocin are administered via the nasal or oral mucous membranes. Unfortunately, until recently, these sites were overlooked as feasible routes for narcotic administration. In the last few years, however, research on alternative routes for drug delivery has been quite active. In addition, new vehicles (i.e., nasal sprays, buccal tablets, lozenges on a handle) are being developed to enable safe, simple, and efficacious transmucosal opioid delivery.

Narcotics have classically been administered parenterally: intravenously (IV), intramuscularly (IM), or subcutaneously (SC). Wide peak and trough plasma concentrations result after intravenous bolus administration of narcotic analgesics, leading to undesired side effects or subtherapeutic action. Erratic absorption from muscle or subcutaneous tissue makes IM and SC routes unreliable for consistent therapeutic action. Furthermore, IM and SC injections are painful, irritating, and unsafe in patients who are anticoagulated or severely thrombocytopenic. Finally, parenteral administration of opioids requires trained personnel for administration and monitoring of drug effect.

While the oral ingestion of drugs overcomes many of the disadvantages of the parenteral route, and is convenient, economical, and generally safe, narcotic analgesics are rarely given orally because their systemic bioavailability is low and erratic. In fact, in cancer patients, the oral bioavailability after a single dose of morphine ranges from 15 to 64%.[3] After oral administration, opioids, which are predominantly organic bases, become ionized in the acid milieu of the stomach and are not readily absorbed through the gastric mucosa. The alkaline pH of the small intestine causes the unionized form to predominate, hastening absorption. Once absorbed, opioids undergo first-pass metabolism in the liver, leaving inactive or less active metabolites. Furthermore, this entire process is slow and erratic because opioids also slow gastrointestinal motility.

Newly developed techniques of transmucosal narcotic delivery combine many of the advantages of both oral and parenteral techniques while eliminating some of the disadvantages. Patients can self-administer buccal tablets, lozenges on a handle (lollipops), or nasal sprays easily and conveniently. The opioid is absorbed directly into the systemic circulation, bypassing the liver, and therefore is more bioavailable than with the oral route. Continuous drug administration, with fewer peaks and valleys in plasma drug concentration, is associated with most transmucosal opioid delivery techniques. Finally, treating pain without injections is not only appealing to children but a practical approach for all patients.

Many transmucosal techniques have applications in anesthesiology. In this chapter, we address these approaches and indicate present and future uses of this new route of drug delivery.

ANATOMY AND PHYSIOLOGY

Unlike the simple columnar epithelium of the gastrointestinal tract, the mucosal surface of the mouth is largely covered by stratified squamous epithelium, similar to that of human skin. Thus, the oral mucosa is not a highly permeable tissue and serves as a barrier to the absorption of potentially dangerous substances.[4] However, absorption through the oral mucosa occurs more readily than through the skin because the mouth is richly supplied with blood and lymphatic vessels and the epidermal lining of the oral mucosa is much thinner than skin.[5] Additionally, the mouth shows less of a depot effect than the skin. In fact, fentanyl can be detected in the blood up to 72 hours following removal of a transdermal fentanyl patch, whereas levels decrease more rapidly and are nondetectable 24 hours after consumption of a fentanyl lozenge.[6,7]

Three sites within the mouth have been characterized for transmucosal drug administration: sublingual, beneath the tongue; buccal, between the gum of the upper molars and the cheek; and gingival, between the gum of the incisors and the upper lip. Although not specifically characterized for opioids, drug permeability is generally highest in the sublingual area and lowest at the gingival site.[4]

Like the mouth, the nasal mucosa is covered with pseudostratified epithelium and is highly vascularized (40 ml/min per 100 grams of tissue);[8] therefore it is suitable for transmucosal drug delivery. However, systemic drug administration via the nasal mucosa is more difficult than via the oral mucosa.[9] Most commonly, drugs are inhaled through the nose as aerosols, drops, or dusts. The inhaled air stream must flow at a high velocity to bypass the anterior area of nose where there exists a constriction known as the nasal valve. Large particles may be deposited anterior to this valve and not be exposed to the area of the nasal mucosa where absorption occurs. Furthermore, insoluble particles are likely to be carried backward by the ciliary stream and dispatched to the stomach. Despite these considerations a myriad of drugs, including sufentanil[10] and butorphenol,[11] can be absorbed systemically through the nose.

DRUG PROPERTIES AND TRANSMUCOSAL PERMEABILITY

Walton, in 1935, pioneered research in oral mucosal permeability, stating that the oil-water solubility coefficient (lipid solubility) was the most important factor in determining whether a drug will pass through biological membranes.[5] Furthermore, he noted that a drug administered in solution will be absorbed to a greater extent than a tablet or powder, as the latter must undergo dissolution in saliva before being directly exposed to the mucosa. Since then, extensive research has been conducted to determine which physiochemical properties are necessary for transmucosal absorption. For a drug to undergo transmucosal absorption, it must possess biphasic solubility, so as first to dissolve in aqueous saliva and then pass through lipoidal membranes. A low molecular weight and a pKa that favors the unionized form also promote mucosal penetration.[5]

Weinberg et al.[12] have recently compared the sublingual absorption of several narcotic analgesics. The opioids that are more lipid-soluble—buprenorphine, fentanyl, and methadone—are absorbed to a significantly greater degree than morphine (Table 20.1, Figure 20.1).[12] Increasing the residence time of the opioid solution in the oral cavity increases the sublingual absorption of fentanyl and methadone but not buprenorphine. As the unionized form of most narcotic analgesics predominates in a basic environment, it is not surprising that increasing the pH of the sublingual solution increases absorption of most narcotics. Even morphine's buccal permeability is raised by increasing the pH of the drug-containing solution (Figure 20.2).[13]

SUBLINGUAL BUPRENORPHINE

Buprenorphine is a long-acting, lipophilic, highly potent mixed opioid agonist-antagonist that is quite suitable for sublingual administration. Because of its high lipophilicity, buprenorphine is well absorbed across biological membranes. Any drug that is accidentally swallowed is effectively cleared and metabo-

TABLE 20.1   The partition coefficient and pKa of selected opioids

Drug	PC	pKa
Morphine	0.00001	7.9
Hydromorphone	0.0001	NA
Levorphanol	0.01	9.4
Heroin	0.04	NA
Fentanyl	19.6	8.4
Methadone	44.6	9.3
Buprenorphine	60.3	NA
Oxycodone	NA	NA
Naloxone	NA	7.9

Source: Reprinted with permission of the publisher from Weinberg D, Inturrisi C, Reidenberg B, et al. Sublingual absorption of selected opioid analgesics. Clin Pharmacol Ther 1988;44:335–342.
PC, partition coefficient; NA, not available.

lized by the liver and does not contribute to drug effect.

Sublingual buprenorphine, though not approved for clinical use in the United States, is utilized in 16 countries.[14] It is established as

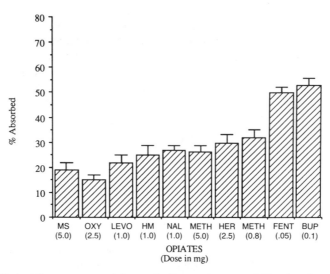

FIGURE 20.1   The mean sublingual absorption (± SE) of selected opioid solutions in normal subjects (MS, morphine sulfate; OXY, oxycodone; LEVO, levorphenol; HM, hydromorphone; NAL, naloxone; METH, methodone; HER, heroin; FENT, fentanyl; BUP, buprenorphine. (Reprinted with permission from Weinberg D, Inturrisi C, Reidenberg B, et al. Sublingual absorption of selected opioid analgesics. Clin Pharmacol Ther 1988;44:335–342.)

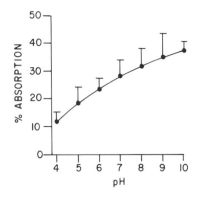

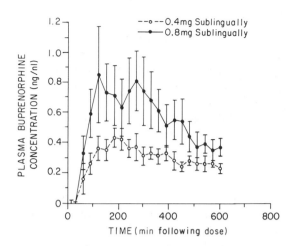

FIGURE 20.2 Mean buccal absorption of morphine sulfate solution in normal volunteers. (Reprinted with permission from Al-Sayed-Omar O, Johnston A, Turner P. Influence of pH on the buccal absorption of morphine sulfate and its major metabolite, morphine-3-glucuronide. J Pharm Pharmacol 1987;39:934–935.)

FIGURE 20.3 Mean buprenorphine plasma concentrations (ng/ml ± SE) following two doses of sublingual buprenorphine. (Reprinted with permission from Bullingham R, McQuay H, Porter E, et al. Sublingual buprenorphine used postoperatively: ten-hour plasma drug concentration analysis. Br J Clin Pharmacol 1982;13:665–673.)

an effective analgesic for treatment of acute postoperative and chronic pain, and is used for premedication and detoxification of narcotic addicts.[15]

Pharmacokinetic Considerations

Clinical analgesic cross-over trials have established sublingual buprenorphine to be 15 times as potent as intramuscular morphine.[16] However, sublingual absorption is slow. Peak buprenorphine plasma concentrations occur approximately 200 minutes after administration (Figure 20.3), but this time varies considerably (range 90 to 360 minutes).[17] Furthermore, there is greater variability in plasma concentrations after sublingual than intramuscular administration.[18] The bioavailability of buprenorphine after sublingual administration is approximately 55% of the dose, more than the bioavailability of any other opioid given sublingually.[17]

Analgesia following a single dose of sublingual buprenorphine, 0.4 mg, lasts approximately 8 hours despite a much shorter plasma terminal elimination half-life (5.2 hours). This unusual finding may be due to buprenorphine's

high affinity with, and very slow dissociation from, the μ and κ opiate receptors.[19] This receptor interaction may also explain the inability of naloxone to easily reverse buprenorphine-induced respiratory depression.[20]

Clinical Experience

Sublingual buprenorphine provides excellent, long-lasting postoperative analgesia with less drowsiness and sedation than comparable doses of intramuscular morphine,[21] meperidine,[22] or buprenorphine.[18,22] In addition, the sublingual route is especially beneficial for children who are sometimes unwilling to accept intramuscular injections of analgesics.[23] Since onset of analgesic action is slow when administered sublingually, clinicians usually give a loading dose of buprenorphine parenterally toward the end of surgery or in the recovery area. Buprenorphine's slow onset of action suggests administration for postoperative pain might best be accomplished on a fixed time schedule.

However, several investigators report excellent analgesia with less sedation and total drug usage when the drug is given on demand.[18,22]

Experience with sublingual buprenorphine for premedication has been mixed. While avoidance of an intramuscular injection is a clear advantage, preoperative anxiolysis and sedation is unreliable.[24,25] Furthermore, hypertension and tachycardia following tracheal intubation and early postoperative respiratory depression is more common after sublingual buprenorphine than after comparable doses of morphine sulfate, or fentanyl administered intramuscularly for premedication.[24,25]

Side effects after sublingual buprenorphine are similar to those of other postoperative analgesics (Table 20.2). Nausea, vomiting, residual sedation, and pruritus lasting 4 to 5 hours are not uncommon after a single dose of sublingual buprenorphine.[26] Several cases of severe respiratory depression, one lasting up to 12.5 hours, is the most alarming side effect reported with sublingual buprenorphine.[20,24]

BUCCAL AND SUBLINGUAL MORPHINE

The need for better methods of morphine administration in cancer patients with chronic pain has stimulated interest in delivering morphine through the oral mucosa. Buccal and sublingual morphine are useful when oral morphine is impractical (patients with nausea and vomiting, a bowel obstruction, or difficulty swallowing) and parenteral injections are difficult and painful (patients with bleeding disorders, inaccessible veins, or muscle wasting).

No special formulations for sublingual (sub) or buccal (buc) morphine have been developed by pharmaceutical companies. Therefore, clinicians use either a tablet (sub) and (buc) or solution (sub) for transmucosal morphine administration.

Pharmacokinetic Considerations

Controversy exists over the systemic bioavailability of morphine when it is administered through the buccal or sublingual mucosal membranes. Representative studies of transmucosal morphine absorption are listed in Table 20.3. The initial studies of Bardgett et al.[27] and Bell et al.[28] found the bioavailability of buccal morphine to be high and slightly greater than that found with the intramuscular route (Figure 20.4). Furthermore, peak plasma concentrations occurred within an hour after administration. Rapid absorption after sublingual

TABLE 20.2 Side effects after intramuscular meperidine, sublingual buprenorphine, or intramuscular buprenorphine when given for postoperative analgesia

	Intramuscular Meperidine (n = 18)	Sublingual Buprenorphine (n = 18)	Intramuscular Buprenorphine (n = 18)
Sedation	12 (66%)	9 (53%)	13 (72%)
Sweating	2 (11%)	1 (6%)	1 (6%)
Nausea	11 (61%)[a]	9 (53%)	6 (33%)[a]
Vomiting	2 (11%)	2 (11%)	2 (11%)
Headache	1 (6%)	3 (18%)	0 (0%)
Dizziness	1 (6%)	2 (11%)	0 (0%)
Urinary retention	1 (6%)	0 (0%)	0 (0%)
Total number with side effects	17 (94%)[a]	13 (72%)	13 (72%)

Source: Reprinted with permission of the publisher from Carl P, Crawford M, Madsen N, et al. Pain relief after major abdominal surgery: a double-blind controlled comparison of sublingual buprenorphine, intramuscular buprenorphine, and intramuscular meperidine. Anesth Analg 1987;66: 142–146.
[a]$p < 0.05$.

TABLE 20.3   Bioavailability of transmucosal morphine

Route of Administration	Dose (mg)	C_{max} (ng/ml)	T_{max} (min)	AUC (ng/min/ml)	Reference No.
Buccal (tab)	10	36.0–61.0	60	15,800	27
Buccal (tab)	10	36.0	60	14,800	28
Buccal (tab)	20	9.1	408	1,615	
Buccal (tab)	25	10.8	284	2,156	43
Buccal (tab)	10	2.5	360	996	30
Sublingual (tab)	15	5.0	30	22% of IM route	12
Sublingual (solution)	10	70.0	3	NA	29
Tracheal mucosa (aerosolized)	10	11.8	46	1,480	44
Intramuscular (for comparison)	10	44.0	60	10,000	28

C_{max}, maximum plasma concentration; T_{max}, time to maximum plasma concentration; AUC, area under the plasma concentration versus time curve; IM, intramuscular; NA, not available.

administration of a morphine solution was also detected by Pannuti et al.[29] The rapid attainment of peak plasma concentrations and high systemic bioavailability present convincing evidence for effective transmucosal absorption.

Unfortunately, studies by Fisher et al.[30] and Hoskin et al.[31] report remarkably conflicting data (Table 20.3). Morphine's bioavailability and peak plasma concentration after a 25-mg (Fisher) or 10-mg (Hoskin) buccal tablet were markedly lower than after a 10-mg intramus-

cular injection (Figure 20.5). Similarly, low bioavailability after sublingual administration was reported by Weinberg et al.[12]

Perhaps moistening the buccal tablet (as Bell did but others did not) to accomplish better adherence and solubilization at the mucosa is important for transmucosal morphine absorption. However, morphine's low lipid solubility, as compared to buprenorphine, fentanyl, and methadone, make it a poor choice for transmucosal absorption.[12]

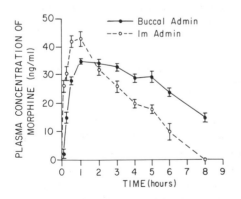

FIGURE 20.4   Plasma concentrations of morphine after intramuscular and buccal administration. (Reprinted with permission from Bell M, Mishra P, Weldon B, et al. Buccal morphine—a new route for analgesia? Lancet 1985; 1:71–73.)

Clinical Experience

Several anecdotal reports suggest that sublingual morphine may play a useful role in controlling chronic cancer pain.[29,32–34] One group believes that a tablet placed under the tongue causes less swallowing and greater bioavailability than a morphine solution.[32] Others feel that the slow administration of drops of a morphine solution will lead to better absorption.[29,34] Irrespective of the formulation administered, many patients complain of morphine's bitter taste when it is given sublingually.[32–34]

Buccal morphine has been used for preoperative sedation and anxiolysis, acute postoperative analgesia, and longer-lasting pain relief

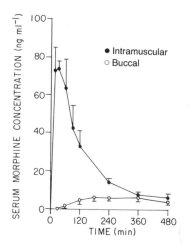

FIGURE 20.5 Change in serum morphine concentration (mean ± SEM) with time after administration of 10 mg intramuscular morphine to surgical patients (•, n = 5) and 25 mg buccal morphine to healthy subjects (○, n = 11). (Reprinted with permission from Fisher A, Fung C, Hanna M. Serum morphine concentrations after buccal and intramuscular morphine administration. Br J Clin Pharmacol 1987;24:685–687.)

in patients with chronic cancer pain.[28,35,36] While most patients find the buccal tablet acceptable, more reliable reductions in anxiety and wakefulness before operation are achieved with intramuscular morphine.[36] When given for postoperative pain, intramuscular morphine provides better pain relief than the buccal route during the first 4 hours after administration, but analgesia lasts longer with buccal morphine.[28]

While initial studies generally employed the sublingual route, the buccal site may ultimately prove superior for transmucosal morphine administration. Enhanced saliva production from the bitter taste of the sublingual tablet causes increased swallowing with drug loss down the esophagus and decreased bioavailability. In addition, since dissolution is more rapid sublingually, the buccal site has gained popularity for long-term therapy.

NASAL SUFENTANIL

The nasal administration of sufentanil has been recently investigated as a preoperative sedative in both children and adults (Table 20.4).[10,37] Sixty children, 6 months to 7 years of age, were given 1.5 to 4.5 μg/kg of undiluted sufentanil nasally over 15 to 20 seconds and compared to 20 children given a saline placebo. Although 61% of the children cried during administration of the nose drops, rapid onset of sedation and anxiolysis was demonstrated by the willing separation from parents in over half the children receiving sufentanil in 4 minutes, and 86% in 10 minutes. Furthermore, children who received nasal sufentanil coughed or moved less frequently during tracheal intubation, needed less intraoperative halothane and postoperative analgesics, and had smoother recoveries than those receiving placebo premedication. Reduced ventilatory compliance (chest wall rigidity) was noted with the higher doses of sufentanil (3 and 4.5 μg/kg), and three children required naloxone at the end of the operation. Nevertheless, this approach may be valuable especially for the frightened or uncooperative child. Vercauteren et al.[37] found that only 10 to 20 μg of nasal sufentanil induced moderate sedation in 79% of adults receiving the premedication. Further clinical experience and pharmacokinetic analysis are needed to establish optimal dosing regimens for nasal sufentanil.

ORAL TRANSMUCOSAL FENTANYL CITRATE (OTFC)

Oral transmucosal fentanyl citrate (OTFC) is a new delivery system for transmucosal fentanyl administration. It consists of a fentanyl-impregnated, bullet-shaped candy lozenge on a handle, sometimes called a lollipop. Patients suck on the lozenge and fentanyl is rapidly released to the oral mucosa for absorption. As onset of action is rapid (15 minutes),[38] the patient or clinician is able to regulate delivery by stopping consumption of OTFC slightly before the desired effect is reached. The optimal

TABLE 20.4   Characteristics of patients receiving nasal sufentanil

		Sufentanil (mg/kg)		
	Placebo (n = 19)	1.5 (n = 20)	3.0 (n = 21)	4.5 (n = 20)
Willing to separate from parents				
At 4 minutes	21[a]	40	57	55
At or before 10 minutes	53[a]	85	86	75
Calm at time of separation from parents	47[a]	85	85	75
Accepts face mask	11	25	29	30
Ventilatory compliance (assessed subjectively)				
Mildly decreased	0[a]	45	52	25
Markedly decreased	0[a]	0	5	25
Airway complication after tracheal extubation				
Laryngospasm	0	5	0	0
Need for airway support	11	15	5	0
Croup	0	0	5	0
Vomiting in PARR[c]	33	25	10	50[b]
Crying in PARR	90[a]	55	38	20
Analgesics in PARR	74[a]	35	19	5
Vomiting after release from PARR[c]	42	25	25	68[b]
Normal appetite one day following surgery[d]	61[a]	77	95	84

Source: Reprinted with permission of the publisher of Henderson J, Brodsky D, Fisher D, et al. Nasally administered sufentanil in children. Anesthesiology 1988;68:671–675.

Data reported as percent. PARR, postanesthesia recovery room.

[a]Different from sufentanil (all doses combined) by chi-square analysis or Fisher's exact test ($p < 0.05$).
[b]Different from other doses of sufentanil by chi-square analysis ($p < 0.05$).
[c]Excludes patients with nasogastric tubes.
[d]Excludes patients who were not by mouth.

dosage range for premedication before operation in children is 15 to 20 μg/kg.[39] OTFC is
currently undergoing clinical trials in the United
States.

Pharmacokinetic Considerations

The 24-hour plasma fentanyl concentration
versus time curve following 15 μg/kg of OTFC
in adult volunteers is shown in Figure 20.6.[7]
Fentanyl absorption through the oral mucosa
is rapid. The maximal rate of fentanyl absorption into the systemic circulation is 12.5 μg/
min, occurring 17 minutes after beginning consumption. This results in peak fentanyl plasma
concentrations that range from 1.4 to 3.8 ng/
ml (mean maximum concentration = 2.5 ng/
ml) 25 minutes after OTFC administration.
While plasma concentrations decrease rapidly,

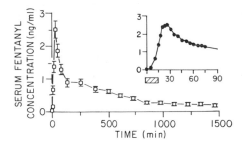

FIGURE 20.6 Serum fentanyl concentrations after oral transmucosal fentanyl citrate
(OTFC) administration (mean ± SEM). The
inset shows the first 90 minutes in detail. The
cross-hatched bar beneath the inset shows
the OTFC consumption time. (Reprinted with
permission from Streisand J, Ashburn M,
LeMaire L, et al. Bioavailability and absorption
of oral transmucosal fentanyl citrate. Anesthesiology 1989;71:A230.)

detectable fentanyl remains in the plasma for as long as 24 hours. The elimination half-life of OTFC is 7.1 hours. It appears as if the pharmacokinetic profile seen after OTFC results from a combination of rapid transmucosal absorption followed by a slower uptake of fentanyl from a depot in the oral mucosa and from slower, hepatically cleared, gastrointestinal absorption.

The systemic bioavailability of OTFC, 49.7%, is similar to sublingual buprenorphine and greater than buccal morphine (18%). This provides further evidence for the importance of lipid solubility in transmucosal absorption, as both fentanyl and buprenorphine have significantly greater lipid solubilities than morphine.[12]

Clinical Experience

Initial clinical trials with OTFC have been targeted toward the pediatric population because of the need for less painful and less frightening methods of narcotic administration in children. Children receiving OTFC for premedication 45 to 60 minutes before surgery are rapidly sedated and show reduced anxiety within 30 minutes. They require less potent inhalation anesthesia during operation and less pain medication in the recovery room.[7,38,40,41] Despite narcotic premedication, recovery times are not prolonged,[7,41] although discharge from the hospital following outpatient surgery may be slightly delayed compared to children who receive no premedication.[40] OTFC produces small, clinically insignificant decreases in respiratory rate and oxygen saturation.

Risk of aspiration is a legitimate concern over the use of OTFC as a premedication. Gastric volume and pH measurements made subsequent to OTFC administration, just after induction of anesthesia, reveal an increase in gastric volume but no change in pH when compared to no premedication (Table 20.5).[38] The percentage of safe (gastric volume < 0.4 ml/kg and pH > 2.5) cases is no different whether children receive OTFC, a placebo lollipop, or no premedication. There are no reports of the aspiration of stomach contents with OTFC administration in over 500 patients.

In addition to being used as a premedication, OTFC is being used in children with leukemia to provide analgesia for lumbar punctures and bone marrow biopsies (no general anesthesia is given for these procedures). It is undergoing clinical trials for use in the emergency room.

Aside from the obvious appeal of OTFC for children, adults may also benefit from this delivery system. Ashburn et al.[42] reported the self-administration of OTFC, on an ambulatory basis, to provide analgesia for breakthrough cancer pain. The utilization of OTFC for breakthrough cancer pain, as well as acute postoperative pain, is currently undergoing clinical investigation.

TABLE 20.5   Gastric volume and pH after oral transmucosal fentanyl citrate (OTFC) premedication

	No Premed	OTFC	Placebo Lozenge
Gastric volume (ml)	7.6 ± 5.3	14.6 ± 10.0[a]	15.6 ± 13.5
Gastric pH	1.69 ± 0.31	1.92 ± 0.53	1.72 ± 0.28

Source: Reprinted with permission of the publisher from Stanley T, Hague B, Mock D, et al. Oral transmucosal fentanyl citrate (lollipop) premedication in human volunteers. Anesth Analg 1989;69: 21–27.

[a]$p < 0.05$ when compared to No premed.

CONCLUSION

Narcotic analgesics are now being administered transmucosally for many different clinical applications. The unique physiology and pharmcokinetic profiles behind transmucosal drug delivery permit reliable drug action previously available only with parenterally administered opioids. Some of these new techniques increase the armamentarium of clinicians who treat acute and chronic pain. As our knowledge of transmucosal absorption increases, new drugs and delivery systems may be specifically developed for utilization of this exciting route of drug delivery.

REFERENCES

1. Murrell W. Nitroglycerine as a remedy for angina pectoris. Lancet 1879;1:234–236, 284–288.
2. Fantus B. The technic of medication. JAMA 1926;86:687–689.
3. Sawe J, Dahlstrom B, Paalzow L, et al. Morphine kinetics in cancer patients. Clin Pharmacol Ther 1981;30:629–635.
4. Squier C, Johnson N. Permeability of oral mucosa. Br Med Bull 1975;31:1969–1975.
5. Gibaldi M, Kanig J. Absorption of drugs through the oral mucosa. J Oral Ther Pharmacol 1965;1:440–450.
6. Varvel J, Shafer S, Hwang S, et al. Absorption characteristics of transdermally administered fentanyl. Anesthesiology 1989;70:928–934.
7. Streisand J, Ashburn M, LeMaire L, et al. Bioavailability and absorption of oral transmucosal fentanyl citrate. Anesthesiology 1989;71:A230.
8. Chien Y, Chang S. Intranasal drug delivery for systemic medications. CRC Crit Rev Ther Drug Carr Syst 1987;4(2):67–194.
9. Brain J, Valberg P. Deposition of aerosol in the respiratory tract. Am Rev Respir Dis 1979;120:1325–1373.
10. Henderson J, Brodsky D, Fisher D, et al. Nasally administered sufentanil in children. Anesthesiology 1988;68:671–675.
11. Abboud T, Zhu J, Gangolly J, et al. Transnasal analgesics: a new method for pain relief in post-cesarean section patients. Anesthesiology 1988;69:A657.
12. Weinberg D, Inturrisi C, Reidenberg B, et al. Sublingual absorption of selected opioid analgesics. Clin Pharmacol Ther 1988;44:335–342.
13. Al-Sayed-Omar O, Johnston A, Turner P. Influence of pH on the buccal absorption of morphine sulfate and its major metabolite, morphine-3-glucuronide. J Pharm Pharmacol 1987;39:934–935.
14. Lewis J. Buprenorphine. Drug Alcohol Depend 1985;14:363–372.
15. Bickel W, Stitzer M, Bigelow G, et al. A clinical trial of buprenorphine: comparison with methadone in the detoxification of heroin addicts. Clin Pharmacol Ther 1988;43:72–78.
16. Wallenstein S, Kaiko R, Rogers A, et al. Crossover trials in clinical analgesic assays: studies of buprenorphine and morphine. Pharmacotherapy 1986;6:228–235.
17. Bullingham R, McQuay H, Porter E, et al. Sublingual buprenorphine used postoperatively: ten-hour plasma drug concentration analysis. Br J Clin Pharmcol 1982;13:665–673.
18. Shah M, Jones D, Rosen M. "Patient demand" postoperative analgesia with buprenorphine: comparison between sublingual and i.m. administration. Br J Anaesth 1986;58:508–511.
19. Boas R, Villiger J. Clinical actions of fentanyl and buprenorphine: the significance of receptor binding. Br J Anaesth 1985;57:192–196.
20. Thorn S, Rawal N, Wennhager M. Prolonged respiratory depression caused by sublingual buprenorphine. Lancet 1988;1:179–180.
21. Cuschieri R, Morran C, McArdle C. Comparison of morphine and sublingual buprenorphine following abdominal surgery. Br J Anaesth 1984;56:855–859.
22. Carl P, Crawford M, Madsen N, et al. Pain relief after major abdominal surgery: a double-blind controlled comparison of sublingual buprenorphine, intramuscular buprenorphine, and intramuscular meperidine. Anesth Analg 1987;66:142–146.
23. Maunuksela E, Korpela R, Olkkola K. Comparison of buprenorphine with morphine in the treatment of postoperative pain in children. Anesth Analg 1988;67:233–239.
24. Korttila K, Hovorka J. Buprenorphine as premedication and as analgesic during and after light isoflurane-N_2O-O_2 anaesthesia: a comparison with oxycodone plus fentanyl. Acta Anaesthesiol Scand 1987;31:673–679.

25. O'Sullivan G, Bullingham R, McQuay H, et al. A comparison of intramuscular and sublingual buprenorphine, intramuscular morphine, and placebo as premedication. Anaesthesia 1983;38:977–984.

26. Woodham M. Pruritus with sublingual buprenorphine. Anaesthesia 1988;43(9):806–807. [Letter]

27. Bardgett D, Howard C, Murray G, et al. Plasma concentration of a buccal preparation of morphine sulfate. Br J Clin Pharmacol 1984;17:198P–199P.

28. Bell M, Mishra P, Weldon B, et al. Buccal morphine—a new route for analgesia? Lancet 1985;1:71–73.

29. Pannuti F, Rossi A, Iafelice G, et al. Control of chronic pain in very advanced cancer patients with morphine hydrochloride administered by oral, rectal, and sublingual route: clinical report and preliminary results on morphine pharmacokinetics. Pharmacol Res Commun 1982;14(4):369–380.

30. Fisher A, Fung C, Hanna M. Serum morphine concentrations after buccal and intramuscular morphine administration. Br J Clin Pharmacol 1987;24:685–687.

31. Hoskin P, Hanks G, Aherne G, et al. The bioavailability and pharmacokinetics of morphine after intravenous, oral, and buccal administration in healthy volunteers. Br J Clin Pharmacol 1989;27:499–505.

32. Pitorak E, Kraus J. Pain control with sublingual morphine: the advantages for hospice care. Am J Hospice Care 1987;4(2):39–41.

33. Hirsch J. Sublingual morphine sulfate in chronic pain management. Clin Pharm 1984;3:585–586.

34. Whitman H. Sublingual morphine: a novel route of narcotic administration. Am J Nurs 1984;84:939–940.

35. Enck R. Mucosal membranes as alternative routes for morphine sulfate administration. Am J Hospice Care 1988;5(4):17–18.

36. Fisher A, Vine P, Whitlock J, et al. Buccal morphine premedication. Anaesthesia 1986;41:1104–1111.

37. Vercauteren M, Boeck E, Hanegreefs G, et al. Intranasal sufentanil for preoperative sedation. Anaesthesia 1988;43:270–273.

38. Stanley T, Hague B, Mock D, et al. Oral transmucosal fentanyl citrate (lollipop) premedication in human volunteers. Anesth Analg 1989;69:21–27.

39. Streisand J, Stanley T, Hague B, et al. Oral transmucosal fentanyl citrate premedication in children. Anesth Analg 1989;69:28–34.

40. Ashburn M, Stephen R, Petelenz T, et al. Controlled iontophoretic delivery of morphine HCl for postoperative pain relief. Anesthesiology 1988;69:A348.

41. Nelson P, Streisand J, Mulder S, et al. Comparison of oral transmucosal fentanyl citrate and an oral solution of meperidine, diazepam, and atropine for premedication in children. Anesthesiology 1989;70:616–621.

42. Ashburn M, Fine P, Stanley T. Oral transmucosal fentanyl citrate for the treatment of breakthrough cancer pain: a case report. Anesthesiology 1989;71:615–617.

43. Fisher A, Fung C, Hanna M. Absorption of buccal morphine: a comparison with slow-release morphine. Anaesthesia 1988;43:552–553.

44. Chrubasik J, Wüst H, Friedrich G, et al. Absorption and bioavailability of nebulized morphine. Br J Anaesth 1988;61:228–230.

21 TRANSDERMAL FENTANYL: AN OVERVIEW OF CLINICAL PROGRESS

Robert A. Caplan and Mary Southam

HISTORICAL PERSPECTIVE

The newest therapies in medicine often have roots in antiquity. This is the case for transdermal narcotic delivery. In the first century BC, the Greek physician Dioscorides of Anazarba described a crushed preparation of opium seeds which was applied to forehead of patients suffering from headache.[1] Based upon our current understanding of skin permeability, we can safely conclude that the benefits of this concoction were largely due to a placebo effect.

The rigorous study of skin permeability is a relatively new activity that was pioneered by Scheuplein[2] in the 1960s. Scheuplein and his coworkers developed experimental techniques that led to the first quantitative understanding of skin as a portal for systemic drug entry. Several key findings emerged. First, drug movement through skin was measured and found consistent with a model of passive diffusion. Second, the outermost layer of skin, or stratum corneum, was convincingly identified as the primary barrier to chemical diffusion. Third, the bulk of drug permeation appeared to take place in and around skin cells, not through dermal appendages such as pores and hair shafts.

A more refined model of drug permeation was developed by Michaels et al.[3] This model incorporated the concept that the stratum corneum is an organized array of interstitial lipids and proteinaceous cells, and that drug transit must therefore require repeated and serial penetration of two distinctly different media. An important outgrowth of this work was the definition of a set of general requirements that candidates for transdermal drug delivery should possess. First, a drug must have physiochemical properties that optimize solubility in the lipid and protein phases of the skin. A relatively small molecular weight ($< 1,000$) is an important aspect of this first requirement. Second, a drug must be potent enough to allow a therapeutic dose to pass through a convenient area of skin. In practical terms, passive transdermal delivery may be feasible if the daily drug requirement is below 2 mg. (Drugs of lesser potency might require extensive and esthetically unappealing skin coverage to achieve adequate dosage.) Finally, the skin itself must be able to tolerate long-term contact with the drug. This last feature can create a frustrating roadblock for otherwise suitable pharmaceuticals.

WHY CHOOSE THE TRANSDERMAL ROUTE?

The unbroken skin offers a number of distinct advantages as a portal for systemic drug delivery. Drugs that are delivered directly through the skin are not subject to gastrointestinal variables such as first-pass hepatic metabolism, unreliable gut absorption, and the inability or unwillingness of the patient to swallow oral medications. Transdermal drug delivery also avoids the discomfort of intramuscular injections and the complexity of sophisticated intravenous infusion devices. These features are particularly attractive in settings that require repeated or prolonged administration of drugs by parenteral routes.

Transdermal delivery offers two important advantages that arise directly from the use of rate-controlling membranes. Rate control is an integral part of most transdermal systems because skin permeability is subject to considerable variation. The presence of a rate-controlling membrane assures predictable delivery by releasing drug more slowly than the skin can absorb it.

The first direct advantage of rate-controlled delivery is that wide variations in serum levels can be minimized, thereby reducing the amount of time that the patient is exposed to serum levels above or below the therapeutic range. In this way, rate-controlling membranes offer an opportunity to select specific, concentration-dependent roles for a given drug. Transdermal scopolamine provides an excellent illustration of this concept. Rate-controlled delivery of scopolamine results in low serum drug levels, which are effective in the treatment of motion sickness, while avoiding higher serum levels, which can lead to excessive drowsiness, tachycardia, or dryness of the mouth.

The second advantage of rate-controlled delivery is the ability to select and maintain a desired serum drug level for an extended period of time. This offers convenience for the patient and the potential for increased compliance with long-term medications. A good example is the antihypertensive agent, clonidine. Oral clonindine is usually administered once or twice each day, whereas transdermal clonidine requires only one application each week. The combination of a rate-controlling membrane and a drug reservoir also offers an opportunity to utilize ultrapotent or short-acting drugs that might otherwise be difficult to manage with conventional delivery systems.

THE CONCEPTUAL BASIS FOR TRANSDERMAL FENTANYL

Inadequacies in pain management have been well recognized for the past two decades.[4-10] Two sources of descriptive evidence helped focus the clinical appreciation of this problem. Once source of evidence was provided by Marks and Sachar,[4] who studied the approaches that physicians adopt in the treatment of pain. These investigators discovered a pervasive pattern of narcotic underdosage, mostly attributable to misconceptions about duration of action and inappropriate fears about addiction. Another important source of evidence emerged from Bonica's inquiries into cancer-related pain.[10] His efforts provided the first clear understanding that inadequately treated cancer pain is a major worldwide health problem.

In parallel with these descriptive findings, important advances took place in the clinical pharmacology of narcotics. Intramuscular injections of narcotics were found to produce up to fivefold variations in peak serum levels.[11-13] Austin and colleagues[14] provided a rigorous demonstration that fluctuating serum levels can be linked to variable pain control in surgical patients. As a logical outgrowth of these studies, interest turned to continuous intravenous infusion as a method for attaining more reliable narcotic levels. This direction proved fruitful. By the mid-1980s, a number of groups had demonstrated that continuous narcotic infusion produced safe and effective analgesia.[15-19] In the context of these clinical and pharmacologic findings, the investigation of transdermal narcotic delivery became especially attractive. Specifically, if a narcotic could be administered by the transdermal route, this would offer an opportunity to provide continuous opioid analgesia without the discomfort, variability, or complexity of other delivery systems.

THE STRUCTURAL COMPONENTS OF TRANSDERMAL FENTANYL

A transdermal delivery system for fentanyl has been developed by ALZA Corporation (Palo Alto, Calif.). This system is a stacked array of five basic components. The outermost layer is a protective backing. The next layer is a concentrated reservoir of fentanyl, which provides the driving force for passive diffusion and a source for sustained delivery. Beneath the reservoir is a rate-controlling element, which regulates the release of fentanyl from the reservoir. This element releases drug from the reservoir at a rate that is less than the average skin flux, thereby ensuring that the transdermal system—not the skin—plays the controlling role in fentanyl delivery. A contact adhesive forms the next layer. After removal of a protective liner, the adhesive is placed in direct contact with the skin. To facilitate release of drug into the skin directly beneath the transdermal system, the contact adhesive contains a priming dose of fentanyl.

Transdermal fentanyl systems are approximately 0.5 mm in thickness and are designed to deliver drug at rates of 25, 50, 75, or 100 µg/hr. To achieve delivery rates in excess of 100 µg/hr, multiple systems can be used simultaneously.

CLINICAL EXPERIENCE

Most studies of transdermal fentanyl have been performed in postoperative patients who have undergone abdominal, orthopedic, or thoracic surgery.[20-35] In these settings, effective postoperative analgesia has been obtained with transdermal systems rated to delivery fentanyl

at 75 or 100 µg/hr. Application times in postoperative patients have ranged from 24 to 72 hours.

Pharmacokinetic analysis indicates that the transdermal fentanyl system releases drug in a predictable and consistent manner.[23,33,36,37] There is no evidence for first-pass metabolism or degradation of fentanyl in the skin.[33] Varvel et al.[33] found that fentanyl blood levels reach a plateau after an application period of 12 to 24 hours. Relatively constant levels are achieved earlier when fentanyl is used intraoperatively.[31] Larajani and coworkers[31] suggest that a single transdermal fentanyl system can function effectively for up to 3 days.

Serum levels produced by transdermal fentanyl systems are comparable to those produced by intravenous infusion,[29,30] although levels rise more slowly with transdermal delivery. The absorption of fentanyl into the skin and then into the systemic circulation contributes to the slow initial rise in serum levels.[23,37] When systems rated to deliver fentanyl at 75 or 100 µg/hr are used, serum fentanyl levels of 1 ng/ml are usually attained by 6 to 12 hours. After removal of the transdermal system, continued absorption from the skin depot contributes to the slow elimination of drug from the body.

Caplan et al.[35] recently conducted a double-blind, placebo-controlled, randomized study of the safety and efficacy of transdermal fentanyl in 42 adult patients undergoing major shoulder surgery with regional anesthesia. This population was chosen to provide a relatively uniform pain stimulus and to avoid the potentially confounding effects of general anesthetics on pain, pain reporting, and side effects. Just prior to administration of regional anesthesia with interscalene block, patients in the active group received a transdermal system rated to deliver fentanyl at 75 µg/hr, while patients in the placebo group received an identical-appearing placebo. The transdermal systems were worn for a total of 24 hours. Intramuscular morphine (5 mg every 2 hours as needed) was available to both groups for supplemental pain control. Morphine requirement was used as the main outcome variable to test efficacy.

REFERENCES

1. Gunther RT. The Greek herbal of Dioscorides. Oxford: Oxford University Press, 1934; 458.
2. Scheuplein RJ, Blank IH. Permeability of the skin. Physiol Rev 1971;51:702–747.
3. Michaels AS, Chandrasekaran SK, Shaw JE. Drug permeation through human skin: theory and in vitro experimental measurement. Am Inst Chem Eng J 1975;21:985–996.
4. Marks RM, Sachar EJ. Undertreatment of medical patients with narcotic analgesics. Ann Intern Med 1973;78:173–181.
5. McCaffrey M, Hart LL. Undertreatment of acute pain with narcotics. Am J Nurs 1976; 76:1586–1591.
6. Utting JE, Smith JM. Postoperative analgesia. Anaesthesia 1979;34:320–332.
7. Cohen FL. Postsurgical pain relief: patients' status and nurses' medication choices. Pain 1980;9:265–274.
8. Mather LE, Mackie J. The incidence of postoperative pain in children. Pain 1983;15:271–282.
9. Donovan M, Dillon P, McGuire L. Incidence and characteristics of pain in a sample of medical-surgical patients. Pain 1987;30:69–78.
10. Cousins MJ. Introduction to acute and chronic pain: implications for neural blockade. In: Cousins MJ, Bridenbaugh PO, eds. Neural blockade in clinical anesthesia and management of pain. 2d ed. Philadelphia: Lippincott, 1988;739–752.
11. Rigg JRA, Browne RA, Davis C, et al. Variation in the disposition of morphine after intramuscular administration in the surgical patient. Br J Anaesth 1978;50:1125–1130.
12. Mather LE, Lindop MJ, Tucker GT, Pflug AE. Pethidine revisited: plasma concentrations and effects after intramuscular injection. Br J Anaesth 1975;47:1269–1275.
13. Stanski DR, Greenblat DJ, Lowenstein E. Kinetics of intravenous and intramuscular morphine. Clin Pharmacol Ther 1978;24:52–59.
14. Austin KL, Stapelton JV, Mather LE. Relationship between blood meperidine concentrations and analgesic response. Anesthesiology 1980;53:460–466.
15. Stapelton JV, Austin KL, Mather LE. A pharmacokinetic approach to postoperative pain: continuous infusion of pethidine. Anaesth Intensive Care 1979;7:25–32.
16. Rutter PC, Murphy F, Dudley HAF. Morphine: controlled trial of different methods of administration for postoperative pain relief. Br Med J 1980;1:12–13.
17. Nimmo WS, Todd JG. Fentanyl by constant rate IV infusion for postoperative analgesia. Br J Anaesth 1985;50:250–254.
18. Duthie DJR, McLaren AD, Nimmo WS. The pharmacokinetics of fentanyl during constant rate IV infusion for the relief of pain after surgery. Br J Anaesth 1986;58:950–956.
19. Mather LE, Gourlay GK. Rate-controlled intravenous administration of analgesics. In: Prescott LF, Nimmo WS, eds. Rate control in drug therapy. New York: Churchill Livingstone, 1985;220–231.
20. Caplan RA, Ready LB, Olsson GL, et al. Transdermal delivery of fentanyl for postoperative pain control. Anesthesiology 1986;65: A196.
21. Holley FO, van Steennis C. Transdermal fentanyl administration of fentanyl for postoperative analgesia. Anesthesiology 1986;65:A548.
22. Nimmo WS, Duthie DJR. Plasma fentanyl concentrations after transdermal or IV infusion of fentanyl. Anesthesiology 1986;65:A559.
23. Plezia PM, Kramer TH, Linford J, et al. Transdermal fentanyl: pharmacokinetics and preliminary clinical evaluation. Pharmacotherapy 1989;9:2–9.
24. Gourlay GK, Kowalski SR, Plummer JL, et al. The transdermal administration of fentanyl in the treatment of postoperative pain: pharmacokinetics and pharmacodynamic effects. Pain 1989;37:193–202.
25. Kramer TH, Plezia PM, Linford J, et al. Pharmacokinetics of transdermally administered fentanyl. Clin Pharmacol Ther 1987;41:181.
26. Oden RV, Caplan RA, Ready LB. Effect on ventilation of transdermal fentanyl compared to intramuscular morphine for postoperative analgesia following upper extremity orthopedic surgery. Pain 1987;4(suppl):S156.
27. Bell SD, Larijani GE, Goldberg ME, et al. Evaluation of transdermal fentanyl for multi-day analgesia in postoperative patients. Anesthesiology 1988;69:A362.
28. Bormann B, Ratthey K, Schwetlick G, et al. Postoperative schmerztherapie durch transdermales fentanyl. Anasth Intensivther Notfallmed 1988;23:3–8.
29. Duthie DJR, Rowbotham DJ, Wyld R, et al. Plasma fentanyl concentrations during trans-

dermal delivery of fentanyl to surgical patients. Br J Anaesth 1988;60:614–618.

30. Holley FO, van Steennis CV. Postoperative analgesia with fentanyl: pharmacokinetics and pharmacodynamics of constant-rate IV and transdermal delivery. Br J Anaesth 1988;60:608–613.

31. Larijani GE, Bell SD, Goldberg ME, et al. Pharmacokinetics of fentanyl following transdermal application. Anesthesiology 1988;69:A363.

32. Plezia PM, Linford J, Kramer TH, et al. Transdermally delivered fentanyl for postoperative pain: a randomized, double-blind, placebo controlled trial. Anesthesiology 1988;69:A364.

33. Varvel JR, Shafer SL, Hwang S, et al. Absorption characteristics of transdermally administered fentanyl. Anesthesiology 1989;70:928–934.

34. Bell SD, Goldberg ME, Larijani GE, et al. Evaluation of transdermal fentanyl for multiday analgesia in postoperative patients. Anesth Analg (Cleve) 1989;68:S22.

35. Caplan RA, Ready LB, Oden RV, et al. Transdermal fentanyl for postoperative pain management: a double-blind placebo study. JAMA 1989;261:1036–1039.

36. Gale RM, Osborne J, Goetz V. In vitro functionality of transdermal therapeutic system (fentanyl). Pharmacol Res 1987;4(suppl):S70.

37. Prather R, Hwang S. Pharmacokinetics of transdermal (TTS) fentanyl in surgical patients. Pharmacol Res 1987;4(suppl):S103.

38. Levy S, Jacobs S, Johnson J, et al. Transdermal fentanyl: pain and quality-of-life effects. Proc Am Soc Clin Oncol 1988;7:292.

39. Simmonds MA, Blain C, Richenbacher J, Southam MA. A new approach to the administration of opiates: TTS (fentanyl) in the management of pain in patients with cancer. J Pain Sympt Man 1988;3:S18.

patient-controlled analgesia devices consisted of electronically controlled infusion pumps connected to timing devices. When patients experienced pain, they would trigger the device by depressing a thumb button located on the end of a cord extending from the machine. The machine then delivered a preset amount of analgesic drug into the patient's indwelling IV catheter. The timer was programmed to preclude administration of additional (supplemental) doses until a specific time period had elapsed (the so-called lockout or delay interval). The purpose of the lockout interval was to prevent the patient from administering a second dose until after the first dose had had time to exert its maximal (peak) pharmacological effect.

Increased concern about inadequacies in the conventional approaches to managing acute postoperative pain has led to renewed interest in the concept of PCA.[5] With an on-demand system for managing postoperative pain, the patient is allowed to self-administer narcotic analgesic medication using a programmable infusion pump, thereby minimizing the effects of pharmacokinetic and pharmacodynamic variability of response to the analgesic medication. Recent advances in infusion pump technology make it possible to safely administer small IV bolus doses of an analgesic using a variety of commercially available PCA devices.

EARLY CLINICAL EXPERIENCE

In 1970, Forrest and colleagues[2] described an instrument (Demand Dropmaster) that automatically administered IV analgesic drugs when activated by pressing a button on a hand grip. In a pilot study involving 30 patients, the investigators reported that both patient and physician acceptance was good and that the failsafe features were reliable. In 1971, Sechzer[3] described his initial experience with an analgesic-demand device. It was concluded that the patient-controlled demand system was a highly satisfactory method for treating acute postoperative pain and that good analgesia could be achieved with relatively low total drug doses.

Using an analgesic-demand device (Deman-alg), Keeri-Szanto[4,6] reported that the use of on-demand analgesia (versus conventional intramuscular therapy) decreased the incidence of substantial postoperative pain from 20–40% to less than 5%. When the demand analgesia group returned to intramuscular (IM) therapy, the incidence of incomplete analgesia increased to 30% even though many of these patients received a larger amount of analgesic medication. More recently, Keeri-Szanto and colleagues[7] reported that demand analgesia improved early mobilization and cooperation with physiotherapy, and was associated with a 22% decrease in the duration of the postoperative hospital stay (versus conventional IM therapy).

Investigators at the Welsh National School of Medicine developed the first commercially available patient-controlled analgesia device, the Cardiff Palliator (Graseby Dynamics Ltd).[8] In subsequent studies,[9–12] they have successfully compared a wide range of analgesic medications for postoperative pain relief using their PCA device. However, investigators in Canada reported that some of their patients found the Cardiff Palliator's demand button hard to operate, and these investigators felt "the technique was too expensive and time-consuming."[13]

Hull and his colleagues[14,15] in the United Kingdom developed a highly sophisticated on-demand analgesia computer (ODAC, Janssen Scientific Instruments). Dosage was limited by a decrease in the patient's respiratory rate and by a series of electronic fail-safe circuits. Using this device, other United Kingdom investigators reported that the postoperative pain relief provided by the on-demand computer was comparable to that produced by epidural bupivacaine.[16] Using an infusion of alfentanil supplemented with bolus injections on demand, Welchew and Hosking[17] recently reported that alfentanil was associated with significantly less sedation than meperidine during the early postoperative period. Lehmann and coworkers[18] in West Germany found that the analgesia provided by the ODAC PCA device was judged superior by 36 to 47% of patients when compared to their previous experiences with conventional postoperative analgesia.

Tamsen and colleagues[19-23] in Sweden performed a series of elegant pharmacokinetic-dynamic studies using a programmable drug injector (Prominject). These investigators reported that age, sex, body weight, and rate of drug elimination did not appear to be directly related to the resulting therapeutic (analgesic) concentrations. Both the analgesic requirement and the resultant therapeutic concentrations were highly variable (four- to sixfold). Although individual drug concentration curves varied, patients maintained relatively constant plasma concentrations when allowed to self-administer meperidine and morphine during the early postoperative period. These investigators reported mean postoperative analgesic requirements of 2.7 ± 1.1 mg/hr and 26 ± 10 mg/hr for morphine and meperidine, respectively.[19] The most frequent complaints were nausea, drowsiness, and dry mouth; however, acute respiratory depression was reported in two hypovolemic patients. Interestingly, Tamsen et al.[23] have reported an inverse relation between cerebrospinal fluid (CSF) endorphin (fraction I) concentrations and the calculated CSF meperidine levels when patients were allowed to achieve satisfactory analgesia using a patient-controlled system. These results suggest a role for the endorphins in the modulation of acute postoperative pain. For example, the presence of high levels of endogenous morphinelike substances in the brain would be expected to minimize the requirement for exogenously administered opioid analgesics during the postoperative period.

Bennett and colleagues[24-30] evaluated the effectiveness of patient-controlled analgesia using the Demanalg device for the management of postoperative pain. They reported that patients maintained "a state of adequate analgesia with minimal sedation throughout their therapeutic course."[24,25] In a study involving morbidly obese patients undergoing gastric bypass surgery, the average PCA morphine requirement was 1.7 mg/hr (with a tenfold variation).[26] Obese patients receiving PCA therapy were reported to have improved postoperative pulmonary function.[27] Compared with a matched group of patients receiving conventional IM therapy, these investigators reported that significantly less medication was required

during the postoperative period in the PCA-treated group.[28] Subjective evaluation of patients following operations involving a flank incision revealed significantly less pain, less sedation, and greater activity in those subjects randomized to PCA therapy.[29] These investigators have also provided evidence for a circadian (cyclical) variation in the postoperative analgesic requirement.[30] Maximal drug usage occurred in the morning (9 a.m.) and was minimal during sleep (3 a.m.). These investigators also report less postoperative pain, greater spontaneous physical activity, and fewer nocturnal sleep disturbances with patient-controlled (versus intramuscular) analgesic therapy.

Unfortunately, many of the PCA studies published in the surgery and anesthesia literature have been poorly controlled clinical reports utilizing subjective endpoints for assessing patient responses to PCA therapy. With attentive nursing care, conventional IM therapy can become on-demand and may be as effective as IV PCA.[31,32] Using a randomized double-blind protocol design for comparing IV PCA therapy with on-demand IM therapy for postoperative pain relief, Welchew[32] reported that the mean pain scores in the two groups were virtually identical. In addition, sedation scores and postoperative pulmonary function tests were not significantly different for the two groups. Although this study has been criticized (e.g., different analgesics were used for the two groups), it emphasized the necessity for carefully controlled studies comparing PCA to conventional IM therapy as well as to other newer approaches to pain management (e.g., epidural narcotics, opioid infusions, transcutaneous opioids).

In a recently published controlled trial, Dahl and colleagues[33] reported that when conventional IV PCA was compared to a "regular" IM dosage regimen (given every 4 hours), which was also supplemented IV on demand, there were no significant differences between the two analgesia regimens with respect to pain scores, morphine dosage requirements, or side effects. Interestingly, these investigators stated that the need for supplemental IV doses in the control (IM) group to ensure optimal treatment is "hardly practicable on a normal ward."

They further suggested that with the standard regular-interval IM regimen, "a large number of patients were either overdosed or underdosed."

More recently, two investigative groups in the United States have compared PCA to conventional IM or epidural opioids for pain control after repeat elective cesarean section.[34,35] Although patients in both the PCA and epidural morphine groups preferred their therapy over the IM regimen administered after their first cesarean section, only those patients receiving epidural morphine reported significantly better pain relief (i.e., analgesia scores) than those in the IM group. In addition, the PCA dosage requirement was similar to the IM treatment group. Patients' perception of sedation and their activity scores did not significantly differ among the three treatment groups. However, epidural morphine produced the highest incidence of pruritus (40 to 45% of the epidural-treated patients required antipruritic therapy), and this group frequently required parenteral opioid supplementation during the first postoperative day.

ALTERNATIVE ROUTES FOR PCA ADMINISTRATION

Conventional PCA therapy involves the administration of small intravenous bolus doses of on-demand analgesic medication. With attentive nursing care, routine intramuscular therapy can become on-demand and may be as effective as IV PCA.[32] Even the longstanding outpatient practice of self-administering oral analgesics on an as-needed basis (i.e., oral PCA) can provide highly effective analgesia in certain postoperative situations. Unfortunately, extensive hepatic metabolism of opioid compounds limits the bioavailability of most orally administered analgesic medication (i.e., the so-called first-pass effect). Recent studies would suggest that PCA therapy can be highly effective when it is administered by a variety of alternative nonparenteral routes of administration (e.g., sublingual,[36] transbuccally,[37] subcutaneously[38]). These newer, simplified

PCA delivery systems would appear to offer advantages over both the oral route of administration and other more complicated drug delivery systems (e.g., spinal or epidural opioids) for patients undergoing superficial noncavitary operations (e.g., ambulatory surgery).

For more extensive operative procedures (e.g., intrathoracic, upper abdominal, major joint replacement), more complex opioid delivery systems (e.g., epidural administration) may offer significant advantages with respect to their ability to improve analgesia and enhance recovery of bodily functions.[39,40] By minimizing residual impairment of central nervous system, respiratory, cardiovascular, and gastrointestinal function, these newer analgesia techniques can contribute to a shorter hospital stay. As a result, the use of intermittent bolus injections of epidural opioids has become a widely accepted technique for managing acute pain after major surgical procedures. Yet the need for subsequent top-up doses has placed an increased burden on physicians and nurses caring for these patients.

While use of epidural opioid or local anesthetic infusions can provide more prolonged analgesia (versus conventional incremental bolus doses),[41-45] determining the optimal infusion rate can also be a time-consuming process. When continuous infusions of epidural local anesthetic solutions were compared to the traditional intermittent bolus technique for maintaining obstetrical analgesia, higher drug dosages were required in the infusion (versus bolus) group, and this appeared to contribute to an increased need for surgical intervention (e.g., outlet forceps).[44] These concerns have limited the more widespread use of this otherwise highly effective therapeutic modality.

The technique of on-demand epidural analgesia using a PCA delivery system can minimize the inconvenience to the staff when the epidural route of administration is chosen for postoperative analgesia. Epidural PCA (versus IV PCA) offers the possibility of improved analgesia with lower drug dosages.[46-48] Combining the inherent analgesic effectiveness of the epidural route of administration with the flexibility in dosage titration offered by PCA therapy would appear to provide advantages over either modality alone. In addition to requiring less analgesic medication with epidural PCA (versus continuous epidural infusion), obstetrical patients were reported to be highly satisfied with their pain relief because they appreciated having "some control over their own pain relief and less reliance on the medical staff."[49] However, outcome studies are needed to evaluate the effect of epidural PCA on postoperative side effects, recovery parameters, and discharge times.

Preliminary studies would suggest that epidural PCA can provide excellent analgesia with lower total narcotic (or local anesthetic) dosages compared to the use of epidural infusions or conventional IV PCA therapy.[44,49,50] Yet, comparative dose-response studies involving narcotic analgesics of differing lipid solubilities are needed to determine the optimal opioid for epidural PCA. The lipophilicity of the narcotic agent is an extremely important determinant of the rate of onset of analgesia as well as the duration of pain relief.

In contrast to morphine and its analogues, the very rapid and short-acting lipophilic opioid compounds (e.g., fentanyl, sufentanil) appear to produce minimal if any dose-sparing effects when injected into the epidural space (versus the intravenous route of administration).[51,52] In fact, Estok et al.[51] reported that there was "no obvious clinical benefit between administering fentanyl epidurally as compared to intravenously using a PCA device." A moderately soluble opioid analgesic (e.g., hydromorphone) can provide for a rapid onset of action (< 10 minutes) and a more prolonged duration of analgesia (2 to 4 hours) when administered epidurally by small incremental (bolus) injections.[50]

Another exciting development in the management of acute pain has been the epidural administration of solutions containing combinations of opioid (narcotic) analgesics and local anesthetics. These drug combinations may be more effective than either drug alone.[43,53] However, additional dose-response studies are required to establish optimal concentrations (dosages) of each drug to minimize potential side effects and untoward drug interactions. Controversy also surrounds the use of epinephrine in this narcotic–local anesthetic combination. Finally, carefully controlled outcome studies are needed to determine the most cost-effective method of PCA therapy in the management of acute pain.

PCA DELIVERY SYSTEMS

In designing patient-controlled analgesia equipment, biomedical engineers have utilized negative feedback control technology.[54,55] When feedback control is applied to the control of pain, the patient self-administers analgesic medication to decrease the error signal [i.e., the difference between the pain experienced and the acceptable (tolerable) level of pain] to zero. Two simplified versions of the PCA feedback loop are shown in Figure 22.1. PCA techniques attempt to close the feedback loop without the necessity of nursing staff intervention, thereby improving the effectiveness of the pain control system.

Since the first widely used PCA device was introduced into clinical practice in the United Kingdom in 1976, several more technologically advanced PCA delivery systems have been introduced in the United States. The major advantages of these newer PCA systems relate to their computerized programming features and fail-safe designs.

Historical PCA Infusion Devices

The Cardiff Palliator (Graseby Dynamics Ltd) (Figure 22.2) is a line-powered syringe pump that can be preprogrammed to deliver the desired dose of medication at a predetermined flow rate with a preselected minimum dose interval. The parameters are adjustable over a wide range to accommodate a variety of drugs and dosage regimens. To minimize the possibility of the button being pressed accidentally, the button must be pressed twice in rapid succession (within 1 second) to achieve a successful demand. A disposable 20-ml sy-

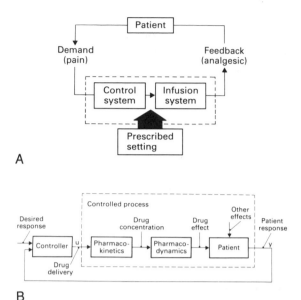

A

B

FIGURE 22.1 Schematic representations of patient-controlled analgesia (PCA) drug delivery as part of a feedback control system. (Reprinted with permission of the authors and publisher from Harmer M, Rosen M, Vickers MD, eds. Patient-controlled analgesia. Oxford: Blackwell Scientific, 1985. A: From McCarthy JP. The Cardiff Palliator, pp. 87–91. B: From Jacobs OLR, Bullingham RES. Modelling, estimation, and control for demand analgesia, pp. 57–82.)

sion pump with three different modes of operation (namely, patient-controlled, consecutive infusions, and constant infusion). The consecutive infusion mode allows for the administration of a loading dose (priming infusion), followed by a constant maintenance infusion. This device is also capable of delivering split incremental doses (e.g., a bolus dose delivered over 1 minute followed by an infusion of the equivalent dose over 1 hour). After selecting the desired operational mode, the operator enters the drug concentration, dose, lockout interval (in PCA mode), and time for infusion of the dose. The alphanumeric message panel guides the operator step by step through the programming procedure. The prescribed drug is delivered from a standard 20-ml B-D luer lock disposable syringe, which is covered by a clear tamperproof plastic cover. This cover is locked with a key, which also electronically locks the keyboard. A hard copy of the drug usage record is produced by a built-in dot matrix printer. The time, date, and accumulated dose are printed simultaneously with the event or retrospectively from the microprocessor memory. Acoustic and diagnostic alarms and status messages will report line occlusion, empty syringe, low battery charge, and improper program settings. The device can be mounted on an infusion stand or placed on a table top.

ringe can be filled with the analgesic of choice. A yellow indicator lamp (which remains on during the lockout interval) and a tone indicate when a bolus dose is successfully infused. An audible alarm sounds whenever the syringe is empty. The thumbwheel switches are accessible on the front and rear of the device for controlling the incremental dose (range 1 to 999 mg), dilution control (range 1 to 99 mg/ml), interval time (range 1 to 99 minutes), and delivery rate (range 1 to 99 ml/hr). Although these thumbwheel switches were not tamperproof on the original Cardiff Palliator, the second-generation device contains the essential safety and security features.

The Pharmacia Prominject pump is a microprocessor-controlled, programmable infu-

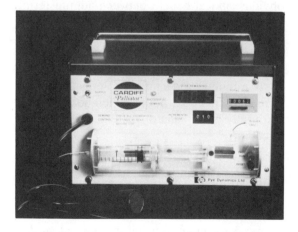

FIGURE 22.2 The original Cardiff Palliator PCA device. (Courtesy of Graseby Dynamics Ltd, United Kingdom.)

The On Demand Analgesia Computer (ODAC, Janssen Scientific Instruments) is a highly innovative experimental PCA device. This infusion device allows the patient to interact directly with the machine using a tape cassette. In addition to demand doses, this device can administer a background infusion based on the amount of analgesic drug the patient demanded during the previous 16-minute interval. An integral pneumograph sensor prevents analgesic administration if the respiratory rate is depressed. With further technical refinement, the ODAC could become a clinically useful device in the management of postoperative pain. However, it would seem unlikely that any of the second-generation pharmacokinetically based, computer-controlled opioid infusion systems currently under investigation will be available for clinical use in the near future.

Commercially Available PCA Infusion Devices

The Abbott Life Care PCA Infusers (Abbott Laboratories, North Chicago, Ill.) combine microprocessor and stepping motor technology for the safe delivery of either intermittent bolus doses or a continuous infusion of narcotic analgesics from disposable cartridges (Figure 22.3). These relatively lightweight, portable, computerized volumetric infusion pumps have lockable security doors that prohibit unauthorized access to the analgesic drug or the controls while the unit is in operation. A liquid crystal display indicates the operational status, total cumulative dose, number of bolus doses administered, and other status and alarm messages. Prefilled (e.g., morphine 1 mg/ml, meperidine 10 mg) or empty drug cartridges are available. After the cartridge has been inserted

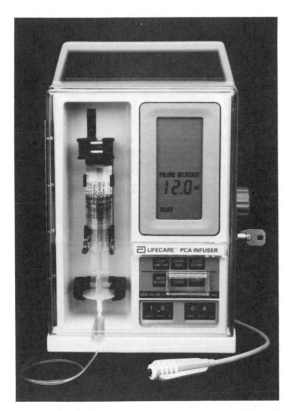
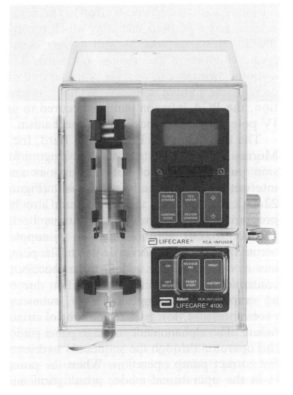

FIGURE 22.3 (A) The Abbott Life Care PCA Infuser 1821, and (B) the Abbott Lifecare PCA Infuser 4100 device. (Courtesy of Abbott Laboratories, North Chicago, Ill.)

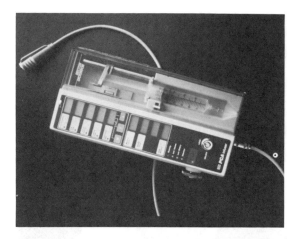

FIGURE 22.5 The Becton-Dickinson PCA Infusor. (Courtesy of B. D. Infusion Systems, Lincoln Park, N.J.)

vice has a 24-hour memory (which remains operational for up to 99 hours even after the device is turned off), and acoustic and diagnostic alarm features, and it can be secured to an IV pole.

The Pharmacia Deltec CADD-PCA (Pharmacia Deltec, St. Paul, Minn.) is a small (15 oz), portable, programmable analgesic infusion device that can provide for the safe delivery of parenteral analgesics both in and outside of the hospital (Figure 22.6). Although this PCA device has not been extensively evaluated for the treatment of acute postoperative pain, its compact size would provide for increased patient activity and mobility during the early postoperative period. The device delivers the analgesic drug on demand, with incremental doses ranging from 0.1 to 99.5 mg and a lockout interval from 5 to 99 minutes. The pump can also be used to continuously infuse analgesics, with a basal infusion rate of 0.1 to 99.5 mg/hr (depending on the concentration of the solution). Analgesic medication is contained in prefilled, sterilized disposable cassettes, which are maintained in a locked compartment. Alarms warn the user when there is a low residual drug volume, low battery power, or a mechanical failure. The updated version of this PCA system has a lockable door and pole clamp, as well as a handheld remote dose button.

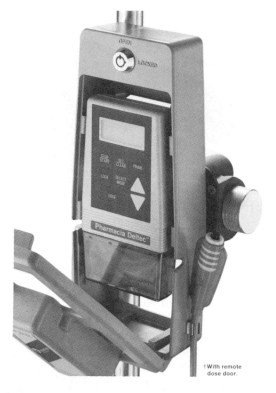

†With remote dose door.

FIGURE 22.6 The Pharmacia Deltec CADD-PCA device. (Courtesy of Pharmacia Deltec, St. Paul, Minn.)

The Baxter (Travenol) PCA Infusor (Baxter Healthcare Corp., Chicago, Ill.) is a small nonelectronic device that is fully disposable (Figure 22.7). It consists of a lightweight plastic cylinder containing the analgesic medication inside an elastic balloon. This drug

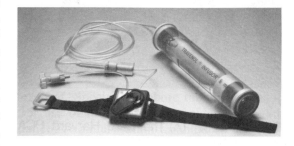

FIGURE 22.7 The Baxter (Travenol) PCA Infusor. (Courtesy of Baxter Healthcare Corp., Chicago, Ill.)

chamber holds a volume of 40 ml, and the amount of drug delivered per injection depends on the opioid concentration. The device is nonprogrammable, delivering a fixed 0.5-ml dose at intervals of 6 minutes or longer. As the balloon reservoir slowly deflates, solution flows through a small orifice (flow restrictor), which determines the time required to fill the 0.5-ml injection reservoir (6 minutes). The injection reservoir is located on a wristband, which is activated by pushing a button. There is no drug infusion between depressions of the medication demand button. Although its simplified design obviates the need for many of the fail-safe features available on the computerized devices, it is somewhat less flexible than the other systems with respect to the administered dose of analgesic medication.

The Pancretec Provider 5000 (Pancretec Inc., San Diego, Calif.) is a lightweight portable PCA pump (14 oz) that can deliver analgesic medication intermittently on demand or by continuous infusion (Figure 22.8). The pumping mechanism consists of a microprocessor-controlled eccentric/rotor peristaltic pump. The power supply consists of two 9-V disposable lithium batteries, which can deliver 4800 ml at a maximum rate of 250 ml/hr. The minimum drug infusion rate of 0.1 ml/hr will maintain the patency of the catheter or the vein. This PCA device has a liquid crystal display, memory function, and audible and visual safety alarms.

These commercially available PCA infusion pumps have been recently evaluated with respect to safety, security, and overall ease of use.[56] All the PCA pumps tested met the accuracy, electrical safety, and performance criteria established by biomedical engineers.[57] The Bard Ambulatory PCA, the Pharmacia Deltec CADD-PCA, and the Baxter PCA Infusor were all judged to be suitable for ambulatory use. Although widely used in many medical centers, the totally disposable Baxter device was not recommended for general hospital use because of its alleged higher costs and lack of dose adjustment features.

In summary, the safe and effective delivery of opioid analgesic medications on demand is

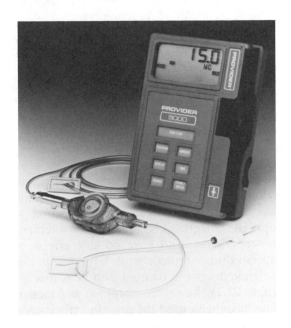

FIGURE 22.8 The Pancretec Provider 5000 device (Courtesy of Pancretec Inc., San Diego, Calif.)

possible using a variety of delivery systems. When utilizing PCA to control acute pain, the physician can choose either a simplified, nonelectronic disposable PCA device or an ultrasophisticated computer-controlled infusion device with a wide variety of delivery modes. It would appear that future generations of PCA devices will be both safer for patients and more cost-effective for the health care system.

MANAGEMENT OF POSTOPERATIVE PAIN

If postoperative PCA therapy is to be successful, it is important that the patient as well as the physician and nursing staff understand the basic concept.[58] As part of their preoperative instructions, patients should be given an explanation of the PCA device; be told not to expect *complete* pain relief but rather to use the device to avoid distressing pain; be encouraged to use the device in a prophylactic manner to avoid the discomfort associated with early ambulation, physical therapy, and dressing changes; and be told that an attempt would be made to minimize the size of the bolus dose during awake hours to avoid excessive sedation, while attempting to maximize the dosing interval during sleeping hours to prevent the patient from awakening repeatedly during the night.

In prescribing postoperative PCA therapy, what pharmacologic properties would be highly desirable in an opioid analgesic? The ideal opioid would have a rapid onset of analgesic action, be highly efficacious in relieving pain, have an intermediate duration of action to improve controllability, not produce tolerance or dependence, and have no side effects or adverse drug interactions. A large number of analgesic drugs can be used with PCA therapy (Table 22.1); however, morphine and meperidine have been used the most in early clinical trials. More recent studies have suggested that both hydromorphone[38] and oxymorphone[59] are excellent alternatives to morphine for acute postoperative pain relief. Unfortunately, all opioid compounds have the same side effect

profile (i.e., nausea, vomiting, ileus, sedation, respiratory depression).

The duration of analgesia produced by methadone and buprenorphine may be too long, while fentanyl and its newer analogues may be too short-acting when administered as incremental bolus doses. However, Gourlay et al.[60] have recently described the blood concentration–analgesic response relation when fentanyl was administered by a continuous (basal) infusion that could be supplemented by bolus injections on demand for postoperative analgesia. Sufentanil and alfentanil can also be effectively administered by continuous infusion or by a continuous plus bolus on-demand delivery mode. Sufentanil (5 to 15 μg IV) has been effectively administered for managing postoperative pain using the traditional intermittent bolus technique.[52] However, the frequency of demands is higher than with the more conventional postoperative analgesic medications. Recently, Chrubasik et al.[47] reported that a continuous plus on-demand epidural infusion of alfentanil produced analgesia that was similar in quality to that of morphine. Because of the more rapid onset of analgesia (and lower requirement for supplemental sedative-tranquilizers), these investigators felt that alfentanil was preferable to morphine. The agonist-antagonist analgesics (e.g., butorphanol, nalbuphine, buprenorphine) produce ceiling or plateau effects with respect to both respiratory depression and analgesia. However, in those situations where an agonist-antagonist can provide adequate pain relief, these drugs would be less likely to produce clinically significant respiratory depression than the pure opioid agonists.

In general, a titrated loading dose of the analgesic is administered to achieve adequate postoperative pain relief prior to initiating maintenance PCA therapy. The loading dose can be administered over 15 to 30 minutes in the postanesthesia care unit. When patients are sufficiently recovered from anesthesia, they are then given the patient control button and allowed to begin self-administering small bolus doses of the analgesic medication using the PCA device. If the size of the bolus dose is

TABLE 22.1 Guidelines regarding the bolus dosages and lockout (delay) intervals for various parenteral analgesics when using a patient-controlled analgesia system

Drug	Bolus Dose (mg or μg)	Lockout Interval (min)
Agonists		
Morphine	0.5–3.0	5–20
Methadone	0.5–3.0	10–20
Hydromorphone	0.1–0.6	5–15
Oxymorphone	0.1–0.6	5–15
Meperidine	5–30	5–15
Fentanyl	15–75	3–10
Sufentanil	2–15	3–10
Agonist-antagonists		
Pentazocine	5–30	5–15
Nalbuphine	1–5	5–15
Buprenorphine	0.03–0.2	5–20

Source: Data from White PF. Patient-controlled analgesia: a new approach to the management of postoperative pain. Semin Anesth 1985; 4:255–266.

inadequate (i.e., pain relief consistently requires one or more bolus injections at frequent intervals), the dose is increased by 25 to 50% until an effective bolus dose is determined. Conversely, if the patient experiences excessive sedation or dizziness after a bolus injection, the dose should be decreased by 25 to 50%. During the night sleeping hours, the size of the bolus dose and lockout interval can be increased or a background (basal) infusion administered in order to maximize the time interval between successive doses.

The overall morphine usage during the first 3 days following major operative procedures will typically range from 1 to 3 mg/hr; however, there is a wide variability in the individual morphine requirements.[58] In this preliminary study, 71% of the patients reported no significant discomfort during the period in which they were using the PCA device. The remaining 29% complained of mild to moderate pain at some point during the study. The patients were awake and alert at least two-thirds of the daytime hours with no episodes of prolonged sedation or sleeping during the day. As expected, the level of physical activity increased with each postoperative day. In general, patients stated a preference for PCA therapy when asked to compare it to their previous experiences with conventional IM injections for the treatment of postoperative pain. However, one patient preferred IM therapy because she was more sedated and therefore had less recall of the early postoperative period.

In a comparative study involving PCA and conventional intramuscular therapy, PCA-treated patients required less narcotic medication to achieve comparable analgesia during the first 48 hours after orthopedic surgery (Figure 22.9).[5] However, the PCA group tended to require parenteral analgesics for a longer period of time after surgery. In a similar comparison of PCA and conventional IM therapy, Bollish et al.[61] reported that comparable dosages of morphine produced superior analgesia in the PCA-treated group. Although they also reported that PCA was no more effective than IM analgesics in relieving pain, Ferrante et al.[62] were able to document a complete cycle

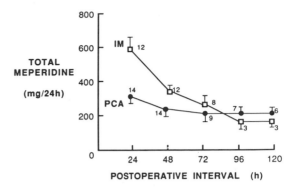

FIGURE 22.9 Meperidine dosage requirements (mg/24 hr) at various intervals after major orthopedic operations. Number of patients in PCA-treated and conventional intramuscularly treated (IM) groups who were receiving parenteral analgesics are indicated at each interval studied. (Data from White PF. Use of patient-controlled analgesia for management of acute pain. JAMA 1988;259:243–247.)

of pain every 5.3 hours in patients receiving IM opioids, but no pain cycle was seen with the use of PCA therapy. Of interest, a preliminary study suggests that continuous infusions of opioid analgesics may be inferior to intermittent bolus administration of narcotic drugs in the relief of postoperative pain because the use of an opioid infusion might facilitate the development of tolerance.[63]

POTENTIAL COMPLICATIONS OF PCA THERAPY

The risk of clinically significant postoperative respiratory depression in a patient receiving PCA therapy is extremely low. Nevertheless, some investigators have suggested that special precautions (e.g., use of pulse oximetry, apnea monitoring) should be considered to minimize the risk of this potentially life-threatening complication. It is important to note that patients undergoing a variety of major operations have maintained normal arterial blood gases

TABLE 22.2 Summary of problems that can occur during patient-controlled analgesia therapy

Operator errors
  Misprogramming PCA device
  Failure to clamp or unclamp tubing
  Improperly loading syringe or cartridge
  Inability to respond to safety alarms
  Failure to adequately monitor patient
  Misplacing PCA pump key
Patient errors
  Failure to understand PCA therapy
  Misunderstanding PCA pump device
  Intentional analgesic abuse
Mechanical errors
  Failure to deliver on demand
  Defective one-way valve at Y connector
  Faulty alarm system
  Malfunctions (e.g., lock, computer program)

Source: White PF. Mishaps with patient-controlled analgesia (PCA). Anesthesiology 1987;66:81–83.

in the early postoperative period while receiving PCA therapy.[16,20]

In a study involving patients undergoing upper abdominal operations, the PCA-treated group had more patients with mildly elevated capillary carbon dioxide levels than patients receiving either IM or epidural narcotics.[64] Yet, postoperative respiratory function in patients receiving PCA therapy was not significantly different from IM-treated patients.[31,32,64] Administration of large bolus doses of analgesics to elderly or hypovolemic patients can produce clinically significant respiratory and cardiovascular depression.[20] Although no respiratory arrests have been reported in the medical literature during PCA therapy,* it is important to assess the drug dose-effect relationship frequently during the early postoperative period. Adjustments in the bolus dose or infusion rate on an individual basis are required in order to optimize the therapy and prevent untoward side effects. The most common problems with PCA therapy are related to operator errors

_____

*Two cases of unexpected deaths in patients using PCA therapy for postoperative analgesia are under active investigation.

(Table 22.2).[65] If errors are to be avoided, the nursing staff must understand the conceptual basis for the therapy. In addition to being knowledgeable about the operational aspects of the PCA pump, the nursing staff should carefully observe the patient after making changes in the opioid dosage regimen.

With repeated or continuous administration of narcotic analgesics, tolerance will develop to the desirable as well as the undesirable pharmacologic effects. As a result, progressively larger narcotic doses may be required to produce the same degree of pain relief during the postoperative period.[63] When narcotic analgesics are discontinued after a prolonged period of treatment, patients may experience withdrawal symptoms as a result of the development of physical dependence. However, addiction or psychological dependence (i.e., compulsive drug-seeking behavior) rarely, if ever, develops in patients receiving narcotics for the treatment of acute postoperative pain.

CONCLUSION

It is impossible to predict accurately how much pain a patient will experience after an operation or how much analgesic medication will be required to provide adequate pain relief. Thus, physicians and nurses necessarily rely on subjective methods to determine the analgesic regimen for patients experiencing postoperative pain. In reviewing the literature, it is clear that "there is a deficient link in the chain that involves the patient who experiences pain and requests medication, the physician prescribing the analgesic drugs, and the nurse who assesses the pain and makes the decision about when to administer analgesics."[66] Problems arise because of the inherent difficulties in determining the appropriate dose and dosing interval, resulting in some patients being overmedicated while others continue to experience unacceptable levels of pain. Given the narrow therapeutic window for an individual patient, a carefully titrated dose of analgesic drug is needed to maintain adequate analgesia without undesirable side effects (Figure 22.10).

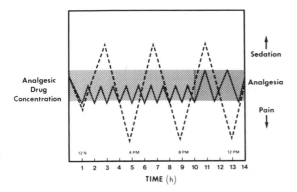

FIGURE 22.10 Theoretical relationship between dosing interval, analgesic (drug) concentration, and clinical effects in patients receiving PCA (solid line) or conventional intramuscular (dashed line) therapy. (Data from White PF. Patient-controlled analgesia: a new approach to the management of postoperative pain. Semin Anesth 1985; 4: 255–266.)

Patient-controlled analgesia is a system designed to accommodate the wide range of analgesic requirements that can be anticipated when managing acute postoperative pain.[58] PCA can also minimize the anxiety resulting from the slow onset of pain relief associated with most commonly used therapeutic modalities. A major psychological advantage with PCA therapy relates to its ability to minimize the time delay between the perception of pain and the administration of analgesic medication. In addition, the increased attention being paid to PCA-treated patients both preoperatively and postoperatively might provide a psychological benefit to patients. The comfort that patients experience as a result of compassionate and attentive nursing and medical care would be expected to significantly decrease their analgesic drug requirement.[67]

Although the concept of patient-controlled analgesic therapy is not new,[2-4] recent progress in the area of infusion pump technology has renewed interest in this concept. Early clinical studies have demonstrated that safe and effective postoperative pain relief can be achieved with a variety of patient-controlled analgesia

infusors. With PCA therapy, Graves et al.[68] have reported that patients experience minimal sedation during awake hours and progressively increase their physical activity during the postoperative period. These investigators suggested that postoperative results are better when patients control their own analgesia.

In the postoperative situation, PCA should be used for maintenance of analgesia. Thus, patients need to receive a titrated loading dose prior to initiating self-administered analgesic therapy. If the therapy is to be successful, it is important that the nurse assess the individual patient's response to the analgesic regimen. Given the marked pharmacodynamic variability that exists among patients with respect to their postoperative analgesic requirements, it will occasionally be necessary to alter the amount of the bolus dose and the duration of the lockout interval in order to optimize the therapeutic regimen. To achieve optimal results with PCA, both patients and staff should understand the basic principles upon which the therapy is based (Figure 22.10). Finally, applications of PCA therapy are not limited to the postsurgical ward. This concept can also be applied to the management of acute and chronic cancer pain on medical and oncology wards. Others have suggested that PCA therapy could be useful in obstetrical suites, intensive care units, coronary care units, and in clinical research.

Individuals with either markedly increased or decreased analgesic requirements can be adequately managed using a PCA delivery system. Thus, the rational use of a PCA infusion device allows patients to titrate the rate of narcotic administration to meet their individual analgesic needs. If recurrent (or intractable) nausea or vomiting develops, patients can be switched to a different narcotic analgesic, or antiemetic therapy can be administered. However, the commonly used antiemetic drugs (e.g., droperidol, hydroxyzine) would be expected to enhance the sedation produced by the opioid analgesics. The use of antihistaminic compounds to treat pruritus would also increase opioid-induced sedation. The agonist-antagonist compounds (e.g., nalbuphine) have been used successfully to treat side effects produced by epidural opioids.

In conclusion, patient-controlled analgesia provides improved titration of analgesic drugs, thereby minimizing the clinical importance of interpatient pharmacokinetic and pharmacodynamic variability in their responses to opioid medication. PCA therapy decreases patient anxiety resulting from delays in receiving pain-relieving medication and from the slow onset of analgesic action when these drugs are administered either intramuscularly or in the extradural space. With PCA therapy, patients are able to maintain an acceptable level of analgesia with minimal sedation and few side effects. The potential for overdose can be minimized if small bolus doses are used with a mandatory lockout interval between successive doses. Finally, additional studies regarding outcome following PCA therapy are important if this therapeutic approach is to achieve even more widespread acceptance.

REFERENCES

1. Sechzer PH. Objective measurement of pain. Anesthesiology 1968;29:209–210.
2. Forrest WH Jr, Smethurst PWR, Kienitz ME. Self-administration of intravenous analgesics. Anesthesiology 1970;33:363–365.
3. Sechzer PH. Studies in pain with analgesic demand system. Anesth Analg (Cleve) 1971; 50:1–10.
4. Keeri-Szanto M. Apparatus for demand analgesia. Can Anaesth Soc J 1971;18:581–582.
5. White PF. Use of patient-controlled analgesia for management of acute pain. JAMA 1988; 259:243–247.
6. Keeri-Szanto M, Heaman S. Postoperative demand analgesia. Surg Gynecol Obstet 1972;134: 647–651.
7. Finley RJ, Keeri-Szanto M, Boyd D. New analgesic agents and techniques shorten postoperative hospital stay. Pain 1984;2:S397.
8. Evans JM, MacCarthy J, Rosen M, et al. Apparatus for patient-controlled administration of intravenous narcotics during labour. Lancet 1976;1:17–18.
9. Chakravaty K, Tucker W, Rosen M, et al. Comparison of buprenorphine and pethidine given intravenously on demand to relieve postoperative pain. Br Med J 1979;2:895–897.
10. Harmer M, Slattery PJ, Rosen M, et al. Comparison between buprenorphine and pentazocine given IV on demand in the control of postoperative pain. Br J Anaesth 1983;55:21–24.
11. Slattery PJ, Harmer M, Rosen M, et al. Comparison of meptazinol and pethidine given IV on demand in the management of postoperative pain. Br J Anaesth 1981;53:927–930.
12. Bahar M, Rosen M, Vickers MD. Self-administered nalbuphine, morphine, and pethidine: comparison by intravenous route following cholecystectomy. Anaesthesia 1985;40:529–532.
13. Sprigge JS, Otton PE. Nalbuphine versus meperidine for postoperative analgesia: a double-blind comparison using the patient-controlled analgesic technique. Can Anaesth Soc J 1983; 30:517–521.
14. Hull CJ, Sibbald A, Johnson MK. Demand analgesia for postoperative pain .Br J Anaesth 1979;51:570–571.
15. Hull CJ, Sibbald A. Control of postoperative pain by interactive demand analgesia. Br J Anaesth 1981;53:385–391.
16. White DC, Pearce DJ, Norman J. Postoperative analgesia: a comparison of intravenous on-demand fentanyl with epidural bupivacaine. Br Med J 1979;2:166–167.
17. Welchew EA, Hosking J. Patient-controlled postoperative analgesia with alfentanil: adaptive, on-demand intravenous alfentanil or pethidine compared double-blind for postoperative pain. Anaesthesia 1985;40:1172–1177.
18. Lehmann KA, Gördes B, Hoeckle W. Postoperative on-demand analgesia with morphine. Anaesthesist 1985;34:494–501.
19. Tamsen A, Hartvig P, Dahlstrom B, et al. Patient-controlled analgesia therapy in the early postoperative period. Acta Anaesthesiol Scand 1979;5:462–470.
20. Tamsen A, Hartvig P, Fagerlund C, et al. Patient-controlled analgesic therapy: clinical experience. Acta Anaesthesiol Scand 1982;74: 157–160.
21. Tamsen A, Hartvig P, Fagerlund C, et al. Patient-controlled analgesic therapy: pharmacokinetics of pethidine in the pre- and postoperative periods. Clin Pharmacokinet 1982;7: 149–163.
22. Dahlstrom B, Tamsen A, Paalzow L, et al.

Patient-controlled analgesic therapy: pharmacokinetics and analgesic plasma concentrations of morphine. Clin Pharmacokinet 1982; 7:266–279.

23. Tamsen A, Sakurada T, Wahlstrom A, et al. Postoperative demand for analgesics in relation to individual levels of endorphins and substance P in cerebrospinal fluid. Pain 1982;13:171–183.

24. Bennett RL, Baumann T, Batenhorst RL, et al. Morphine titration in postoperative laparotomy patients using patient-controlled analgesia. Curr Ther Res 1982;32:45–52.

25. Bennett RL, Batenhorst RL, Graves D, et al. Patient-controlled analgesia: a new concept of postoperative relief. Ann Surg 1982;195:700–705.

26. Bennett RL, Batenhorst RL, Graves D, et al. Variation in postoperative analgesic requirements in the morbidly obese following gastric bypass surgery. Pharmacotherapy 1982;2:43–49.

27. Bennett RL, Batenhorst RL, Foster TS, et al. Postoperative pulmonary function with patient-controlled analgesia. Anesth Analg 1982; 6:171.

28. Bennett RL, Batenhorst RL, Graves D, et al. Drug use pattern in patient-controlled analgesia. Anesthesiology 1982;57:A210.

29. Atwell JR, Flanigan RC, Bennett RL, et al. The efficacy of patient-controlled analgesia in patients recovering from flank incisions. J Urol 1984;132:701–703.

30. Graves DA, Batenhorst RL, Bennett RL, et al. Morphine requirements using patient-controlled analgesia: influence of diurnal variation and morbid obesity. Clin Pharm 1983;2:49–53.

31. Ellis R, Haines D, Shah R, et al. Pain relief after abdominal surgery: comparison of IM morphine, sublingual buprenorphine, and self-administered IV pethidine. Br J Anaesth 1982; 54:421–428.

32. Welchew EA. On-demand analgesia: a double-blind comparison of on-demand intravenous fentanyl with regular intramuscular morphine. Anaesthesia 1983;38:19–25.

33. Dahl JB, Daugaard JJ, Larsen HV, et al. Patient-controlled analgesia: a controlled trial. Acta Anaesthesiol Scand 1987;31:744–747.

34. Eisenach JC, Grice SC, Dewan DM. Patient-controlled analgesia following cesarean section: a comparison with epidural and intra-

muscular narcotics. Anesthesiology 1988;68: 444–448.

35. Harrison DM, Sinatra R, Morgese L, et al. Epidural narcotic and patient-controlled analgesia for post-cesarean section pain relief. Anesthesiology 1988;68:454–457.

36. Shah MV, Jones DI, Rosen M. "Patient demand" postoperative analgesia with buprenorphine: comparison between sublingual and intramuscular administration. Br J Anaesth 1986;58:508–511.

37. Bell MDD, Mishra P, Weldon BD, et al. Buccal morphine—a new route for analgesia? Lancet 1985;1:71–73.

38. Urquhart ML, Klapp K, White PF. Patient-controlled analgesia: a comparison of intravenous versus subcutaneous hydromorphone. Anesthesiology 1988;69:428–432.

39. Rawal N, Sjostrand U, Christoffersson E, et al. Comparison of intramuscular and epidural morphine for postoperative analgesia in the grossly obese: influence on postoperative ambulation and pulmonary function. Anesth Analg 1984;63:583.

40. Yeager MP, Glass DD, Neff RK, et al. Epidural anesthesia and analgesia in high-risk surgical patients. Anesthesiology 1987;66:729–736.

41. El-Baz NM, Faber LP, Jensik RJ. Continuous epidural infusion of morphine for treatment of pain after thoracic surgery: a new technique. Anesth Analg 1984;63:757–764.

42. Fischer RL, Lubenow TR, Liceaga A, et al. Comparison of continuous epidural infusion of fentanyl-bupivacaine and morphine-bupivacaine in management of postoperative pain. Anesth Analg 1988;67:559–563.

43. Phillips G. Continuous infusion epidural analgesia in labor: the effect of adding sufentanil to 0.125% bupivacaine. Anesth Analg 1988; 67:462–465.

44. Smedstad KG, Morison DH. A comparative study of continuous and intermittent epidural analgesia for labour and delivery. Can Anaesth Soc J 1988;35:234–241.

45. Mitchell RWD, Scott DB, Holmquist E, et al. Continuous extradural infusion of 0.125% bupivacaine for pain relief after lower abdominal surgery. Br J Anaesth 1988;60:851–853.

46. Chrubasik J, Wiemers K. Continuous-plus-on-demand epidural infusion of morphine for postoperative pain relief by means of a small, externally worn infusion device. Anesthesiology 1985;62:263–267.

47. Chrubasik J, Wüst H, Schulte-Mönting J, et al. Relative analgesic potency of epidural fentanyl, alfentanil, and morphine in treatment of postoperative pain. Anesthesiology 1988;68: 929–933.
48. Sjostrom S, Hartvig D, Tamsen A. Patient-controlled analgesia with extradural morphine or pethidine. Br J Anaesth 1988;60:358–366.
49. Gambling DR, Yu P, Cole C, et al. A comparative study of patient-controlled epidural analgesia (PCEA) and continuous infusion epidural analgesia (CIEA) during labour. Can Anaesth Soc J 1988;35:249–254.
50. Marlowe S, Engstrom R, White PF. Epidural PCA: An alternative to continuous epidural infusions. Pain 1989;37:97–101.
51. Estok PM, Glass PSA, Goldberg JS, et al. Use of patient-controlled analgesia to compare intravenous to epidural administration of fentanyl in the postoperative patient. Anesthesiology 1987;67:A230.
52. Cohen SE, Tan S, White PF. Sufentanil analgesia following cesarean section: epidural versus intravenous administration. Anesthesiology 1988;68:129–134.
53. Lee A, Simpson D, Whitfield A, et al. Postoperative analgesia by continuous extradural infusion of bupivacaine and diamorphine. Br J Anaesth 1988;60:845–850.
54. McCarthy JP. The Cardiff Palliator. In: Harmer M, Rosen M, Vickers MD, eds. Patient-controlled analgesia. Oxford: Blackwell Scientific Publications, 1985;87–91.
55. Jacobs OLR, Bullingham RES. Modelling, estimation, and control for demand analgesia. In: Harmer M, Rosen M, Vickers MD, eds. Patient-controlled analgesia. Oxford: Blackwell Scientific Publications, 1985;57–72.
56. Patient-controlled analgesic infusion pumps (I). Health Devices 1988;17:137–167. (Editorial)
57. Patient-controlled analgesic infusion pumps (II). Health Devices 1988;17:368–370. (Editorial)
58. White PF. Patient-controlled analgesia: a new approach to the management of postoperative pain. Semin Anesth 1985;4:255–266.
59. Harrison DM, Sinatra RS, Lodge K, et al. A comparison of meperidine, morphine, and oxymorphone for use in patient-controlled analgesia following cesarean delivery. Anesthesiology 1987;67:A462.
60. Gourlay GK, Kowalski SR, Plummer JL, et al. Fentanyl blood concentration–analgesic response relationship in the treatment of postoperative pain. Anesth Analg 1988;67:329–337.
61. Bollish SJ, Collins CL, Kirking DM, et al. Efficacy of patient-controlled versus conventional analgesia for postoperative pain. Clin Pharm 1985;4:48–52.
62. Ferrante FM, Orav EJ, Rocco AG, et al. A statistical model for pain in patient-controlled analgesia and conventional intramuscular opioid regimens. Anesth Analg 1988;67:457–461.
63. Marshall H, Porteous C, McMillan I, et al. Relief of pain by infusion of morphine after operation: does tolerance develop? Br Med J 1985;291:19–21.
64. Rosenberg PH, Heino A, Scheinin B. Comparison of intramuscular analgesia, intercostal block, epidural morphine, and on-demand IV fentanyl in the control of pain after upper abdominal surgery. Acta Anaesthesiol Scand 1984;28:603–607.
65. White PF. Mishaps with patient-controlled analgesia (PCA). Anesthesiology 1987;66:81–83.
66. Weis OF, Sriwatanakul K, Alloza JL, et al. Attitudes of patients, housestaff, and nurses toward postoperative analgesic care. Anesth Analg 1983;62:70–74.
67. Egbert LD, Battit GE, Welch CE, et al. Reduction of postoperative pain by encouragement and instruction of patients. N Engl J Med 1964;270:825–827.
68. Graves DA, Foster TS, Batenhorst RL, et al. Patient-controlled analgesia. Ann Intern Med 1983;99:360–366.

Part III Discussion

DR. REAM: I'm indebted to Nathan Pace for this slide; he wanted to make the point that in trying to reach our immediate goals, we could lose our ultimate goals. Nathan also pointed out that the temptation to alter data can occasionally become overwhelming. But it's equally true that biological and individual variability often prevent an adequate level of control.

We can identify two important aspects about the delivery of opioid anesthesia. One is the delivery mechanism (the delivery system and the transition from a single bolus dose to continuous infusions), and delivery routes (dermal, buccal, ocular, and so on). The second is the concept of control. We started our training as anesthesia residents with an idea of an open loop, and then we progressed to the point where we have a mental model of the patient. Finally, we begin to observe some of the problems of kinetic models because of biological variability, but at some point we choose true endpoints, and that's where monitoring begins.

The two endpoints of narcotics are respiratory depression and addiction. In the short term, we worry about respiratory depression. And yet, the casual list that I made of the papers in this section left me with 30 to 40 indices of endpoint control. The topics so elegantly discussed in these chapters lead to methods for making the system safer and more tractable and predictable. Take that statistic of anesthetic mortality, 1 in 8,000 or something in that range, which has often been quoted as an academic number—perhaps, we make greater contributions but don't get credit for them.

And so it's time we learn the vocabulary. We begin with a mental model. We then use a kinetic model, for example, and the physician modifies it to anticipate the dynamic aspects. Or we develop a baseline by using patch or oral absorption rates. What we're doing in most of these cases is taking a very intractable mental model, as Dr. Reves so aptly pointed out, and we're reducing it to a system that we can easily visualize, which provides us with safe and effective procedures. It seems to me that if we take this process to the logical endpoint, ultimately a computer with a very sophisticated method of calculation will be handling this technique. This system will still need to be checked, so that the patient status is intuitively obvious. We won't be dependent on the Oracle of Delphi. We won't be helpless. We will have, in fact, considerable insight into whether or not the system is working properly.

Some years ago, Stanford University had a tremendous leak in the library system pipes, destroying a number of very rare books. The librarians, faced with a limited budget, had elected to buy rare books rather than replace the building. This comment was made by one of the trustees of the University, and I think it applies very well to what we're doing here. On the one end we have this very sophisticated concern about the actual mode of action of these drugs, how they work, and what our endpoints should be. On the other hand, we have a very justifiable obsession with modes of delivery, rates of delivery, mental models and so on. My perception is that, in the long run, we will find adequate endpoints for our monitoring and still perform closed loop anesthesia with each patient determining his or her own endpoint.

23 OPIATE ADDICTION IN ANESTHESIOLOGISTS

William J. Farley

The specialty of anesthesiology presents distinct stresses and simultaneously offers access to some of the most highly addictive opiates available today. Consequently, the incidence of drug abuse and addiction among anesthesiologists is growing. Studies continue to show that anesthesiology is over-represented among medical specialties with regard to the number of addicted physicians in treatment programs.[1] This chapter discusses ways of recognizing potential substance abusers, the drugs of choice, and treatment options available.

DEFINITIONS OF ABUSE AND ADDICTION

In order to understand the incidence and meaning of alcohol and drug abuse in anesthesiology, we must begin with a discussion of the nature of abuse and addiction themselves. The terms *drug abuse* and *drug addiction* are often used interchangeably to describe excessive drug use, but they are not synonymous. Drug abuse may be defined as the use of a psychoactive chemical up to the point that it interferes with a person's physical, economic, or social functioning. Drug addiction is characterized by compulsion, loss of control, and continued use of the drug in spite of adverse consequences.[2] Addiction is a complex illness with physical, psychological, and social components. Biochemical, genetic, and environmental factors all play roles in its onset. It is chronic and progressive, with stages of the disease being readily observable. Its primary dynamic—denial—is always present.

THE INCIDENCE OF ADDICTION IN ANESTHESIOLOGISTS

In spite of our increased understanding of the disease process, addiction often goes unrecognized, undiagnosed, and unreported. Recent studies concerning a shift in the most commonly abused drug among anesthesiologists suggest that abuse and addiction present true danger to our profession and to our patients.

As early as 1973, the American Medical Association Council on Mental Health officially recognized drug and alcohol abuse among physicians as a problem. The state medical societies in all 50 states now have impaired physician committees, and 17 state medical societies now have full- or part-time medical directors whose sole job is to deal with the problem of chemical dependence among the physicians in their state. In addition, the American Medical Association now holds a yearly four-day conference devoted entirely to the topic of the impaired physician.

Anesthesiologists seem to have a higher incidence of abuse and addiction than the general physician population; studies cited here bear out that fact. Certain factors concerning the practice of anesthesiology probably account for this higher incidence; concomitant with those factors, the reality of the practice of anesthesiology often makes identification of the abuser difficult.

As reported by Gallegos et al.[1] in 1988, of the 1,225 physicians seen by the Medical Association of Georgia (MAG) Impaired Physicians Program (IPP) between July 1975 and September 1987, 146 (11.9%) were anesthesiologists. By comparison, fewer than 4.0% of all United States physicians are anesthesiologists.

The MAG-IPP data also reveal specific findings that point to a shift in the population of chemically dependent anesthesiologists: Compared to all U.S. anesthesiologists and all U.S. physicians, the impaired anesthesiologists (IA) were younger; women, blacks, and other minority members were significantly underrepresented among IAs; residents and fellows (physicians who have completed residency and are taking further training) appeared to be significantly over-represented; and IAs were more frequently retired or unemployed as a direct result of chemical addiction.

With regard to their patterns of substance abuse, the IAs also showed specific differences from the other groups: the IAs were significantly more likely to be polydrug addicted (81.5% reported the abuse of two or more substances); were significantly less likely to abuse alcohol exclusively; were more likely to use only drugs, to abuse narcotics, and to use their drug of choice parenterally; and more frequently abused drugs taken from the workplace. After alcohol, first fentanyl citrate and then meperidine hydrochloride were the drugs most frequently abused by IAs.

The problem seems to have started during residency. Approximately 85% of the IAs who were residents reported during the course of treatment that one of the reasons they were attracted to the practice of anesthesiology was access to drugs. In my own ongoing followup of 155 anesthesiologists treated for chemical addiction, 67 (43%) were residents.

The evidence would clearly suggest that abuse and addiction are realities within our profession and that the problem of impaired anesthesiologists requires specific attention.

THE VULNERABILITY OF ANESTHESIOLOGISTS

Physicians in general tend to share personality traits that make them vulnerable to becoming chemically dependent. Being a physician often requires a certain detachment in dealing with others. Physicians carry this detachment into marriages and relationships with their children. Trained to keep their feelings at bay, addicted physicians use chemicals to sedate themselves and entrench their detachment.

For all physicians, stress is an ever-present reality. For anesthesiologists, the stress is even higher. When a problem arises in the operating room, time becomes a luxury. Decisions must be made instantaneously and rapid action taken. There is no time for peer consultation. In addition, the knowledge of chemicals, of their effects and usage, combined with easy access to drugs, places anesthesiologists in a particularly vulnerable position. Anesthesiologists tend to believe that their highly specialized knowledge of drugs and drug effects will enable them to use drugs themselves without becoming drug-dependent. Research contradicts this belief and, in fact, shows it to be the typical mindset of any addictive personality.[3]

TRIGGER MECHANISMS

In-depth assessments of anesthesiologists in treatment programs have identified several trigger mechanisms that initially precipitated abuse and then sustained addictive use of these drugs. Five trigger mechanisms specific to anesthesiology have been identified. First is the availability of drugs. In addition to having easy access to drugs in the operating room and in the hospital, the U.S. physician usually lives in a moderate to heavy drinking culture where alcoholic beverages are a way of life. Second is the tendency among anesthesiologists to experiment with mood-altering drugs. This is more common and quite prevalent among the younger generation of anesthesiologists, who have grown up at a time when our society was particularly tolerant of experimentation with drugs. The next factor is job stress. There is no question that anesthesiology is one of the most highly skilled and most highly stressed specialties in medicine today, with instant disaster an ever-present threat in the operating room.

Anesthesiologists must also contend with the "Rodney Dangerfield—I don't get no respect" syndrome. Although the anesthesiologist is a key person in the operating room, the awards and applause often go to the surgeon and the surgeon's assistants. Finally, anesthesiology itself promotes a chemical way of life. The instant drug relief ambiance that the anesthesiologist constantly practices, preaches, and teaches produces an almost rote or mechanical way of dealing with psychological pain, stress, fatigue, worry, and physical discomfort. It becomes second nature for anesthesiologists to seek instant chemical relief. This chemical way of life is set against a background of the established scientific fact that now one out of every five abusers will develop the disease of chemical addiction.[4]

DRUGS OF CHOICE AND DOSAGES

The drugs of choice among anesthesiologists have shifted during recent years. I am currently following 155 anesthesiologists who have gone through extended treatment for addiction between May 1982 and April 1989. Virtually all abused more than one chemical. For the seven-year period, 60% (93 cases) said they had used fentanyl. From 1982 to 1984, the two most commonly used drugs were alcohol and meperidine. From 1985 until the present, however, the drugs of choice have been fentanyl and sufentanil. Of the 50 most recent anesthesiologists in treatment, 80% (40 cases) used fentanyl or sufentanil.

The drug of choice is affected by the age group of the impaired anesthesiologist. For anesthesiologists over 50, alcohol is the drug most frequently abused; more younger physicians and residents, however, are being seen in treatment programs, and their drugs of choice have clearly shifted to fentanyl and its analogues. In my current study, 60% (93 cases) of the impaired anesthesiologists abused fentanyl; 53% (82 cases) abused alcohol. The next most commonly abused drug was meperidine, with 33% (52 cases) reporting, followed by the benzodiazepines, with 20% (31 cases), and cocaine, with 19% (29 cases). We rarely see anesthesiologists addicted to inhalation agents, although nitrous oxide is a common drug of abuse for dentists.

Many addicted anesthesiologists report that they initially used the narcotics by squirting the fluid into their mouths or noses, allowing the opiate to be absorbed through the mucous membrane. One anesthesiologist reported initial administration by rectal catheter. They believed that if they took the drug parenterally, they would soon become addicted. In reality, the tolerance to the opiates rose so rapidly that in no time the transmucosal route no longer provided the large concentration of opiate needed to give the desired effect. Intravenous injections soon followed.

The dosages that have been reported most commonly fluctuate between a 3 and 10 ml fentanyl bolus, although two anesthesiologists were able to tolerate 50 ml injections and continue working. For sufentanil, 1 to 3 ml is the average bolus size, but we have treated anesthesiologists who tolerated 8 ml. Addicted anesthesiologists have reported using a 200 to 300 mg meperidine bolus, and two have tolerated a "1-gram push." Clearly the tolerance to these drugs builds very rapidly.

HOW AND WHY DRUG ABUSE AND ADDICTION EVOLVE WITHOUT DETECTION IN ANESTHESIOLOGISTS

A variety of factors contribute to the difficulty of identifying chemical abusers among anesthesiologists. For many years, the medical community has been ignorant of the symptoms of abuse and addiction, among patients as well as themselves. The nature of abuse and addiction are such that secrecy and manipulation are an integral part of the disease, adding to the difficulty of diagnosis.

Identifying chemically dependent individuals is often difficult in the general population; because of the continuing "conspiracy of silence" in the medical community, it is even more difficult among physicians. Alcoholism, in particular, may take many years to progress to a level where impairment is readily detectable, and with most chemical addictions the job is the last area to be affected by the addiction. An addict's personal, financial, and inner life may be in chaos before professional relationships or performance are affected.

The use of drugs like fentanyl, sufentanil, and meperidine actually make identification of chemical addiction easier, since these more potent drugs cause quicker and more obvious symptoms.

Because tolerance develops so rapidly, in a relatively short period of time the addicted anesthesiologist is compelled to take increasingly greater risks of being detected in order to obtain the amount of narcotic needed to surpass the body's tolerance level. As a result, detection usually occurs quite early when these drugs are being abused.

In my experience, most anesthesiologists addicted to fentanyl are detected within six to nine months of the onset of usage. Anesthesiologists addicted to sufentanil are usually detected within three to four months of onset of use. This contrasts with several years' undetected abuse of alcohol, benzodiazepines, or oral opiates such as hydrocodone before addiction is detected.

The major symptom of addiction is the compulsive, irrational, and inappropriate continued use of the drug in spite of negative consequences. The dynamic that justifies this continued use is denial. That denial affects not only the chemically addicted person but also the people with whom he or she comes into contact. Drug addiction must often be blatantly overt before family members, close friends, and coworkers will acknowledge that it exists.

Because anesthesiologists have easy access to drugs, their method of usage is distinct. In our experience with abusers of fentanyl and sufentanil, in particular, their methods of obtaining and using these drugs have been shown to be quite innovative. As noted earlier, many addicted anesthesiologists initially use potent opiates by nasal or oral routes before finally switching to intravenous use.

Since anesthesiologists are ultimately responsible for the record keeping of drug administration, this provides one avenue of relatively easy abuse. They can record that they are administering fentanyl to a patient when, in fact, the patient is receiving butorphanol, nalbuphine, or a strong inhalation anesthetic while the anesthesiologist keeps the fentanyl for personal use.

Recently, we have assessed anesthesiologists who obtained fentanyl by using a small diamond drill and making a small hole in the bottom of the ampule, into which they then inserted a 30-gauge needle. They withdrew the drug from the ampule and replaced it with a saline solution or sterile water, resealing the ampule with a spot of glue. We are also seeing some anesthesiologists who snapped the tops off opiate ampules, removed the drug, replaced it with saline or water, and then glued the tops back on.

Many addicted anesthesiologists, while relieving their colleagues for lunch, will switch syringes, replacing the fentanyl with a syringe labeled fentanyl, but containing less potent chemicals.

Also, addicted anesthesiologists can obtain their drugs through any of the numerous hospitals in the United States where the accountability system for opiates is almost nonexistent.

In these cases, they simply sign out all they need or pick what is left over and lying around in the other operating rooms at the end of the day. Addicted persons will go to any lengths to obtain their drug of choice because when withdrawals begin they truly believe death is inevitable.

IDENTIFYING ANESTHESIOLOGISTS WHO ARE ADDICTED TO CHEMICALS

The nature of chemical addiction is such that addicts believe they are still in control of the drug even when it is becoming apparent to others that this is not the case. Anesthesiologists are particularly vulnerable to the paradox of abuse and addiction because, even at the point where they may begin to realize they are chemically dependent, they fear professional reprisal and thus are unwilling to ask for help. Also, they feel that to admit to out-of-control drug use is to admit failure.

Certain behavioral patterns are readily observable and may indicate chemical addiction. Table 23.1 contains the commonest factors, signs, and symptoms that lead to suspicion.

According to Ward et al.,[5] 50% of questions concerning substance abuse were initially raised by other staff anesthesiologists, followed by 28% from staff nurse anesthetists. Operating room nurses raised the question of abuse in 9% of the cases, while students accounted for the remainder.

Confirmation of addiction most often results from confrontation and admission; incapacitation, obvious intoxication, witnessed drug administration, and entrapment are almost evenly distributed in accounting for the remainder of the confirmations. The time lapse between initial suspicion by other staff members and confirmation of drug addiction was less than 1 month in 39% of the cases, between 1 and 3 months in 24% of the cases, and divided evenly between 3 to 6 months and 6 to 12 months for the remainder.[5]

It is worthwhile to reiterate that on-the-job symptoms are traditionally the last to be ap-

TABLE 23.1 Signs of chemical addiction

Changes in behavior as exhibited by wide mood swings, including irritability, depression, euphoria, and isolation.
Signing out increasing quantities of narcotics.
Sloppy charting.
Exhibiting a desire to work alone (so as not to leave personal drug supply for very long).
Offering to relieve others frequently, affording increased access to drug supply.
Often wearing long-sleeved gowns, indicative not of hiding needle tracks but of compensation for altered internal temperature control caused by large doses of narcotics.
Frequent requests for bathroom relief. Most overdose victims are discovered in the bathroom.
Often refusing lunch relief in order to have continued access to drugs.
A desire to do the long cases, since these usually provide more access to potent opiates.
Physical changes, including loss of weight, tremors, and diphoresis, indicating withdrawal symptoms. Pinpoint pupils may also be observed.

parent and that chemical addiction in the general population as well as in physicians may be deeply entrenched before it becomes apparent in the workplace.

INTERVENING FOR ADDICTED ANESTHESIOLOGISTS

All states now have impaired physicians committees, and many hospitals also have their own committees to address chemical impairment problems in their medical staff. If there is suspicion that an anesthesiologist may be abusing drugs, it is recommended that the department director be informed, evidence noted, and the state impaired physician committee contacted.

Confidentiality must be protected. The state impaired physicians committee is composed of physicians knowledgeable about the disease and practiced in the art of identification and intervention. It is their role to examine the

Chapter 23 Discussion

STEVEN SHAFER: Dr. Farley has elegantly addressed the health problem that represents the anesthesiologist's greatest occupational risk. I would like to add a few thoughts about government regulation and chemical dependence in physicians that were not addressed in Dr. Farley's excellent monograph and Dr. Swift's discussion.

Addicted physicians steal drugs and shoot up, just like any other addict. They need the kind of therapy Dr. Farley proposes. However, our society is increasingly intolerant of drug abuse. Drug abuse by physicians represents an easy target for legislative grandstanding by elected officials.

If we want to give our colleagues compassionate care, we must demonstrate aggressive attempts to identify and treat addicted physicians, or the government will do it for us. Every hospital should have an effective impaired physicians committee, as outlined by Dr. Swift, to demonstrate that we are tackling the problem of chemical dependence in health professionals, and those committees should have appropriate monitors to prove effectiveness. My fear is that if we can't demonstrate that we can identify and treat addicted physicians, government legislation may lead to criminal charges against addicted physicians, just like those that currently await most other addicts.

PETER S.A. GLASS: The current attitudes toward drug abuse and addiction in the United States, coupled with the alarming number of impaired physicians in the specialty of anesthesia, demands an education plan directed towards anesthesiologists and anesthetists. Dr. Farley has provided a clear outline of what such an education plan should incorporate: (1) awareness of trigger mechanisms and the dangers of nonparenteral experimentation with opiates, (2) knowledge of characteristics that identify chemically dependent persons, (3) available treatment and the knowledge that the disease is reversible, and (4) acceptance that addiction is a disease and that it respects no social, cultural, or racial barriers.

There are several other issues related to opiate addiction in anesthesiologists that need to be addressed: (1) Is there a role for random drug testing within the profession? Anesthesiologists play a critical role in the perioperative care of patients, and therefore the impaired physician is a major risk to patients. Random testing of anesthesia professionals not only faces all the ethical issues but also the technical difficulties of detecting potent opiates in urine. (2) Should previously addicted anesthesia professionals be allowed to practice anesthesia with its ever-present temptations? (3) Besides education, where do we need to direct resources? Toward prevention (such as better policing and accounting of opiates used by anesthesia professionals), or toward treatment?

Opiate addiction is not a simple disease with a simple cure. However, the fact that it is now recognized as a curable disease is at least a move in the correct direction.

24 IMPAIRMENT AND DISABILITY: THE YALE DEPARTMENT OF ANESTHESIOLOGY PROGRAM

Clyde A. Swift, Byung Y. Kim, Luke M. Kitahata, and Paul G. Barash

Medicine recognizes that impairment and disability (I/D) can exist in physicians[1] and in anesthesiology personnel.[2-5] The stresses of everyday practice may be eased with self-treatment, self-prescription, and the use of alcohol.[6-8] In recent years, an increase in illegal synthesis,[9] self-experimentation, recreational use, and easy availability of chemical substances have added to the problem. Thus, physicians and anesthesiology personnel who may eventually become either impaired or disabled may be unable to practice medicine with reasonable skill and safety.[10-20]

Major emphasis concerning I/D has focused on chemical use, abuse, and dependence, although physical injury and illness, mental illness,[21-23] aging, and psychosocial disorders are included.[24] Also, the ethical codes of medicine obligate the physician to a high level of professional, social, and moral integrity.[25]

In recognition of these facts, the chairperson of the Department of Anesthesiology at Yale University School of Medicine appointed a department member to select a committee to develop an I/D program appropriate to the department. Without an I/D program, the personnel presenting with I/D, and especially those with chemical use, abuse, or dependence, may suddenly thrust the parent institution into precarious and uncompromising professional and legal turmoil.[26,27] The "guilty until proven innocent" approach often compelled immediate resignation and possible loss of medical licensure for the implicated individual. These drastic measures are, unfortunately, still frequently instituted as the only immediate, obviously punitive, recourses. The inability to effectively direct personnel with I/D may also indicate a lack of understanding and recognition of I/D as a treatable illness.[28-31]

The I/D committee developed a departmental program with specific and intricate management guidelines and policies. This program could be easily adapted to other anesthesia departments, hospitals,[32] other specialties, and various professional organizations with substitution of titles and other appropriate modifications. Included in the program are depart-

Composition

PAC members are physicians, one of whom is appointed as director by the Department of Anesthesiology chairperson.

Responsibilities

PAC members' duties include

- Prevention of I/D with participation in educational programs
- Identification of I/D by receiving reports of alleged I/D from resident advisors, pharmacy personnel, security department personnel, other physicians, spouse and family, medical societies, hospital personnel, patients, and other sources
- Documentation of allegations
- Determination of validity of allegations
- Formulation of guidelines
- Maintaining confidential and accurate records
- Attending PAC meetings

The PAC director is responsible for

- Intervention. The PAC director and a committee member meet with the identified individual to explain allegations, document responses, and report to the department chairperson. Action may include, but is not limited to, exoneration, limitation of duties, supervision of duties, referral to a mental health care professional, referral to some other health care professional, suspension from duty, discharge from the department, reporting to the hospital administrator, reporting to the legal department, reporting to the state department of health services, and reporting to the Drug Enforcement Administration.
- Rehabilitation monitoring, which includes receiving monthly reports from the treating professional and documenting progress.
- Re-entry action, which consists of informing the department chairperson for delineation of professional responsibilities, receiving monthly reports from the treating professional, and reporting recurrence of I/D to the department chairperson.
- Additional activities, which include documenting all PAC proceedings, reporting PAC activities to the department chairperson, delegating responsibilities to other PAC members, functioning as a tie-breaker, presiding at PAC meetings using Roberts' Rules of Order, reviewing the current literature, and preparing an annual report.

Prevention

There is primary and secondary prevention. Primary prevention includes the promotion of well being, educational programs, emotional support for participants and their families, recognition of good performance, and encouraging physical activities and hobbies. Secondary prevention allows persons with I/D to seek help through the I/D program without fear of immediate dismissal and possible loss of medical licensure.

Identification

Identification of possible I/D occurs through reports from resident advisors, pharmacy personnel, the security department, peers, spouses, patients, the impaired or disabled person, and others. All communications are confidential. Review of reports and pertinent material determines the need for intervention.

Intervention

Intervention is the initial meeting where allegations are presented. It is held in a private setting with two or more committee members. Their role is to establish confidence, present allegations, collect information, and determine validity. Allegations are often denied. Complete exoneration may be recommended. After receiving PAC reports, the department chairperson indicates the action prescribed.

Rehabilitation

Rehabilitation is coordinated with the treating professional. The legal rights of the identified individual are observed, respected, and preserved. A clear understanding of specific rehabilitation goals, expected costs, arrangements for payment, and alternative plans are included.

Re-entry

Re-entry requires realistic goals for therapy with expected time off, future leaves of absences, and other potential disruptions. The re-entered person may be returned to active practice, but a part-time practice, an alternative career, or retirement remain as viable options. Aid from colleagues is needed to provide for a dignified re-entry. Followup as appropriate is continuous and discreet.

Immunity

It is a person's legal and moral responsibility to report to the PAC any individual suspected of I/D. As long as the report is made in good faith, and not maliciously, the person reporting is generally protected.

Financial Considerations

Financial assistance may be available through personal insurance plans and through the department.

DISCUSSION

The professional assistance committee (PAC), the executive body of the impairment and disability program (I/D program) has, since November 1, 1983, investigated personnel with alleged I/D. Included were instances indicating potential use, abuse, or dependence on cocaine, nitrous oxide, fentanyl, pentobarbital, and sufentanil. Additional allegations involved aberrant psychosocial behavior and recording inaccuracies.

Prospective attending and resident candidates are apprised of the program through the department annual report. Recognition of potential I/D by resident, fellow, and attending staffs is periodically reinforced with seminars and literature. These activities have fostered an attitude of mature concern for I/D as a potential personal and professional disaster. Those who subsequently accept outside professional positions are familiar with I/D and are therefore able to make positive contributions to colleagues and to their institutions.

Implementation of a strict accountability plan for controlled substances documents the requisition of medications for patient use and accounts for unused portions. Surveillance and cooperation with the pharmacy and security department permits spot-checks of records, with qualitative and quantitative tests of returned substances as necessary.

Department policy does not mandate urine testing.[45] Personnel with I/D are referred to the appropriate health professionals, whose diagnosis and treatment determines the necessity and frequency of required tests. Unlike personnel in other departments, anesthesiology personnel usually practice in close proximity to one another. Variations in behavior, appearance, and professional conduct become quickly apparent to perceptive colleagues.[46] The conceived and adopted approach to recognition of I/D encompassing all aspects of the stated definition is one of sincere concern by colleagues for their peers.

Telephone calls from outside physicians, who seek advice on the management of I/D in a colleague, are frequently received and often illustrate the turmoil created in the absence of a workable I/D program.

A supportive department chairperson is crucial to the successful inception, development, and perpetuation of an I/D program. Interested department members are necessary to develop the I/D program; receive incoming reports; respond quickly, humanely, and maturely; and persevere to resolution.

CONCLUSION

It is our opinion that the I/D program at the Yale Department of Anesthesiology has proved effective and has possibly served as a deter-

25 LEGAL EXPOSURE AND OPIOID ANESTHESIA

George Gore

Accusations of medical malpractice in anesthesia cases continue to increase annually. The introduction of potent and ultrapotent opioid anesthetic agents, while adding significantly to the therapeutic armamentarium of anesthesiologists, has increased the opportunity for significant anesthetic injuries resulting from careless acts of both omission and commission.

The basic legal principles applicable to cases involving opioid anesthesia are essentially the same as those involved in virtually all anesthesia cases. In this chapter, I first discuss these principles, reviewing the basic anatomy of an anesthesia lawsuit. I then assess how those principles apply to several aspects of anesthesia care and treatment, with particular emphasis on cases involving opioids.

ESTABLISHING LIABILITY

Negligence

In these tort (civil injury) cases, the plaintiff (usually the former patient or the patient's next of kin) must present evidence to prove three essential elements in order to establish liability. First and foremost, the plaintiff must prove negligence, a deviation from the requisite medical standard of care. Generally speaking, to establish negligence the plaintiff must present evidence that in the care and treatment rendered to the patient the defendant did something that anesthesiologists of ordinary skill, care, and diligence would not have done under the same or similar circumstances—or that the defendant failed or omitted to do some particular thing that anesthesiologists of ordinary skill, care, and diligence would have done under the same or similar circumstances.

Applying this basic standard of care, the phrase "under the same or similar circumstances" is extremely important. It is, as it must be, a subjective standard. The adequacy and propriety of the actions of the anesthesiologist must always be judged in the context of the specific facts and circumstances under which care was rendered.

One of the most important factors to be considered in applying this standard of care is time. There have been many beneficial developments in anesthesia practice in recent years. However, the courts have consistently held that it is inappropriate and essentially unfair to consider such new developments in judging the actions of an anesthesiologist that occurred prior thereto.

The law judges the defendant based upon the standard of care, the state of the art, the state of science, and the state of the development of the practices and procedures of the profession extant at the time of the incident that gave rise to the lawsuit. The law will not, therefore, judge the defendant physician through the infamous retrospectoscope. Unfortunately, many of these cases take years to come to trial. Consequently, if, for example, the incident giving rise to the lawsuit occurred in 1986 but the trial does not occur until 1990, the court will not permit any evidence to be presented regarding new agents, monitoring devices, or standards developed subsequent to 1986.

To establish the standard of care by which the defendant is to be judged, in the great majority of cases the plaintiff must present the testimony of a qualified expert witness. A number of years ago, almost any physician would be considered qualified to testify as to the requisite standard of care. Fortunately, the law has evolved so that in virtually every case against an anesthesiologist the plaintiff would be required to present this testimony through a trained, qualified (and in some states, a currently practicing) anesthesiologist. Such an expert would be required to testify not only as to what the standard of care was at the time in question but also as to precisely how the defendant anesthesiologist deviated from or fell below that standard of care and was therefore negligent.

One exception to the requirement of expert testimony in this regard can be found in cases in which the doctrine of res ipsa loquitur (the thing speaks for itself) is applicable. However, this doctrine is available to the plaintiff only in instances in which the thing really does speak for itself—the negligence is cognizable by a layman. For example, if a surgeon inadvertently removes the wrong leg, the doctrine applies, and plaintiff does not need an expert witness to testify as to the standard of care and the deviation therefrom. However, because of the scientific complexities of anesthesia procedures and techniques, applicability of the doctrine of res ipsa loquitur in such cases is extremely rare, indeed practically nonexistent.

Consequently, in almost every case, to establish this first element of negligence the plaintiff must prove (1) the requisite medi-cal standard of care, (2) extant at the time of the incident that gave rise to the lawsuit, (3) through the testimony of a qualified anesthesiologist.

Causation

The second element of the plaintiff's case involves causation. To establish liability on the part of the defendant, it is not enough simply to prove that there was negligence. The plaintiff must also prove that the specific act of negligence, the deviation from the requisite standard of care, proximately caused or contributed to the claimed injury. Here, again, appropriately qualified expert testimony must be presented as to how the established negligence directly caused or contributed to the injury.

Extent of Injuries

The final element for the plaintiff to prove includes the extent of the claimed injuries and all compensable damages (past, present, and future) claimed to result therefrom.

CASE STUDY: DR. W.

With those basic principles in mind, I now review the facts and the findings of the jury in the most recent opioid anesthesia case we tried. This case, *Rounsaville v. Dr. W. et al.,*[1] provides an incredible number of examples of what can (and did) go wrong in an opioid anesthesia case.

The *Rounsaville* case was tried for three months in Fort Worth, Texas, from February to May 1989. The jury returned a verdict in favor of Mr. Rounsaville and his family in the amount of $13.6 million dollars, against five defendants. Fortunately, our client, the manufacturer of the opioid sufentanil, was found not liable.

This was the first sufentanil case ever tried. We were defending the manufacturer, Janssen, against whom there were a variety of allegations regarding safety, efficacy, and adequacy of warnings. Clearly, the jury did not find any of the allegations well taken. The five defendants who were held liable for $13.6 million dollars were the anesthesiologist who did the case; his anesthesia department chairman, who had no direct involvement in the case; his former partner, who also had nothing to do with the case; the hospital's chief of staff, a neurologist; and the hospital itself.

In April 1985, John Rounsaville was a 44-year-old estimator for General Dynamics earning $50,000 a year; he was on a fast track in his profession, having progressed rapidly through the ranks and being apparently destined for a vice presidency.

A myelogram performed about a week before the operation in question confirmed the need for a lumbar laminectomy. The patient had some problems following the myelogram, including an apparent untoward reaction to the dye used for the procedure, an adverse reaction to meperidine, and some adverse reaction to diazepam. Consequently, the scheduled surgery was postponed, and Mr. Rounsaville was discharged from the hospital to give him some time to overcome these reactions and prepare for surgery.

After readmission, Dr. W., the anesthesiologist, met with Mr. Rounsaville the night before the scheduled surgery. Among other things, he learned that Mr. Rounsaville had no prior history of surgery. He did, however, learn about the prior problems with drugs (including the apparent reactions to meperidine and diazepam) as well as some possible difficulty with nitrous oxide. There was ample evidence to indicate to the anesthesiologist that this patient was what is sometimes referred to as "a light touch."

The patient indicated to Dr. W. that although he had never had surgery previously he wanted to be put to sleep and didn't want to know anything about the operation. There was no question that he desired and requested general anesthesia.

Nevertheless, the following morning Dr. W. administered tetracaine as a spinal anesthetic.

Apparently an insufficient amount was administered, or the tetracaine was administered in the wrong place, because when the surgeon tugged on the S2 nerve root, Mr. Rounsaville moaned. They paused for a moment. Then the surgeon went ahead and attempted to resume the operation. Mr. Rounsaville moaned again and it was obvious that he was in significant discomfort. Thus, Dr. W. decided to convert to general anesthesia.

At this stage, we have a 190-lb man with an unknown amount of tetracaine, in the prone position, with no intubation or assisted ventilation, and with the drug history outlined above.

Dr. W. decided, in spite of the foregoing, to administer 10 mg diazepam and 1, 2, or 5 ml sufentanil. We are uncertain as to exactly how much sufentanil was administered. Dr. W. testified that he thinks he supplied 1 ml; the anesthesia record shows 2 ml; the hospital pharmacy records shows that a 5-ml ampule was checked out for the case, and there are no wastage records to document disposal of any of those 5 ml. One of the many questions raised during this trial was whether some of the 5 ml sufentanil checked out of the pharmacy was administered to the doctor rather than to the patient.

Understandably, under the foregoing set of circumstances, Mr. Rounsaville became totally apneic. After some discussion between Dr. W. and the surgeon, the patient was turned over, intubated and ventilated as he should have been much earlier, and resuscitated to a limited extent. Tragically, Mr. Rounsaville was left with devastating brain damage, awake and aware, trapped in his body, totally cognizant of his pitiful plight.

At this stage, there should be no doubt as to why Dr. W. was held liable. But why all the other defendants? There was substantial evidence presented during the three-month trial that Dr. W. had sustained some permanent neurological deficit as a result of a stroke experienced a few years earlier. The evidence showed that Dr. W. had consulted the chief of staff, a neurologist, at the request of his former partner and his chairman (both anesthesiologists) about six months prior to Mr. Rounsaville's operation. The chief of staff had sent Dr. W. to New York to a neurological specialist to be examined and tested. In point of fact, he was not fully checked out and additional tests were required and planned, but everyone involved knew that Dr. W. had a neurological problem of some significant potential.

In addition, there was evidence that six weeks prior to Mr. Rounsaville's operation Dr. W. had major problems with another anesthetic case. He did not properly monitor a young patient, as a result of which that patient died. Within days after that prior tragedy, Dr. W.'s two former partners (one of whom was the chairman of the department) professionally disassociated themselves from him.

Compelling evidence was also presented that at the time of Mr. Rounsaville's operation Dr. W. was chemically dependent—unquestionably alcoholic and possibly involved with other substances. Some or all of this was known to the chief of staff, the hospital administration, the chairman of the anesthesia department, and the other anesthesiologist who was Dr. W.'s former partner.

Originally only Dr. W. and his hospital were sued. They happened to have the same insurance carrier, which, during the pendency of the litigation, became insolvent. Subsequently the plaintiff added a substantial number of new parties defendant, including the chief of staff, the anesthesia department chairman, Dr. W.'s former partner, and Janssen (the manufacturer of sufentanil).

Ironically, while Dr. W. and the hospital were the only defendants in the case Dr. W. testified that before Mr. Rounsaville's operation he was completely familiar with sufentanil, very experienced in its use, well aware of its potential side effects (including respiratory depression and apnea), and entirely familiar with all the warnings and precautions set forth in the labeling for sufentanil.

On the morning the trial commenced, Dr. W. filed for personal bankruptcy. With the exception of a cameo appearance during the first day of jury selection, Dr. W. did not

attend the trial. His pretrial deposition was read into evidence. (Within months after the verdict was rendered, Dr. W. died.)

As we indicated earlier, the *Rounsaville* case provides numerous examples of acts and omissions that can expose anesthesiologists to legal liability. Clearly, the jury found Dr. W. liable based upon his own gross negligence. The hospital, the chief of staff, the anesthesia department chairman, and the other anesthesiologist who was Dr. W.'s former partner (and also a former chairman of the department of anesthesia) were all held liable for what might be termed administrative negligence. The jury found that based upon what these parties knew prior to Mr. Rounsaville's surgery about Dr. W.'s personal health problems and professional incompetence, they should have taken action to preclude Dr. W. from administering anesthesia to any patient and should have barred him from practicing anesthesia until he resolved his own problems.

ERRORS IN ANESTHESIA CARE

I would now like to review a number of aspects of anesthesia care and treatment to point out how various anesthesia practitioners have become mired (as was Dr. W.) in some of the pitfalls of medical malpractice. First, a few comments about the preinduction phase.

Patient History and Input

Here a number of problems seem to stem from the anesthesiologist's either being unaware of or giving insufficient consideration to the patient's history, current condition, and wishes regarding the anesthesia to be administered. For example, in the *Rounsaville* case, despite the fact that Dr. W. was aware of some apparent prior sensitivity of Mr. Rounsaville to both meperidine and diazepam, meperidine was administered pursuant to Dr. W.'s order as part of the preanesthetic medication. Then, when the patient got into trouble during the procedure, one of the drugs administered by Dr. W. was diazepam.

Also, Mr. Rounsaville told Dr. W. the night before the operation that he wanted to be put to sleep—he obviously wanted general anesthesia. With no discussion whatsoever about why spinal anesthesia might be preferred, Dr. W. the following morning, directly contrary to the expressed wishes of the patient, administered a spinal.

A similar problem was presented in another case involving a relatively short, 240-lb man scheduled for a lumbar laminectomy.[2] This patient was extremely apprehensive and anxious during the preanesthetic visit. He told his anesthesiologist that he did not want to know anything at all about his operation: "Just put me to sleep and get it over with." The anesthesiologist knew that the neurosurgeon who was going to perform the operation preferred to do so with the patient under spinal anesthesia, so with no further discussion with the patient, the anesthesiologist simply administered a spinal. Despite substantial doses of preoperative medications, the patient was apprehensive, crying, and actively moving on the table in the operating room. Several attempts at spinal punctures were necessary. Perhaps those factors contributed to cause the high spinal, the respiratory arrest, and the resultant brain damage. Clearly it would have been preferable during the preanesthetic visit to discuss the situation with the patient, explain the value of the proposed spinal anesthetic technique, and attempt to allay the patient's concerns, perhaps thereby avoiding the terrible injury that occurred.

In the preinduction phase, the anesthesiologist must give careful consideration to the current condition of the patient as reflected not only in the examination he conducts but, probably more significantly, in the medical chart. Of particular concern here is what the chart reflects with regard to preoperative medications, administration of blood and other fluids, and the patient's laboratory picture. Consider, for example, a 24-year-old woman who underwent a cholecystectomy without incident, was found to have postoperative bleeding the following morning, and had to be returned to surgery to resolve that problem.[3] The patient never fully awakened from the second procedure and suffered severe, irreversible brain damage. Several problems were presented in that case that could have been easily avoided by careful consideration of the patient's condition and the notations in the chart.

In the first place, after the surgeon determined that there was postoperative bleeding and that reoperation was required, he ordered two units of blood to be administered as fast as possible prior to the second operation. The first unit was started without a pump about half an hour before the patient was taken to the operating room. The second unit was started after induction. No doubt, anesthesia was induced while the patient was anemic and at least relatively hypovolemic.

Second, the patient had a ten-year history of hypoparathyroidism, which required administration of calcium. Her internist had ordered calcium subsequent to the cholecystectomy and prior to the second operation, but that order was not carried out. This contributed to some degree to the calcium level of 6.0 reported in the chemical profile for blood drawn approximately six hours prior to the second operation.

Finally, that chemistry profile never found its way to the chart until some time after the second operation. When anesthesia was induced for that procedure, the anesthesiologist did not know that virtually all the chemistry values reported were significantly abnormal. He testified that if he had known what the situation really was he would not have induced anesthesia without at least resolving the calcium problem and perhaps some of the others. He also testified that he did not know that the patient was hypoparathyroid because the surgeon had not told him. However, hypoparathyroidism was well documented throughout the patient's chart, and if the anesthesiologist had looked, he would have known this.

Equipment

As we move into the operating room to consider perioperative problems, one of our first considerations must be the equipment utilized by the anesthesiologist. Many problems have arisen over the years with such equipment, and many of them are the responsibility of the anesthesiologist. These are the tools of the trade, and the anesthesiologist must be concerned about their appropriateness and operative condition. In many instances, it simply will not do to say that the hospital owns the equipment and provides it to the anesthesia personnel and therefore its condition is the hospital's responsibility. Legally, it is often the anesthesiologist's responsibility to make certain, to the extent practicable, that the equipment is appropriate and functioning well.

Certainly in some instances the hospital that owns the equipment, or the manufacturer of the equipment, may be held liable for injuries caused by defects therein. However, that does not always absolve the anesthesiologist. If the defect in the equipment that causes the injury is patent, one about which the anesthesiologist knew or should have known, then the anesthesiologist too will be held liable.

A 43-year-old attorney with a long history of bleeding ulcers was scheduled for a subtotal gastrectomy in New York a number of years ago.[4] Prior to induction the anesthesiologist knew that hospital personnel had placed an improper, makeshift oxygen hose on the anesthesia machine. The hose was too long and was not properly connected. The anesthesiologist had had problems with this in the past. In the middle of this procedure, when the anesthesiologist got up to hang a bag of blood, he inadvertently kicked this long hose and disconnected it from the machine, interrupting the oxygen flow. He did not discover that interruption until it was too late and the patient had suffered significant hypoxia and cardiac arrest. This equipment was patently improper and defective, and the anesthesiologist knew that. He should not have used it. Both the hospital and the anesthesiologist were exposed to liability there. (Incidentally, in this particular case, a small amount of fentanyl was administered to the patient, and an effort was made by the plaintiff's attorney and his independent expert anesthesia witness to attribute the patient's arrest to the opioid. That argument was unsuccessful.)

Anesthetic Agents

Among the most important concerns for the anesthesiologist intraoperatively are the anesthetic agents to be administered. In making the clinical judgment as to which agents to use and when and by what route and in what dosage, the anesthesiologist must bring to bear the knowledge of the scientific community about these agents as well as his or her own clinical experience. We realize that even today we do not know exactly how each anesthetic agent works. However, we do know a great deal about what they do, generally how quickly they act, and for how long. We also know a lot about agent interactions, including those that potentiate the effect of other anesthetic agents. All these factors must be taken into consideration.

We know that many anesthesiologists recommend "balanced anesthesia," including the administration of opioids as a valuable technique in some cases. However, balanced anesthesia is one thing and polypharmacy is quite another. In one of our cases, no fewer than 23 different agents were administered in the operating room during the course of a long procedure, cardiac arrest, and resuscitation.

Anesthesiologists are expected to keep up to date and know the currently available information about the agents they use. We recognize that there are controversies in the literature about how certain drugs should be used and whether to use a particular agent under certain circumstances. However, as long as anesthesiologists are up-to-date on the literature and take into consideration their own clinical experience, they should be in a good defensible position in using a particular agent.

Among the many sources of information about anesthetic agents, anesthesiologists should rely on peers, journals, seminar presentations, and symposia (particularly with regard to new agents). Another basic and important source of information is the manufacturer's package insert containing the FDA-approved

Too much reliance upon monitoring equipment can be dangerous to both the patient and the anesthesiologist. The importance of personal, clinical observation cannot be overemphasized. It is surprising how many cases we have encountered in which at the time of the patient's arrest, or some other crucial event, the anesthesiologist was out of the room. Clearly, such practice cannot be tolerated or defended.

Even if the anesthesiologist is in the operating room, it does not help the patient if the anesthesiologist is not aware and alert. In one of our cases, the surgeon was being cross-examined during a pretrial deposition as to whether he had observed the anesthesiologist reading journals or papers at the head of the table. While there was no specific evidence that the anesthesiologist had been reading during that particular operation, he did admit to leaving the operating table (after at least two significant episodes of "very dark blood" that required treatment to restore proper oxygenation) to go to the back of the operating room to clean his laryngoscope for the next procedure. Shortly after he returned to the table, the patient was, in the words of the surgeon "very blue."[7]

Being present and alert and monitoring properly are essential. However, if the patient gets into trouble and the anesthesiologist does not act quickly and decisively to resolve the problem, all the monitoring is for naught. Anesthesia personnel cannot afford to be reticent. They must take whatever definitive action is necessary, even if it includes aborting the procedure.

Monitoring and the anesthesiologist's responsibility therefore continue even into the postoperative period. Despite the fact that the surgeon and perhaps one or more of the assistants might accompany the patient from the operating room to the recovery room, it is absolutely essential that the anesthesiologist go with the patient to the recovery room and continuously observe and monitor the patient en route. Neither medical nor legal responsibility ends at the operating room door. A myriad of events can and have occurred en route to the recovery room where the patient needed the anesthesiologist immediately available to respond.

Once the patient is in the recovery room, it is proper and appropriate for the anesthesiologist to turn the patient's care over to the recovery room staff, provided that it is safe and reasonable to do so. It is not appropriate to leave a patient in a recovery room that is obviously understaffed. A surprising number of cases have involved incidents that occurred in the recovery room during the lunch hour, when a number of operative procedures are ending, a number of patients are being taken to the recovery room, and half or more of the regular recovery room nurses are at lunch or elsewhere.[8] There is no legally mandated ratio of recovery room nurses to patients. But if it is clear that the recovery room is insufficiently staffed, the anesthesiologist owes it to the patient to stay with the patient and make whatever arrangements (by telephone or otherwise) are necessary to resolve any problem before leaving.

It is also important to communicate directly and verbally with the recovery room personnel and advise them of any special concerns or problems that they should anticipate. If unusual agents with which they might not be familiar were utilized, it is not sufficient to simply leave the chart with the patient and expect the recovery room personnel to review it, analyze it, and act upon it. Direct, personal communication is essential for the well being of the patient.

CONCLUSION

These are just some of the medico-legal problems that can be encountered in anesthesia cases, opioid or otherwise. While it is important for all anesthesia personnel to be aware of and, to some extent, to be concerned about the legal aspects of medical care and potential exposure to legal liability, it is more important that they not permit such concerns to control or interfere with administration of proper anesthesia care. If anesthesiologists are consumed with concern about potential legal problems, if they try to practice what some have referred to as defensive medicine, they will inevitably practice inadequate or improper anesthesia, to the detriment of both patient and anesthesiologist. If problems occur in the operating room, the smartest thing anesthesiologists can do is to simply practice the best anesthesia they know how and let the lawyers worry about potential legal problems later on.

REFERENCES

1. *Rounsaville v. Dr. W. et al.* (1989), unreported.
2. *Kries v. McNeil et al.* (1975), unreported.
3. *Norwest v. Presbyterian Intercommunity Hospital et al.* (1979), unreported.
4. *Apicella v. McNeil et al.* (1975), unreported.
5. *Hollingsworth v. Akron City Hospital et al.* (1982), unreported.
6. *Swayze v. McNeil,* 807 F.2d 464 (1987).
7. *Dubinsky v. St. John's Hospital et al.* (1976), unreported.
8. *Foster v. St. John's Hospital et al.* (1975), unreported.

INDEX